An Evidence-Based Approach to Dietary Phytochemicals

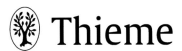

An Evidence-Based Approach to Dietary Phytochemicals

Jane Higdon, Ph.D.
Research Associate
Linus Pauling Institute
Oregon State University
Corvallis, Oregon

Thieme
New York · Stuttgart

Thieme Medical Publishers, Inc.
333 Seventh Ave.
New York, NY 10001

Associate Editor: Birgitta Brandenburg
Assistant Editor: Ivy Ip
Vice-President, Production and Electronic Publishing: Anne T. Vinnicombe
Production Editor: Becky Dille
Sales Director: Ross Lumpkin
Chief Financial Officer: Peter van Woerden
President: Brian D. Scanlan
Compositor: primustype Hurler

Library of Congress Cataloging-in-Publication Data
Higdon, Jane.
   An evidence-based approach to dietary phytochemicals / Jane Higdon.
     p. ; cm.
   Includes bibliographical references and index.
   ISBN-13: 978-1-58890-408-9 (alk. paper)
   ISBN-10: 1-58890-408-3 (alk. paper)
   ISBN-13: 978-3-13-141841-8 (alk. paper)
   ISBN-10: 3-13-141841-9 (alk. paper)
1. Phytochemicals—Physiological effect. 2. Evidence-based medicine. I. Title.
   [DNLM: 1. Plant Extracts—therapeutic use. 2. Dietary Supplements. 3. Phytotherapy.
4. Plants, Edible—chemistry. QV 766 H634e 2006]   QP144.V44H54 2006
   615'.32—dc22   2006017925

Important note: Medical knowledge is ever-changing. As new research and clinical experience broaden our knowledge, changes in treatment and drug therapy may be required. The authors and editors of the material herein have consulted sources believed to be reliable in their efforts to provide information that is complete and in accord with the standards accepted at the time of publication. However, in the view of the possibility of human error by the authors, editors, or publisher of the work herein or changes in medical knowledge, neither the authors, editors, or publisher, nor any other party who has been involved in the preparation of this work, warrants that the information contained herein is in every respect accurate or complete, and they are not responsible for any errors or omissions or for the results obtained from use of such information. Readers are encouraged to confirm the information contained herein with other sources. For example, readers are advised to check the product information sheet included in the package of each drug they plan to administer to be certain that the information contained in this publication is accurate and that changes have not been made in the recommended dose or in the contraindications for administration. This recommendation is of particular importance in connection with new or infrequently used drugs.

Some of the product names, patents, and registered designs referred to in this book are in fact registered trademarks or proprietary names even though specific reference to this fact is not always made in the text. Therefore, the appearance of a name without designation as proprietary is not to be construed as a representation by the publisher that it is in the public domain.

5 4 3 2
TMP ISBN 1–58890–408–3
TMP ISBN 978–1–58890–408–9
GTV ISBN 3 13 141841 9
GTV ISBN 978–3 13 141841 8

Dedicated to the memory of Jane Higdon (1958–2006), scholar, athlete, and compassionate advocate of healthful eating and exercise.

Table of Contents

Foreword

Accuse not Nature! She has done her part;
Do Thou but Thine!
John Milton, *Paradise Lost*, 1667

Archeology reveals that ancient peoples recognized certain foods could provide health-promoting and disease-treating properties. The use of decoctions, distillates, extracts, and infusions of plant foods, spices, and related botanicals in apothecary, Ayurvedic, Chinese, Native American, and other traditional medicines reflect the early application of this knowledge regarding their bioactive constituents. Today, exciting advances in nutrition and medicine as well as numerous reports in popular books and the media have stimulated a general interest in phytochemicals. New recipes emphasizing phytochemical-rich dishes, common foods fortified with these "functional" ingredients, and dietary supplements formulated with a variety of these compounds seem to be appearing every month.

We now appreciate that our evolution in a world of edible plants allowed our bodies not only to forego the requirement for synthesizing many critical compounds (that we now call "essential nutrients") but also to take advantage of other natural constituents in these foods beyond their provision of basic nutritive value. For example, it is interesting to note how our retina employs the carotenoid lutein to filter phototoxic blue light and near-ultraviolet radiation in the same way it protects the plants from which we obtain it. Nutrition scientists are now working to understand the enormous complexity and health implications for thousands of phytochemicals, including their bioavailability, distribution, metabolism, excretion, mechanisms of action, and interactions with one another within individual foods and whole diets. It is worth noting that recent research indicates that some flavonoids have the potential to influence the expression of mammalian genes, suggesting phytochemicals can influence fundamental aspects of our cellular function despite their not being "essential" to us. Understanding the myriad of fruits, grains, legumes, nuts, seeds, and vegetables in our diets and the ways in which they serve to support our physical well-being as well as our mental state can appear an overwhelming challenge. However, Dr. Jane Higdon makes this task much easier by providing here a concise synthesis of the basic scientific, observational, and clinical data now available and organizing the material in a practical fashion both by foods and by phytochemicals and their applications to health promotion and treatment.

The worldwide demographic imperative of the aging population is readily reflected in the shift during the last century of the greatest mortality resulting from communicable diseases to the greatest, resulting from chronic disease. The promise of the power of nutrition lies in our being able to understand the benefits offered not only by essential macro- and micronutrients but also by other dietary constituents, especially phytochemicals like carotenoids, chlorophylls, fiber, glucosinolates, organosulfurs, phytosterols, and polyphenols (including subclasses like flavonoids, lignans, and stilbenes). All of these compounds, and the foods that contain them, are described in this book. In addition to her own expertise, Dr. Higdon has ensured her accuracy by having each chapter reviewed by an authority in that field.

The application of this knowledge about phytochemicals will provide a sound foundation for new dietary guidelines and requisite scientific substantiation for the development of new food products—sometimes called designer foods, functional foods, pharmafoods, or nutraceuticals—and for dietary supplements. However, a great deal of research must be done to demonstrate the efficacy and the safety of new dietary guidelines and of specific products that offer to enhance our biological defense mechanisms, promote optimal physiologic responses, reduce the risk of specific diseases, and slow processes associated with aging.

There is no doubt that evaluating the emerging scientific information with sound judgment as is done in this book will help healthcare providers, especially dietitians, nurses, and physicians, and policymakers and researchers.

Whether counseling patients about their diets or developing more healthful food products, a two-pronged approach is required, that is, reducing ingredients with negative attributes, such as refined sugars, saturated and trans-fatty acids, and sodium and increasing ingredients with positive attributes. However, this opportunity is difficult not only because issues of convenience, cost, and taste must be considered but also because our knowledge of exactly which are healthful and safe ingredients and in what doses and combinations, including most phytochemicals, is still quite limited. Nonetheless, many factors are now converging to assure these challenges will be met: the requirement of both the private and public sectors to reduce healthcare costs, the demands of consumers for "natural" solutions to live longer and better, and the drive of food companies and the stores that sell their products to respond to their customers needs. Dr. Higdon has given us an authoritative but easy-to-read book providing a solid background for those wanting to understand how phytochemicals may offer some solutions to these problems.

Jeffrey Blumberg, Ph.D., F.A.C.N., C.N.S.
Director, Antioxidants Research Laboratory
Jean Mayer USDA Human Nutrition
Research Center on Aging
Professor, Friedman School of
Nutrition Science and Policy
Tufts University
Boston, MA

Preface

Plant foods, including fruits, vegetables, legumes, whole grains, and nuts, are prominent features of healthy dietary patterns. In addition to providing energy and essential micronutrients (vitamins and minerals), plant foods contribute thousands of phytochemicals to the human diet. Although the term "phytochemicals" literally means plant chemicals, it is often used to describe plant-derived compounds that may affect health but are not essential nutrients. Although there is ample evidence to support the health benefits of diets rich in plant foods, evidence that these benefits are due to specific phytochemicals is more limited. Because plant foods are complex packages of biologically active compounds, the health benefits of individual phytochemicals cannot always be separated from those of the foods that contain them. Consequently, the first section of the book discusses the evidence for the health benefits of plant foods and beverages, including fruits and vegetables, legumes, nuts, whole grains, coffee, and tea.

Scientific research on the potential for specific dietary phytochemicals or classes of dietary phytochemicals to prevent and treat chronic diseases has expanded rapidly over the past decade. In some cases, the results of preclinical research have been promising enough to warrant clinical trials designed to examine the bioavailability, safety, and efficacy of high doses of isolated phytochemicals in humans. In the United States and other countries, supplements and extracts containing concentrated doses of isolated phytochemicals are available to the public as dietary supplements without a prescription. The market for functional foods, such as phytosterol-enriched margarines, is also rapidly expanding. As the popularity of these products increases, health and nutrition professionals need accurate information about potential health benefits, risks, and interactions associated with these phytochemicals. The second section of this book reviews the scientific and clinical evidence for the health benefits of individual dietary phytochemicals and classes of phytochemicals. Because high doses of isolated phytochemicals may have unexpected effects, the available evidence regarding the safety of these compounds is also reviewed.

My goal in writing this book was to synthesize and organize the results of thousands of experimental, clinical, and epidemiological studies to provide an overview of current scientific and clinical knowledge regarding the role of plant foods and phytochemicals in human health and disease. An expert in the field covered in each chapter has reviewed the text to ensure its accuracy. The names and affiliations of these scientists are listed in the Editorial Advisory Board. Throughout this book, human research published in peer-reviewed journals is emphasized. Where relevant, the results of experimental studies in cell culture or animal models are included. Although randomized controlled trials provide the strongest support for the efficacy of phytochemicals, it is not always ethical or practical to perform a randomized, double-blind, placebo-controlled trial. Observational studies also provide important information about relationships between plant food and phytochemical intakes and human health and disease. In reviewing the epidemiological research, more weight is given to the results of large prospective cohort studies, such as the Nurses' Health Study and Health Professionals Follow-up Study, than retrospective case-control or cross-sectional studies. When available, the results of systematic reviews and meta-analyses, which summarize information on the findings of many similar studies, are also included.

This book could not have been written without the collaboration and support of the scientists and staff of the Linus Pauling Institute at Oregon State University. The Institute was founded in 1973 by Linus Pauling, Ph.D., the only individual ever to win two, unshared Nobel Prizes (Chemistry, 1954; Peace, 1962). In

1996, the Linus Pauling Institute moved to the campus of Oregon State University (Dr. Pauling's undergraduate alma mater) and now operates as one of the University's Research Centers and Institutes. More than 35 years ago, Dr. Pauling proposed that dietary factors, such as vitamin C, could play a significant role in enhancing human health and preventing chronic disease. The basic premise that an optimum diet is the key to optimum health continues today as the foundation of the Linus Pauling Institute at Oregon State University. Scientists at the Linus Pauling Institute investigate the roles that micronutrients and phytochemicals play in human aging and chronic diseases, particularly cancer, cardiovascular disease, and neurodegenerative disease. The goals of the research at the Linus Pauling Institute are to understand the molecular mechanisms behind the effects of nutrition on health and to determine how micronutrients and phytochemicals can be used in the prevention and treatment of diseases. In particular, scientists at the Linus Pauling Institute's Cancer Chemoprotection Program are working to understand the mechanisms by which dietary phytochemicals may prevent or treat cancer and to identify novel dietary phytochemicals that may protect against cancer. The Linus Pauling Institute is also dedicated to training and supporting new researchers in the interdisciplinary science of nutrition and optimum health, as well as to educating the public about the science of optimum nutrition.

Acknowledgments

First and foremost, I wish to thank the faculty, staff, and students of the Linus Pauling Institute for providing me with the impetus and the opportunity to write this book. Balz Frei, Ph.D., Director of the Linus Pauling Institute, Roderick Dashwood, Ph.D., Chief of the Institute's Cancer Chemoprotection Program, and David Williams, Ph.D., were especially generous with their expertise and advice throughout the project. I would also like to thank each of the distinguished scientists listed in the Editorial Advisory Board for taking the time to carefully review each chapter of this book and provide insightful and constructive comments. I owe special thanks to Bruce Ames, Ph.D., who originally conceived the Web site that inspired this book and to Jeffrey Blumberg, Ph.D., for his eloquent foreword. I am indebted to the Linus Pauling Institute's superb administrative team, Barbara McVicar, Tracy Oddson, Cathy Abney, and Stephen Lawson, who provided invaluable support throughout the preparation of this book. Heartfelt thanks go to my colleagues, Gayle Orner, Ph.D., Silvina Lotito, Ph.D., Angela Mastaloudis, Ph.D., and Mindy Myzak, Ph.D., who were ready with suggestions and resources whenever I consulted them. I am also grateful to Melissa Von Rohr for encouraging me to submit the proposal for this book to Thieme and Birgitta Brandenburg for patiently and efficiently answering each of my many questions about the manuscript. Of course, this project would not have been possible without the generous support of the many donors to the Linus Pauling Institute. Finally, I would like to thank my husband, Tom Jefferson, and my friends, including the folks at Emerald Aquatics, the Eugene Running Club, and the Wednesday P.M. Ride, for their enthusiasm, understanding, and willingness to listen.

Jane Higdon, Ph.D.
The Linus Pauling Institute
Oregon State University
Corvallis, OR

Editorial Advisory Board

How to Use This Book

Chapter Organization

Information on the health benefits of various classes of plant foods can be found in Chapters 1 to 5. Chapters 6 and 7 provide information on the phytochemical-rich beverages coffee and tea. Information on individual dietary phytochemicals or classes of dietary phytochemicals can be found in Chapters 8 to 20.

Plant Foods (Chapters 1 to 5)

Each chapter on plant foods contains the following sections:
- Introduction
- Prevention—A review of the evidence that diets rich in certain plant foods play a role in chronic disease prevention.
- Intake Recommendations—A review of intake recommendations from government or health-oriented agencies, for example, the 2005 Dietary Guidelines for Americans or recommendations by the National Cancer Institute.
- Summary
- References

Coffee and Tea (Chapters 6 and 7)

Chapters on coffee and tea contain the following sections:
- Introduction
- Bioactive Compounds—A discussion of some of the phytochemicals thought to contribute to the health effects of these beverages.
- Prevention—A review of the evidence that these beverages play a role in disease prevention.
- Safety—A discussion of potential adverse effects of high intakes of these beverages, including drug and nutrient interactions.
- Summary
- References

Phytochemicals (Chapters 8 to 20)

Each chapter on phytochemicals contains the following sections:
- Introduction
- Metabolism and Bioavailability—A review of the available information on absorption, metabolism, and elimination as it relates to bioavailability in humans.
- Biological Activities—A discussion of the biological activities, often identified in cell culture or animal experiments, which may contribute to the health effects of a phytochemical.
- Prevention—A review of the evidence that specific phytochemicals play a role in disease prevention.
- Treatment—A review of the evidence that specific phytochemicals may be useful in disease treatment.
- Sources—Information about foods and supplements that contain the phytochemical of interest. When available, information about supplement doses is included.
- Safety—Information about adverse effects and drug and nutrient interactions.
- Intake recommendation.
- Summary
- References

Appendices

Several appendices have been included to facilitate the use of this book.
- Glycemic Index and Glycemic Load—A review of the evidence that the blood glucose-raising potential of carbohydrate in different foods plays a role in their health effects.
- Quick Reference to Diseases—A chart that allows the reader to locate information on plant foods or phytochemicals by disease or health condition.

- Drug Interactions—A table summarizing drug-phytochemical interactions discussed in this book.
- Nutrient Interactions—A table summarizing nutrient-phytochemical interactions discussed in this book.
- Quick Reference to Phytochemical-Rich Foods—A chart that allows the reader to identify plant foods, which are rich in a variety of phytochemicals.
- Glossary

1 Fruits and Vegetables

Despite the controversy surrounding the optimal ingredients of a healthy diet, there is little disagreement among scientists regarding the importance of fruits and vegetables. The results of literally hundreds of epidemiological studies and recent clinical trials provide strong and consistent evidence that diets rich in fruits and vegetables can reduce the risk of chronic disease.[1] On the other hand, evidence that pharmacological doses of individual micronutrients or phytochemicals can do the same is inconsistent and relatively weak. Fruits and vegetables contain thousands of biologically active phytochemicals that are likely to interact in a number of ways to prevent disease and promote health.[2] The best way to take advantage of these complex interactions is to eat a variety of fruits and vegetables.

Prevention

Cardiovascular Disease

Dietary patterns characterized by relatively high intakes of fruits and vegetables are consistently associated with significant reductions in the risk of coronary heart disease (CHD) and stroke. A meta-analysis that combined the results of 11 prospective cohort studies found that people in the 90th percentile of fruit and vegetable intake (~ 5 servings/d or more) had a risk of myocardial infarction (MI) that was ~ 15 % lower than those in the 10th percentile of intake.[3] Among more than 126,000 men and women participating in the Health Professionals Follow-up Study and the Nurses' Health Study, those who consumed 8 or more servings of fruits and vegetables daily had a risk of developing CHD over the next 8 to 14 years that was 20 % lower than those who consumed less than 3 servings daily.[4] In the same men and women, the risk of ischemic stroke was 30 % lower in those who consumed at least 5 servings of fruits and vegetables daily than in those who consumed less than 3 servings daily.[5] Based on the results of Health Professionals Follow-up Study and the Nurses' Health Study, eating one extra serving of fruits or vegetables daily would decrease one's risk of CHD by ~ 4 % and the risk of ischemic stroke by 6 %. In a meta-analysis designed to estimate the global burden of disease attributable to low fruit and vegetable consumption, epidemiologists concluded that increasing individual fruit and vegetable consumption to 600 g/d (~ 7 servings/d) could decrease the risk of CHD by 31 % and the risk of ischemic stroke by 19 %.[1]

Hypertension increases the risk of heart disease and stroke.[6] Adding more fruits and vegetables to a sensible diet is one potential way to lower blood pressure. In the Dietary Approaches to Stop Hypertension (DASH) study, 459 people with and without high blood pressure were randomly assigned to one of three diets: (1) a typical American diet that provided ~ 3 servings/d of fruits and vegetables and one serving/d of a low-fat dairy product, (2) a fruit and vegetable diet that provided 8 servings/d of fruits and vegetables and one serving/d of a low-fat dairy product, or (3) a combination diet (now called the DASH diet) that provided 9 servings/d of fruits and vegetables and 3 servings/d of low-fat dairy products.[7] After 8 weeks, the blood pressures of those on the fruit and vegetable diet were significantly lower than those on the typical American diet, whereas the blood pressures of those on the combination (DASH) diet were lower still.

Several compounds may contribute to the cardioprotective effects of fruits and vegetables, including vitamin C, folate, potassium, fiber, and other phytochemicals.[8] However, supplementation of individual micronutrients or phytochemicals has not generally resulted in significantly decreased incidence of cardiovascular events in randomized controlled trials. Thus, in the case of fruits and vegetables, the "benefit of the whole may be greater than the sum of its parts."

Type 2 Diabetes Mellitus

In addition to its other complications, type 2 diabetes mellitus (DM) is associated with increased risk of cardiovascular disease, the leading cause of death in type 2 diabetics.[9] Although the evidence for a beneficial effect of a diet rich in fruits and vegetables on diabetes is not as consistent as it is for heart disease, the results of a small number of studies suggest that higher intakes of fruits and vegetables are associated with improved blood glucose control and lower risk of developing type 2 DM. In a cohort of almost 10,000 adults in the United States, the risk of developing type 2 DM over the next 20 years was ~20% lower in those who reported consuming at least 5 servings/d of fruits and vegetables compared with those who reported consuming none.[10] In another U.S. prospective cohort study that followed more than 40,000 women for an average of 9 years, fruit and vegetable intake was not associated with the risk of developing type 2 DM in the entire cohort, but higher intakes of green leafy and yellow vegetables were associated with significant reductions in the risk of type 2 DM in overweight women.[11] In a cross-sectional study of more than 6,000 nondiabetic adults in the United Kingdom, those with higher fruit and vegetable intakes had significantly lower levels of glycosylated hemoglobin (HbA1c), a measure of long-term blood glucose control.[12] Possible compounds in fruits and vegetables that may enhance glucose control include fiber and magnesium.

Cancer

The results of numerous case-control studies indicate that eating a diet rich in fruits and vegetables decreases the risk of developing several different types of cancer, particularly cancers of the digestive tract (oropharynx, esophagus, stomach, colon, and rectum) and lung.[13,14] The results of these studies are the foundation for the National Cancer Institute's "5 a Day" program, which is aimed at increasing the fruit and vegetable consumption of the American public to a minimum of 5 servings daily. In contrast to the results of case-control studies, many recent prospective cohort studies have found little or no association between total fruit and vegetable intake and the risk of various cancers.[15-26] There are several possible explanations for this discrepancy. Case-control studies, in which the past diets of people diagnosed with a particular type of cancer are compared with the diets of people without cancer, are more susceptible to bias in the selection of participants and dietary recall than prospective cohort studies, which collect information on the diets of large cohorts of healthy people and follow the development of disease in the cohort over time.[27] Although prospective cohort studies provide weak support for an association between total fruit and vegetable consumption and cancer risk, they provide some evidence that high intakes of certain classes of fruits or vegetables are associated with reduced risk of individual cancers. Higher intakes of fruits were associated with modest but significant reductions in lung cancer risk in a pooled analysis of eight prospective cohort studies.[21] In men, higher intakes of cruciferous vegetables were associated with significant reductions in the risk of bladder cancer,[28] and higher intakes of tomato products were associated with significant reductions in the risk of prostate cancer.[29] See Chapters 2 and 3 for more information on specific classes of vegetables and cancer risk.

Osteoporosis

Several cross-sectional studies have reported that higher intakes of fruits and vegetables are associated with significantly higher bone mineral density (BMD) and lower levels of bone resorption (loss) in men and women.[30-32] In a study that followed BMD over 4 years, higher fruit and vegetable intakes were associated with significantly less decline in BMD at the hip in elderly men but not elderly women.[30] Fruits and vegetables are rich in precursors to bicarbonate ions, which serve to buffer acids in the body. When the quantity of bicarbonate ions is insufficient to maintain normal pH, the body is capable of mobilizing alkaline calcium salts from bone to neutralize acids consumed in the diet and generated by metabolism.[33] Increased consumption of fruits and vegetables reduces the net acid content of the diet and may preserve calcium in bones, which might otherwise be mobilized to maintain normal pH. Results from the DASH study also support a beneficial link between fruit and vegetable intake and bone health. In addition to decreasing blood pressure, increasing fruit and vegetable intakes from ~ 3 servings to 9 servings daily decreased urinary calcium loss by almost 50 mg/d[7] and lowered biochemical markers of bone turnover, particularly bone resorption.[34] Taken together, the results of epidemiological and controlled clinical trials suggest that a diet rich in fruits and vegetables can help prevent bone loss.

Cataracts

Cataracts are caused by oxidative damage of proteins in the eye's lens induced by long-term exposure to ultraviolet (UV) light. The resulting cloudiness and discoloration of the lens leads to vision loss that becomes more severe with age. The results of several large prospective cohort studies suggest that diets rich in fruits and vegetables, especially carotenoid- and vitamin C-rich fruits and vegetables, are associated with decreased incidence and severity of cataracts.[35-38] In a study of male health professionals in the United States, high intakes of both broccoli and spinach were associated with fewer cataract extractions.[35]

Age-Related Macular Degeneration

Degeneration of the macula, the center of the retina, is the leading cause of blindness in people over the age of 65 in the United States.[39] Lutein and zeaxanthin are carotenoids that are found in relatively high concentrations in the retina, and may play a role in preventing damage to the retina caused by light or oxidants.[40] In two case-control studies, high intakes of carotenoid-rich vegetables, especially those rich in lutein and zeaxanthin, were associated with a significantly lower risk of developing age-related macular degeneration.[41,42] A prospective cohort study of more than 118,000 men and women found that those who consumed 3 or more servings of fruits daily had a risk of developing age-related macular degeneration over the next 12 to 18 years that was 36% lower than those who consumed less than 1.5 servings.[43] Interestingly, vegetable intake was not associated with the risk of macular degeneration in this cohort.

Chronic Obstructive Pulmonary Disease

Chronic obstructive pulmonary disease (COPD) is a term that includes emphysema and chronic bronchitis, two chronic lung diseases that are characterized by airway obstruction. Although smoking is by far the most important risk factor for COPD, the results of several epidemiological studies suggest beneficial associations between vegetable and, particularly, fruit intakes and COPD risk.[44] The results of several cross-sectional studies in Europe indicate that higher fruit intakes, especially apple intakes, are associated with higher forced expiratory volume (FEV1) values, indicative of better lung function.[45-47] In a study of 2500 middle-aged Welsh men, those who ate at least five apples weekly had significantly slower declines in lung function than those who did not eat apples over a 5-year period.[46] In a study of 2917 European men followed over 20 years, each 100 g (3.5 oz) increase in daily fruit consumption was associated with a 24% decrease in the risk of death from COPD.[48] The reasons for the beneficial association between fruit intake and lung health are not yet known. Because oxidative stress plays a role in the etiology of chronic obstructive lung disease, scientists are currently investigating the possibility that antioxidants found in fruits, such as vitamin C or flavonoids, could play a protective role.

Neurodegenerative Disease

Although it is not yet clear whether a diet rich in fruits and vegetables will decrease the risk of neurodegenerative diseases such as Alzheimer's disease and Parkinson's disease in humans, recent studies in animal models of these diseases suggest that diets high in fruits such as blueberries[49] or tomatoes may be protective.[50]

Intake Recommendations

The National Cancer Institute recommends a range of 5 to 9 servings of fruits and vegetables daily.[51] Specifically, adolescent and adult women should aim for 7 daily servings, whereas adolescent and adult men should aim

Table 1–1   Examples of One Serving of Fruits or Vegetables

Fruit or Vegetable	Amount in One Serving
Fruit or vegetable juice	$3/4$ cup (6 fl oz)
Apple	1 medium
Orange	1 medium
Banana	1 small
Salad greens, raw	1 cup
Chopped fruit or vegetables	$1/2$ cup
Cooked vegetables	$1/2$ cup
Cooked beans, peas, or lentils	$1/2$ cup
Dried fruit	$1/4$ cup

for 9 daily servings. **Table 1–1** provides some examples of a single serving of fruits or vegetables. The 2005 Dietary Guidelines for Americans are similar with respect to fruit and vegetable intake recommendations, but they are tied to energy (caloric) intake rather than age and gender.[52] Daily consumption of 2 cups (4 servings) of fruit and $2^1/2$ cups (5 servings) of vegetables are recommended for people who consume 8368 kJ/d (2000 kcal/d), 1.5 cups of fruit (3 servings) and 2 cups (4 servings) of vegetables are recommended for people who consume 6693.4 kJ/d (1600 kcal/d). In both cases, consumption of a variety of different fruits and vegetables is recommended, including dark green, red, orange, yellow, blue, and purple fruits and vegetables, as well as legumes (peas and beans), onions, and garlic.

Summary

- Dietary patterns characterized by high intakes of fruits and vegetables are consistently associated with significant reductions in cardiovascular disease risk.
- Although prospective cohort studies provide weak support for an association between total fruit and vegetable consumption and cancer risk, they provide some evidence that high intakes of certain classes of fruits or vegetables are associated with reduced risk of individual cancers.
- The results of epidemiological and controlled clinical trials suggest that diets rich in fruits and vegetables can help prevent bone loss.
- The results of prospective cohort studies suggest that high intakes of vitamin C- and carotenoid-rich fruits and vegetables may be associated with decreased risk of age-related eye diseases, such as macular degeneration or cataracts.
- The National Cancer Institute and Dietary Guidelines for Americans recommend that adults consume 7 to 9 servings ($3^1/2$ to $4^1/2$ cups) of fruits and vegetables daily.

References

1. Lock K, Pomerleau J, Causer L, Altmann DR, McKee M. The global burden of disease attributable to low consumption of fruit and vegetables: implications for the global strategy on diet. Bull World Health Organ 2005;83(2):100–108
2. Liu RH. Potential synergy of phytochemicals in cancer prevention: mechanism of action. J Nutr 2004;134(12 Suppl):3479S–3485S
3. Law MR, Morris JK. By how much does fruit and vegetable consumption reduce the risk of ischaemic heart disease? Eur J Clin Nutr 1998;52(8):549–556
4. Joshipura KJ, Hu FB, Manson JE, et al. The effect of fruit and vegetable intake on risk for coronary heart disease. Ann Intern Med 2001;134(12):1106–1114
5. Joshipura KJ, Ascherio A, Manson JE, et al. Fruit and vegetable intake in relation to risk of ischemic stroke. JAMA 1999;282(13):1233–1239
6. Chobanian AV, Bakris GL, Black HR, et al. The Seventh Report of the Joint National Committee on Prevention, Detection, Evaluation, and Treatment of High Blood Pressure: the JNC 7 report. JAMA 2003;289(19):2560–2572
7. Appel LJ, Moore TJ, Obarzanek E, et al. A clinical trial of the effects of dietary patterns on blood pressure. DASH Collaborative Research Group. N Engl J Med 1997;336(16):1117–1124
8. Bazzano LA, Serdula MK, Liu S. Dietary intake of fruits and vegetables and risk of cardiovascular disease. Curr Atheroscler Rep 2003;5(6):492–499
9. Winer N, Sowers JR. Epidemiology of diabetes. J Clin Pharmacol 2004;44(4):397–405
10. Ford ES, Mokdad AH. Fruit and vegetable consumption and diabetes mellitus incidence among U.S. adults. Prev Med 2001;32(1):33–39
11. Liu S, Serdula M, Janket SJ, et al. A prospective study of fruit and vegetable intake and the risk of type 2 diabetes in women. Diabetes Care 2004;27(12):2993–2996
12. Sargeant LA, Khaw KT, Bingham S, et al. Fruit and vegetable intake and population glycosylated haemoglobin levels: the EPIC-Norfolk Study. Eur J Clin Nutr 2001;55(5):342–348
13. Block G, Patterson B, Subar A. Fruit, vegetables, and cancer prevention: a review of the epidemiological evidence. Nutr Cancer 1992;18(1):1–29

14. World Cancer Research Fund. Food, Nutrition, and the Prevention of Cancer: A Global Perspective. Washington, DC: American Institute for Cancer Research; 1997
15. van Gils CH, Peeters PH, Bueno-de-Mesquita HB, et al. Consumption of vegetables and fruits and risk of breast cancer. JAMA 2005;293(2):183–193
16. Tsubono Y, Otani T, Kobayashi M, Yamamoto S, Sobue T, Tsugane S. No association between fruit or vegetable consumption and the risk of colorectal cancer in Japan. Br J Cancer 2005;92(9):1782–1784
17. Sato Y, Tsubono Y, Nakaya N, et al. Fruit and vegetable consumption and risk of colorectal cancer in Japan: The Miyagi Cohort Study. Public Health Nutr 2005;8 (3):309–314
18. Lin J, Zhang SM, Cook NR, et al. Dietary intakes of fruit, vegetables, and fiber, and risk of colorectal cancer in a prospective cohort of women (United States). Cancer Causes Control 2005;16(3):225–233
19. Key TJ, Allen N, Appleby P, et al. Fruits and vegetables and prostate cancer: no association among 1104 cases in a prospective study of 130544 men in the European Prospective Investigation into Cancer and Nutrition (EPIC). Int J Cancer 2004;109(1):119–124
20. Hung HC, Joshipura KJ, Jiang R, et al. Fruit and vegetable intake and risk of major chronic disease. J Natl Cancer Inst 2004;96(21):1577–1584
21. Smith-Warner SA, Spiegelman D, Yaun SS, et al. Fruits, vegetables and lung cancer: a pooled analysis of cohort studies. Int J Cancer 2003;107(6):1001–1011
22. McCullough ML, Robertson AS, Chao A, et al. A prospective study of whole grains, fruits, vegetables and colon cancer risk. Cancer Causes Control 2003;14 (10):959–970
23. Michaud DS, Pietinen P, Taylor PR, Virtanen M, Virtamo J, Albanes D. Intakes of fruits and vegetables, carotenoids and vitamins A, E, C in relation to the risk of bladder cancer in the ATBC cohort study. Br J Cancer 2002;87(9):960–965
24. Flood A, Velie EM, Chaterjee N, et al. Fruit and vegetable intakes and the risk of colorectal cancer in the Breast Cancer Detection Demonstration Project follow-up cohort. Am J Clin Nutr 2002;75(5):936–943
25. Smith-Warner SA, Spiegelman D, Yaun SS, et al. Intake of fruits and vegetables and risk of breast cancer: a pooled analysis of cohort studies. JAMA 2001;285 (6):769–776
26. Michels KB, Edward G, Joshipura KJ, et al. Prospective study of fruit and vegetable consumption and incidence of colon and rectal cancers. J Natl Cancer Inst 2000;92(21):1740–1752
27. Willett W. Nutritional Epidemiology. 2nd ed. New York: Oxford University Press; 1998
28. Michaud DS, Spiegelman D, Clinton SK, Rimm EB, Willett WC, Giovannucci EL. Fruit and vegetable intake and incidence of bladder cancer in a male prospective cohort. J Natl Cancer Inst 1999;91(7):605–613
29. Giovannucci E, Rimm EB, Liu Y, Stampfer MJ, Willett WC. A prospective study of tomato products, lycopene, and prostate cancer risk. J Natl Cancer Inst 2002;94(5):391–398
30. Tucker KL, Hannan MT, Chen H, Cupples LA, Wilson PW, Kiel DP. Potassium, magnesium, and fruit and vegetable intakes are associated with greater bone mineral density in elderly men and women. Am J Clin Nutr 1999;69(4):727–736
31. New SA, Bolton-Smith C, Grubb DA, Reid DM. Nutritional influences on bone mineral density: a cross-sectional study in premenopausal women. Am J Clin Nutr 1997;65(6):1831–1839
32. New SA, Robins SP, Campbell MK, et al. Dietary influences on bone mass and bone metabolism: further evidence of a positive link between fruit and vegetable consumption and bone health? Am J Clin Nutr 2000;71(1):142–151
33. New SA. Nutrition Society Medal lecture. The role of the skeleton in acid-base homeostasis. Proc Nutr Soc 2002;61(2):151–164
34. Lin PH, Ginty F, Appel LJ, et al. The DASH diet and sodium reduction improve markers of bone turnover and calcium metabolism in adults. J Nutr 2003;133 (10):3130–3136
35. Brown L, Rimm EB, Seddon JM, et al. A prospective study of carotenoid intake and risk of cataract extraction in US men. Am J Clin Nutr 1999;70(4):517–524
36. Christen WG, Liu S, Schaumberg DA, Buring JE. Fruit and vegetable intake and the risk of cataract in women. Am J Clin Nutr 2005;81(6):1417–1422
37. Jacques PF, Chylack LT Jr, Hankinson SE, et al. Long-term nutrient intake and early age-related nuclear lens opacities. Arch Ophthalmol 2001;119(7):1009–1019
38. Lyle BJ, Mares-Perlman JA, Klein BE, Klein R, Greger JL. Antioxidant intake and risk of incident age-related nuclear cataracts in the Beaver Dam Eye Study. Am J Epidemiol 1999;149(9):801–809
39. Cooper DA, Eldridge AL, Peters JC. Dietary carotenoids and certain cancers, heart disease, and age-related macular degeneration: a review of recent research. Nutr Rev 1999;57(7):201–214
40. Mares-Perlman JA, Millen AE, Ficek TL, Hankinson SE. The body of evidence to support a protective role for lutein and zeaxanthin in delaying chronic disease. Overview. J Nutr 2002;132(3):518S–524S
41. Seddon JM, Ajani UA, Sperduto RD, et al. Dietary carotenoids, vitamins A, C, and E, and advanced age-related macular degeneration. Eye Disease Case-Control Study Group. JAMA 1994;272(18):1413–1420
42. Snellen EL, Verbeek AL, Van Den Hoogen GW, Cruysberg JR, Hoyng CB. Neovascular age-related macular degeneration and its relationship to antioxidant intake. Acta Ophthalmol Scand 2002;80(4):368–371
43. Cho E, Seddon JM, Rosner B, Willett WC, Hankinson SE. Prospective study of intake of fruits, vegetables, vitamins, and carotenoids and risk of age-related maculopathy. Arch Ophthalmol 2004;122(6):883–892
44. Romieu I, Trenga C. Diet and obstructive lung diseases. Epidemiol Rev 2001;23(2):268–287
45. Tabak C, Smit HA, Rasanen L, et al. Dietary factors and pulmonary function: a cross sectional study in middle aged men from three European countries. Thorax 1999;54(11):1021–1026
46. Butland BK, Fehily AM, Elwood PC. Diet, lung function, and lung function decline in a cohort of 2512 middle aged men. Thorax 2000;55(2):102–108
47. Tabak C, Arts IC, Smit HA, Heederik D, Kromhout D. Chronic obstructive pulmonary disease and intake of catechins, flavonols, and flavones: the MORGEN Study. Am J Respir Crit Care Med 2001;164(1):61–64
48. Walda IC, Tabak C, Smit HA, et al. Diet and 20-year chronic obstructive pulmonary disease mortality in middle-aged men from three European countries. Eur J Clin Nutr 2002;56(7):638–643

49. Joseph JA, Denisova NA, Arendash G, et al. Blueberry supplementation enhances signaling and prevents behavioral deficits in an Alzheimer disease model. Nutr Neurosci 2003;6(3):153–162

50. Suganuma H, Hirano T, Arimoto Y, Inakuma T. Effect of tomato intake on striatal monoamine level in a mouse model of experimental Parkinson's disease. J Nutr Sci Vitaminol (Tokyo) 2002;48(3):251–254

51. National Cancer Institute. Eat 5 to 9 servings of fruits and vegetables a day for better health. 2005. Available at: http://www.5aday.gov/homepage/index_content. html. Accessed 8/1/06

52. U.S. Department of Health and Human Services, US Department of Agriculture. Dietary Guidelines for Americans. 2005. Available at: http://www.health-ierus.gov/dietaryguidelines/. Accessed 8/1/06

2 Cruciferous Vegetables

Cruciferous or *Brassica* vegetables are plants in the family known as Cruciferae (Brassicaceae). Many commonly consumed cruciferous vegetables come from the *Brassica* genus, including broccoli, Brussels sprouts, cabbage, cauliflower, collard greens, kale, kohlrabi, mustard, rutabaga, turnips, bok choy, and Chinese cabbage.[1] Arugula, horseradish, radish, wasabi, and watercress are also cruciferous vegetables. Cruciferous vegetables are unique in that they are rich sources of glucosinolates, sulfur-containing compounds that are responsible for their pungent aromas and spicy (or bitter) taste.[2] The hydrolysis (breakdown) of glucosinolates by a class of plant enzymes called myrosinase results in the formation of biologically active compounds, such as indoles and isothiocyanates.[3] Myrosinase is physically separated from glucosinolates in intact plant cells. However, when cruciferous vegetables are chopped or chewed, myrosinase comes in contact with glucosinolates and catalyzes their hydrolysis. Scientists are currently investigating the potential for high intakes of cruciferous vegetables as well as several glucosinolate hydrolysis products to prevent cancer (see Chapters 15 and 16).

Prevention

Cancer

Like most other vegetables, cruciferous vegetables are good sources of a variety of nutrients and phytochemicals that may work synergistically to help prevent cancer.[4] One challenge in studying the relationships between cruciferous vegetable intake and cancer risk in humans is separating the benefits of diets that are generally rich in vegetables from those that are specifically rich in cruciferous vegetables.[5] One characteristic that sets cruciferous vegetables apart from other vegetables is their high glucosinolate content.[6] Glucosinolate hydrolysis products could help prevent cancer by enhancing the elimination of carcinogens before they can damage DNA or by altering cell signaling pathways in ways that help prevent normal cells from being transformed into cancerous cells.[7] Some glucosinolate hydrolysis products may alter the metabolism or activity of hormones like estrogen in ways that inhibit the development of hormone-sensitive cancers.[8]

In an extensive review of epidemiological studies published prior to 1996, the authors reported that the majority (67%) of 87 case-control studies found an inverse association between some type of cruciferous vegetable intake and cancer risk.[9] At that time, the inverse association appeared to be most consistent for cancers of the lung and digestive tract. The results of retrospective case-control studies are more likely to be distorted by bias in the selection of participants (cases and controls) and dietary recall than prospective cohort studies, which collect dietary information from participants before they are diagnosed with cancer.[10] In the past decade, results of large prospective cohort studies and studies taking into account individual genetic variation suggest that the relationship between cruciferous vegetable intake and the risk of several types of cancer is more complex than previously thought.

Lung Cancer

When evaluating the effect of cruciferous vegetable consumption on lung cancer risk, it is important to remember that the benefit of increasing cruciferous vegetable intake is likely to be small compared with the benefit of smoking cessation.[11,12] Although several case-control studies found that people diagnosed with lung cancer had significantly lower intakes of cruciferous vegetables than people in cancer-free control groups,[9] the findings of more recent prospective cohort studies have been mixed. Prospective studies of Dutch men and women,[13] American women,[14] and Finnish men[15] found that higher intakes of cruciferous vegetables (more than 3 weekly servings) were associated with significant reductions in lung cancer risk, but prospective studies of American men[14] and European men and women[11] found no inverse association. The results of several studies suggest that genetic factors affecting the metabolism of glucosinolate hydrolysis products may influence the effects of cruciferous vegetable consumption on lung cancer risk[16–19] (see the Genetic Influences section below).

Colorectal Cancer

A small clinical trial found that the consumption of 250 g/d (9 oz/d) of broccoli and 250 g/d of Brussels sprouts significantly increased the urinary excretion of a potential carcinogen found in well-done meat, suggesting that high cruciferous vegetable intakes might decrease colorectal cancer risk by enhancing the elimination of some dietary carcinogens.[20] Although several case-control studies conducted prior to 1990 found that people diagnosed with colorectal cancer were more likely to have lower intakes of various cruciferous vegetables than people without colorectal cancer,[21–24] most prospective cohort studies have not found significant inverse associations between cruciferous vegetable intake and the risk of developing colorectal cancer over time.[25–28] One exception was a prospective study of Dutch adults, which found that men and women with the highest intakes of cruciferous vegetables (averaging 58 g/d) were significantly less likely to develop colon cancer than those with the lowest intakes (averaging 11 g/d).[29] Surprisingly, higher intakes of cruciferous vegetables were associated with increased risk of rectal cancer in women in that study. As in lung cancer, the relationship between cruciferous vegetable consumption and colorectal cancer risk may be complicated by genetic factors. The results of several recent epidemiological studies suggest that the protective effects of cruciferous vegetable consumption may be influenced by inherited differences in the capacity of individuals to metabolize and eliminate glucosinolate hydrolysis products[30–33] (see the Genetic Influences section below).

Genetic Influences

There is increasing evidence that genetic differences in humans may influence the effects of cruciferous vegetable intake on cancer risk.[34] Isothiocyanates are glucosinolate hydrolysis products that play a role in the cancer-preventive effects associated with cruciferous vegetable consumption. Glutathione S-transferases (GSTs) are a family of enzymes that metabolize a variety of compounds, including isothiocyanates, in a way that promotes their elimination from the body. Genetic variations (polymorphisms) that affect the activity of GST enzymes have been identified in humans. Null variants of the GSTM1 gene and GSTT1 gene contain large deletions, and individuals who inherit two copies of the GSTM1-null or GSTT1-null gene cannot produce the corresponding GST enzyme.[35] Lower GST activity in such individuals could result in slower elimination and longer exposure to isothiocyanates after cruciferous vegetable consumption.[36] In support of this idea, several epidemiological studies have found that inverse associations between isothiocyanate intake from cruciferous vegetables and the risk of lung cancer[16–19] or colon cancer[30–32] were more pronounced in GSTM1-null and/or GSTT1-null individuals. These findings suggest that the protective effects of high intakes of cruciferous vegetables may be enhanced in individuals who eliminate potentially protective compounds like isothiocyanates more slowly.

Breast Cancer

The endogenous estrogen 17β-estradiol can be irreversibly metabolized to 16α-hydroxyestrone (16αOHE1) or 2-hydroxyestrone (2OHE1). In contrast to 2OHE1, 16αOHE1 is highly estrogenic and has been found to enhance the proliferation of estrogen-sensitive breast cancer cells in culture.[37,38] It has been hypothesized that shifting the metabolism of 17β-estradiol toward 2OHE1 and away from 16αOHE1 could decrease the risk of estrogen-sensitive cancers, such as breast cancer.[39] In a small clinical trial, increasing cruciferous vegetable intake of healthy postmenopausal women for 4 weeks increased urinary 2OHE1:16αOHE1 ratios, suggesting that high intakes of cruciferous vegetables can shift estrogen metabolism. However, the relationship between urinary 2OHE1:16αOHE1 ratios and breast cancer risk is not clear. Several small case-control studies found that women with breast cancer had lower urinary ratios of 2OHE1:16αOHE1,[40–42] but larger case-control and prospective cohort studies did not find significant associations between urinary 2OHE1:16αOHE1 ratios and breast cancer risk.[43–45] The results of epidemiological studies of cruciferous vegetable intake and breast cancer risk are also inconsistent. Several recent case-control studies in the United States, Sweden, and China found that measures of cruciferous vegetable intake were significantly lower in women diagnosed with breast cancer than in cancer-free control groups,[46–48] but cruciferous vegetable intake was not associated with breast cancer risk in a pooled analysis of seven large prospective cohort studies.[49]

Prostate Cancer

Although glucosinolate hydrolysis products have been found to inhibit growth and promote death (apoptosis) of cultured prostate cancer cells,[50,51] the results of epidemiological studies of cruciferous vegetable intake and prostate cancer risk are inconsistent. Four out of eight case-control studies published since 1990 found that some measure of cruciferous vegetable intake was significantly lower in men diagnosed with prostate cancer than in a control group of cancer-free men.[52–55] Of the four prospective cohort studies that have examined associations between cruciferous vegetable intake and the risk of prostate cancer, none found statistically significant inverse associations overall.[56–59] However, the prospective study that included the longest follow-up period and the most cases of prostate cancer found a significant inverse association between cruciferous vegetable intake and the risk of prostate cancer when the analysis was limited to men who had a prostate-specific antigen (PSA) test.[56] Because men who have PSA screening are more likely to be diagnosed with prostate cancer, limiting the analysis in this way is one way to reduce detection bias.[60] Presently, epidemiological studies pro-

vide only modest support for the hypothesis that high intakes of cruciferous vegetables reduce prostate cancer risk.[1]

Nutrient Interactions

Iodine and Thyroid Function

Very high intakes of cruciferous vegetables, such as cabbage and turnips, have been found to cause hypothyroidism in animals.[61] Two mechanisms have been identified to explain this effect. The hydrolysis of some glucosinolates found in cruciferous vegetables (e. g., progoitrin) may yield a compound known as goitrin, which has been found to interfere with thyroid hormone synthesis. The hydrolysis of another class of glucosinolates, known as indole glucosinolates, results in the release of thiocyanate ions, which can compete with iodine for uptake by the thyroid gland. Increased exposure to thiocyanate ions from cruciferous vegetable consumption or, more commonly, cigarette smoking does not appear to increase the risk of hypothyroidism unless accompanied by iodine deficiency. One study in humans found that the consumption of 150 g/d (5 oz/d) of cooked Brussels sprouts for 4 weeks had no adverse effects on thyroid function.[62]

Intake Recommendations

Although many organizations, including the National Cancer Institute, recommend the consumption of 5 to 9 servings (2$\frac{1}{2}$ to 4$\frac{1}{2}$ cups) of fruits and vegetables daily,[63] separate recommendations for cruciferous vegetables have not been established. Much remains to be learned regarding cruciferous vegetable consumption and cancer prevention, but the results of some prospective cohort studies suggest that adults should aim for at least 5 weekly servings of cruciferous vegetables.[14,56,64]

Summary

- Cruciferous vegetables are unique in that they are rich sources of sulfur-containing compounds known as glucosinolates.

- Chopping or chewing cruciferous vegetables results in the formation of bioactive glucosinolate hydrolysis products, such as isothiocyanates and indole-3-carbinol.
- High intakes of cruciferous vegetables have been associated with lower risk of lung and colorectal cancer in some epidemiological studies, but there is evidence that genetic differences may influence the effect of cruciferous vegetables on human cancer risk.
- Although glucosinolate hydrolysis products may alter the metabolism or activity of sex hormones in ways that could inhibit the development of hormone-sensitive cancers, evidence of an inverse association between cruciferous vegetable intake and breast or prostate cancer in humans is limited and inconsistent.
- Many organizations, including the National Cancer Institute, recommend the consumption of 5 to 9 servings ($2^1/_2$ to 4 $^1/_2$ cups) of fruits and vegetables daily, but separate recommendations for cruciferous vegetables have not been established.

References

1. Kristal AR, Lampe JW. Brassica vegetables and prostate cancer risk: a review of the epidemiological evidence. Nutr Cancer 2002;42(1):1–9
2. Drewnowski A, Gomez-Carneros C. Bitter taste, phytonutrients, and the consumer: a review. Am J Clin Nutr 2000;72(6):1424–1435
3. Holst B, Williamson G. A critical review of the bioavailability of glucosinolates and related compounds. Nat Prod Rep 2004;21(3):425–447
4. Liu RH. Potential synergy of phytochemicals in cancer prevention: mechanism of action. J Nutr 2004;134(12 Suppl):3479S–3485S
5. McNaughton SA, Marks GC. Development of a food composition database for the estimation of dietary intakes of glucosinolates, the biologically active constituents of cruciferous vegetables. Br J Nutr 2003;90(3):687–697
6. van Poppel G, Verhoeven DT, Verhagen H, Goldbohm RA. Brassica vegetables and cancer prevention. Epidemiology and mechanisms. Adv Exp Med Biol 1999;472:159–168
7. Zhang Y. Cancer-preventive isothiocyanates: measurement of human exposure and mechanism of action. Mutat Res 2004;555(1–2):173–190
8. Auborn KJ, Fan S, Rosen EM, et al. Indole-3-carbinol is a negative regulator of estrogen. J Nutr 2003;133(7 Suppl):2470S–2475S
9. Verhoeven DT, Goldbohm RA, van Poppel G, Verhagen H, van den Brandt PA. Epidemiological studies on brassica vegetables and cancer risk. Cancer Epidemiol Biomarkers Prev 1996;5(9):733–748
10. Willett W. Nutritional Epidemiology. 2nd ed. New York: Oxford University Press; 1998
11. Miller AB, Altenburg HP, Bueno-de-Mesquita B, et al. Fruits and vegetables and lung cancer: findings from the European Prospective Investigation into Cancer and Nutrition. Int J Cancer 2004;108(2):269–276
12. Smith-Warner SA, Spiegelman D, Yaun SS, et al. Fruits, vegetables and lung cancer: a pooled analysis of cohort studies. Int J Cancer 2003;107(6):1001–1011
13. Voorrips LE, Goldbohm RA, Verhoeven DT, et al. Vegetable and fruit consumption and lung cancer risk in the Netherlands Cohort Study on diet and cancer. Cancer Causes Control 2000;11(2):101–115
14. Feskanich D, Ziegler RG, Michaud DS, et al. Prospective study of fruit and vegetable consumption and risk of lung cancer among men and women. J Natl Cancer Inst 2000;92(22):1812–1823
15. Neuhouser ML, Patterson RE, Thornquist MD, Omenn GS, King IB, Goodman GE. Fruits and vegetables are associated with lower lung cancer risk only in the placebo arm of the beta-carotene and retinol efficacy trial (CARET). Cancer Epidemiol Biomarkers Prev 2003;12(4):350–358
16. Zhao B, Seow A, Lee EJ, et al. Dietary isothiocyanates, glutathione S-transferase-M1, -T1 polymorphisms and lung cancer risk among Chinese women in Singapore. Cancer Epidemiol Biomarkers Prev 2001;10(10):1063–1067
17. Lewis S, Brennan P, Nyberg F, et al. Re: Spitz, M. R., Duphorne, C. M., Detry, M. A., Pillow, P. C., Amos, C. I., Lei, L., de Andrade, M., Gu, X., Hong, W. K., and Wu, X. Dietary intake of isothiocyanates: evidence of a joint effect with glutathione S-transferase polymorphisms in lung cancer risk. Cancer Epidemiol Biomarkers Prev 2001;10(10):1105–1106
18. Spitz MR, Duphorne CM, Detry MA, et al. Dietary intake of isothiocyanates: evidence of a joint effect with glutathione S-transferase polymorphisms in lung cancer risk. Cancer Epidemiol Biomarkers Prev 2000;9(10):1017–1020
19. London SJ, Yuan JM, Chung FL, et al. Isothiocyanates, glutathione S-transferase M1 and T1 polymorphisms, and lung-cancer risk: a prospective study of men in Shanghai, China. Lancet 2000;356(9231):724–729
20. Walters DG, Young PJ, Agus C, et al. Cruciferous vegetable consumption alters the metabolism of the dietary carcinogen 2-amino-1-methyl-6-phenylimidazo[4,5-b]pyridine (PhIP) in humans. Carcinogenesis 2004;25(9):1659–1669
21. Benito E, Obrador A, Stiggelbout A, et al. A population-based case-control study of colorectal cancer in Majorca. I. Dietary factors. Int J Cancer 1990;45(1):69–76
22. West DW, Slattery ML, Robison LM, et al. Dietary intake and colon cancer: sex- and anatomic site-specific associations. Am J Epidemiol 1989;130(5):883–894
23. Young TB, Wolf DA. Case-control study of proximal and distal colon cancer and diet in Wisconsin. Int J Cancer 1988;42(2):167–175
24. Graham S, Dayal H, Swanson M, Mittelman A, Wilkinson G. Diet in the epidemiology of cancer of the colon and rectum. J Natl Cancer Inst 1978;61(3):709–714
25. Kojima M, Wakai K, Tamakoshi K, et al. Diet and colorectal cancer mortality: results from the Japan Collaborative Cohort Study. Nutr Cancer 2004;50(1):23–32

26. McCullough ML, Robertson AS, Chao A, et al. A prospective study of whole grains, fruits, vegetables and colon cancer risk. Cancer Causes Control 2003;14 (10):959–970

27. Michels KB, Edward G, Joshipura KJ, et al. Prospective study of fruit and vegetable consumption and incidence of colon and rectal cancers. J Natl Cancer Inst 2000;92(21):1740–1752

28. Steinmetz KA, Kushi LH, Bostick RM, Folsom AR, Potter JD. Vegetables, fruit, and colon cancer in the Iowa Women's Health Study. Am J Epidemiol 1994;139(1): 1–15

29. Voorrips LE, Goldbohm RA, van Poppel G, Sturmans F, Hermus RJ, van den Brandt PA. Vegetable and fruit consumption and risks of colon and rectal cancer in a prospective cohort study: The Netherlands Cohort Study on Diet and Cancer. Am J Epidemiol 2000; 152(11):1081–1092

30. Turner F, Smith G, Sachse C, et al. Vegetable, fruit and meat consumption and potential risk modifying genes in relation to colorectal cancer. Int J Cancer 2004;112(2):259–264

31. Seow A, Yuan JM, Sun CL, Van Den Berg D, Lee HP, Yu MC. Dietary isothiocyanates, glutathione S-transferase polymorphisms and colorectal cancer risk in the Singapore Chinese Health Study. Carcinogenesis 2002;23(12):2055–2061

32. Slattery ML, Kampman E, Samowitz W, Caan BJ, Potter JD. Interplay between dietary inducers of GST and the GSTM-1 genotype in colon cancer. Int J Cancer 2000;87(5):728–733

33. Lin HJ, Probst-Hensch NM, Louie AD, et al. Glutathione transferase null genotype, broccoli, and lower prevalence of colorectal adenomas. Cancer Epidemiol Biomarkers Prev 1998;7(8):647–652

34. Lampe JW, Peterson S. Brassica, biotransformation and cancer risk: genetic polymorphisms alter the preventive effects of cruciferous vegetables. J Nutr 2002; 132(10):2991–2994

35. Coles BF, Kadlubar FF. Detoxification of electrophilic compounds by glutathione S-transferase catalysis: determinants of individual response to chemical carcinogens and chemotherapeutic drugs? Biofactors 2003;17(1–4):115–130

36. Seow A, Shi CY, Chung FL, et al. Urinary total isothiocyanate (ITC) in a population-based sample of middle-aged and older Chinese in Singapore: relationship with dietary total ITC and glutathione S-transferase M1/T1/P1 genotypes. Cancer Epidemiol Biomarkers Prev 1998;7(9):775–781

37. Telang NT, Suto A, Wong GY, Osborne MP, Bradlow HL. Induction by estrogen metabolite 16 alpha-hydroxyestrone of genotoxic damage and aberrant proliferation in mouse mammary epithelial cells. J Natl Cancer Inst 1992;84(8):634–638

38. Yuan F, Chen DZ, Liu K, Sepkovic DW, Bradlow HL, Auborn K. Anti-estrogenic activities of indole-3-carbinol in cervical cells: implication for prevention of cervical cancer. Anticancer Res 1999;19(3A):1673–1680

39. Bradlow HL, Telang NT, Sepkovic DW, Osborne MP. 2-hydroxyestrone: the 'good' estrogen. J Endocrinol 1996;150(Suppl):S259–S265

40. Ho GH, Luo XW, Ji CY, Foo SC, Ng EH. Urinary 2/16 alpha-hydroxyestrone ratio: correlation with serum insulin-like growth factor binding protein-3 and a potential biomarker of breast cancer risk. Ann Acad Med Singapore 1998;27(2):294–299

41. Kabat GC, Chang CJ, Sparano JA, et al. Urinary estrogen metabolites and breast cancer: a case-control study. Cancer Epidemiol Biomarkers Prev 1997;6(7):505–509

42. Schneider J, Kinne D, Fracchia A, et al. Abnormal oxidative metabolism of estradiol in women with breast cancer. Proc Natl Acad Sci U S A 1982;79(9):3047–3051

43. Cauley JA, Zmuda JM, Danielson ME, et al. Estrogen metabolites and the risk of breast cancer in older women. Epidemiology 2003;14(6):740–744

44. Meilahn EN, De Stavola B, Allen DS, et al. Do urinary oestrogen metabolites predict breast cancer? Guernsey III cohort follow-up. Br J Cancer 1998;78(9):1250–1255

45. Ursin G, London S, Stanczyk FZ, et al. Urinary 2-hydroxyestrone/16alpha-hydroxyestrone ratio and risk of breast cancer in postmenopausal women. J Natl Cancer Inst 1999;91(12):1067–1072

46. Ambrosone CB, McCann SE, Freudenheim JL, Marshall JR, Zhang Y, Shields PG. Breast cancer risk in premenopausal women is inversely associated with consumption of broccoli, a source of isothiocyanates, but is not modified by GST genotype. J Nutr 2004;134(5): 1134–1138

47. Fowke JH, Chung FL, Jin F, et al. Urinary isothiocyanate levels, brassica, and human breast cancer. Cancer Res 2003;63(14):3980–3986

48. Terry P, Wolk A, Persson I, Magnusson C. Brassica vegetables and breast cancer risk. JAMA 2001; 285(23):2975–2977

49. Smith-Warner SA, Spiegelman D, Yaun SS, et al. Intake of fruits and vegetables and risk of breast cancer: a pooled analysis of cohort studies. JAMA 2001; 285(6):769–776

50. Singh AV, Xiao D, Lew KL, Dhir R, Singh SV. Sulforaphane induces caspase-mediated apoptosis in cultured PC-3 human prostate cancer cells and retards growth of PC-3 xenografts in vivo. Carcinogenesis 2004;25(1):83–90

51. Sarkar FH, Li Y. Indole-3-carbinol and prostate cancer. J Nutr 2004;134(12 Suppl):3493S–3498S

52. Cohen JH, Kristal AR, Stanford JL. Fruit and vegetable intakes and prostate cancer risk. J Natl Cancer Inst 2000;92(1):61–68

53. Jain MG, Hislop GT, Howe GR, Ghadirian P. Plant foods, antioxidants, and prostate cancer risk: findings from case-control studies in Canada. Nutr Cancer 1999; 34(2):173–184

54. Joseph MA, Moysich KB, Freudenheim JL, et al. Cruciferous vegetables, genetic polymorphisms in glutathione s-transferases m1 and t1, and prostate cancer risk. Nutr Cancer 2004;50(2):206–213

55. Kolonel LN, Hankin JH, Whittemore AS, et al. Vegetables, fruits, legumes and prostate cancer: a multiethnic case-control study. Cancer Epidemiol Biomarkers Prev 2000;9(8):795–804

56. Giovannucci E, Rimm EB, Liu Y, Stampfer MJ, Willett WC. A prospective study of cruciferous vegetables and prostate cancer. Cancer Epidemiol Biomarkers Prev 2003;12(12):1403–1409

57. Hsing AW, McLaughlin JK, Schuman LM, et al. Diet, tobacco use, and fatal prostate cancer: results from the Lutheran Brotherhood Cohort Study. Cancer Res 1990;50(21):6836–6840

58. Key TJ, Allen N, Appleby P, et al. Fruits and vegetables and prostate cancer: no association among 1104 cases in a prospective study of 130544 men in the European Prospective Investigation into Cancer and Nutrition (EPIC). Int J Cancer 2004;109(1):119–124

59. Schuurman AG, Goldbohm RA, Dorant E, van den Brandt PA. Vegetable and fruit consumption and prostate cancer risk: a cohort study in The Netherlands. Cancer Epidemiol Biomarkers Prev 1998;7(8):673–680

60. Kristal AR, Stanford JL. Cruciferous vegetables and prostate cancer risk: confounding by PSA screening. Cancer Epidemiol Biomarkers Prev 2004;13(7):1265

61. Fenwick GR, Heaney RK, Mullin WJ. Glucosinolates and their breakdown products in food and food plants. Crit Rev Food Sci Nutr 1983;18(2):123–201

62. McMillan M, Spinks EA, Fenwick GR. Preliminary observations on the effect of dietary brussels sprouts on thyroid function. Hum Toxicol 1986;5(1):15–19

63. National Cancer Institute. Eat 5 to 9 servings of fruits and vegetables a day for better health. 2005. Available at: http://www.5aday.gov/homepage/index_content.html. Accessed 8/1/06

64. Michaud DS, Spiegelman D, Clinton SK, Rimm EB, Willett WC, Giovannucci EL. Fruit and vegetable intake and incidence of bladder cancer in a male prospective cohort. J Natl Cancer Inst 1999;91(7):605–613

3 Legumes

Legumes are plants with seedpods that split into two halves. Edible seeds from plants in the legume family include beans, peas, lentils, soybeans, and peanuts. Peanuts are nutritionally similar to tree nuts; therefore, information on the health benefits of peanuts is presented in Chapter 4. Although legumes are an important part of traditional diets around the world, they are often neglected in typical Western diets. Legumes are inexpensive, nutrient-dense sources of plant protein that can be substituted for dietary animal protein.[1] Whereas sources of animal protein are often rich in saturated fats, the small quantities of fats in legumes are mostly unsaturated fats. Not only are legumes excellent sources of essential minerals, they are rich in dietary fiber and other phytochemicals that may affect health. Soybeans have attracted the most scientific interest, mainly because they are a unique source of phytoestrogens known as isoflavones.[2] Although other legumes lack isoflavones, they also represent unique packages of nutrients and phytochemicals that may work synergistically to reduce chronic disease risk. In this chapter the health effects of diets rich in legumes and soy foods are summarized. Research on the health effects of soy isoflavones is discussed in Chapter 14.

Prevention

Type 2 Diabetes Mellitus

Dry Beans, Peas, and Lentils

The glycemic index is a measure of the potential for carbohydrates in different foods to raise blood glucose levels. In general, consuming foods with high-glycemic index values causes blood glucose levels to rise more rapidly, resulting in greater insulin secretion by the pancreas than consuming foods with low-glycemic index values. Chronically elevated blood glucose levels and excessive insulin secretion are thought to play important roles in the development of type 2 diabetes mellitus (DM).[3] Because legumes generally have low-glycemic index values, substituting legumes for high-glycemic index foods like white rice or potatoes lowers the glycemic load of one's diet. Low dietary glycemic loads have been associated with reduced risk of developing type 2 DM in several large prospective studies.[4,5] Obesity is another important risk factor for type 2 DM. Numerous clinical trials have shown that the consumption of low-glycemic index foods delays the return of hunger, decreases subsequent food intake, and increases the sensation of fullness compared with high-glycemic index foods.[6] The results of several small short-term trials of a few months suggest that low-glycemic index diets result in significantly more weight or fat loss than high-glycemic index diets.[7–9] Thus, diets rich in legumes may decrease the risk of type 2 DM by improving blood glucose control, decreasing insulin secretion, and delaying the return of hunger after a meal. For more information on glycemic index values and glycemic load, see Appendix 1.

Cardiovascular Disease

Dry Beans, Peas, and Lentils

The only prospective cohort study to examine the effect of legume intake on cardiovascular disease risk found that after 19 years of follow-up, men and women who ate dry beans, peas, or peanuts at least 4 times weekly had a risk of coronary heart disease (CHD) that was 21% lower than those who ate them less than once weekly.[10] When compared with a typical Western diet, legume intake as part of a healthy dietary pattern that included higher intakes of vegetables, fruits, whole grains, fish, and poultry, was associated with a risk of CHD that was 30% lower in men[11] and 24% lower in women.[12] The results of controlled clinical trials suggest that increasing dry bean consumption improves serum lipid and lipoprotein profiles. A meta-analysis that combined the results of 11 clinical trials found that increasing the consumption of dry beans resulted in modest (6 to 7%) decreases in total cholesterol and low-density lipoprotein (LDL) cholesterol.[13] Several characteristics of dry beans may contribute to their cardioprotective effects. Dry beans are rich in soluble fiber, which is known to have a cholesterol-lowering effect (see Chapter 12). Elevated plasma homocysteine levels are associated with increased cardiovascular disease risk, and dry beans are good sources of folate, which helps to lower homocysteine levels. Dry beans are also good sources of magnesium and potassium, which may decrease cardiovascular disease risk by helping to lower blood pressure.[13] The low glycemic index values of dry beans means that they are less likely to raise blood glucose and insulin levels, which may also decrease cardiovascular disease risk. For more information on glycemic index values, see Appendix 1.

Soy

In 1999, the U.S. Food and Drug Administration (FDA) approved the following health claim: "Diets low in saturated fat and cholesterol that include 25 grams of soy protein a day may reduce the risk of heart disease."[14] Most of the evidence to support this health claim was included in a 1995 meta-analysis of 38 controlled clinical trials, which found that an average intake of 47 g/d of soy protein decreased total serum cholesterol levels by an average of 9% and LDL-cholesterol levels by 13%.[15] However, the results of clinical trials conducted since 1995 suggest that the LDL-cholesterol-lowering effect of soy protein is more modest.[16] Only 8 out of 22 controlled clinical trials conducted since 1998 found that supplementation with soy protein significantly lowered LDL cholesterol compared with milk or animal protein, and the overall reduction in LDL cholesterol was ~ 3%.[17] A meta-analysis of 10 controlled clinical trials of soy protein conducted from 1995 to 2002 found a comparably modest overall reduction in serum LDL cholesterol.[18] The consumption of isolated soy isoflavones (as supplements or extracts) does not appear to have favorable effects on serum lipid profiles.[18-20] A recent science advisory from the Nutrition Committee of the American Heart Association concluded that earlier research indicating soy protein consumption resulted in clinically important reductions in LDL cholesterol compared with other proteins has not been confirmed.[17] However, many soy products may be beneficial for overall cardiovascular health due to their relatively high content of polyunsaturated fat, fiber, and phytosterols compared with animal products.[21]

Cancer

Dry Beans, Peas, and Lentils

Although dry beans, peas, and lentils are rich in several compounds that could potentially reduce the risk of certain cancers, the results of epidemiological studies are too inconsistent to draw any firm conclusions regarding dry bean intake and cancer risk in general.[22,23]

Prostate Cancer

There is limited evidence from observational studies that legume intake is inversely related to the risk of prostate cancer. In a 6-year prospective study of more than 14,000 Seventh Day Adventist men living in the United States, those with the highest intakes of legumes (beans, lentils, or split peas) had a significantly lower risk of prostate cancer.[24] A prospective study of more than 58,000 men in the Netherlands found that those with the highest intakes of legumes had a risk of prostate cancer that was 29% lower than those with the lowest intakes.[25] Similarly, in a case-control study of 1619 North American men diagnosed with prostate cancer and 1618 healthy men matched for age and ethnicity, those with the highest legume intakes had a risk of prostate cancer that was 38% lower than those with the lowest intakes.[26] Excluding the intake of soy foods from the analysis did not weaken the inverse association between legume intake and prostate cancer, suggesting that soy was not the only legume that conferred protection against prostate cancer.

Soy

Prostate Cancer

Although there is considerable scientific interest in the potential for soy products to prevent prostate cancer, evidence that higher intakes of soy foods can reduce the risk of prostate cancer in humans is limited. Only two out of six case-control studies found that higher intakes of soy products were associated with significantly lower prostate cancer risk. In the largest case-control study, North American men who consumed an average of at least 1.4 oz of soy foods daily were 38% less likely to have prostate cancer than men who did not consume soy foods.[26] A much smaller case-control study of Chinese men found that men who consumed at least 4 oz of soy foods daily were only half as likely to have prostate cancer as those who consumed less than 1 oz daily.[27] However, case-control studies conducted among North American,[28,29] Japanese,[30] and Taiwanese men[31] did not find that higher soy intakes were associated with significantly lower prostate cancer risk. A 6-year prospective cohort study of more than 12,000 Seventh Day Adventist men in the United States found that those who drank soy milk more than once daily had a risk of prostate cancer that was 70% lower than those who never drank soy milk;[32] however, a 23-year study of more than 5000 Japanese American men found no association between tofu consumption and prostate cancer risk.[33]

Breast Cancer

At least 15 epidemiological studies have assessed the relationship between soy food intake and the risk of breast cancer. Only one out of four prospective studies (three in Asian populations and one in the U.S. population) found that higher intakes of a soy food were associated with a significant reduction in breast cancer risk. In that 9-year study of more than 21,000 Japanese women, higher intakes of miso soup, but not other soy foods, were inversely associated with breast cancer risk.[34] Most case-control studies did not find that women with higher soy intakes were at lower risk of breast cancer, except for women who had higher soy intakes during adolescence.[35,36] Two case-control studies, one of Chinese women[37] and one of Asian American women[38] found that women with higher soy intakes during adolescence were significantly less likely to develop breast cancer later in life.

Intake Recommendations

Substituting beans, peas, and lentils for foods that are high in saturated fat or refined carbohydrates is likely to help lower the risk of type 2 DM and cardiovascular disease. Soybeans and foods made from soybeans (soy foods) are excellent sources of protein. In fact, soy protein is complete protein, meaning it provides all of the essential amino acids in adequate amounts for human health.[2] As with beans, peas, and lentils, soy foods are also excellent substitutes for protein sources that are high in saturated fat like red meat or cheese. Although several health-related organizations recommend daily consumption of 5 to 9 servings ($2^1/_2$ to $4^1/_2$ cups) of fruits and vegetables daily (see Chapter 1), few make specific recommendations for legumes. In the 2005 Dietary Guidelines for Americans, an intake of 3 cups (6 servings) of legumes weekly is recommended for people who consume $\sim$8368 kJ ($\sim$2000 kcal/d).[39] A serving of legumes is equal to $^1/_2$ cup of cooked beans, peas, lentils, or tofu.

Summary

- Plant foods from the legume family include dry beans, peas, lentils, and soybeans.
- Legumes are excellent sources of protein, low-glycemic index carbohydrates, essential micronutrients, and fiber.
- Substituting legumes for foods that are high in saturated fats or refined carbohydrates is likely to lower the risk of cardiovascular disease and type 2 DM.
- Although legumes are rich in several compounds that could potentially reduce the risk of certain cancers, the results of epidemiological studies are too inconsistent to draw any firm conclusions regarding legume intake and cancer risk in general.
- The most recent Dietary Guidelines for Americans recommend a weekly intake of 6 servings (3 cups) of legumes for people who consume $\sim$8368 kJ (2000 kcal/d.[39]

References

1. Anderson JW, Smith BM, Washnock CS. Cardiovascular and renal benefits of dry bean and soybean intake. Am J Clin Nutr 1999;70(3 Suppl):464S–474S
2. Messina MJ. Legumes and soybeans: overview of their nutritional profiles and health effects. Am J Clin Nutr 1999;70(3 Suppl):439S–450S
3. Willett W, Manson J, Liu S. Glycemic index, glycemic load, and risk of type 2 diabetes. Am J Clin Nutr 2002;76(1):274S–280S
4. Salmeron J, Ascherio A, Rimm EB, et al. Dietary fiber, glycemic load, and risk of NIDDM in men. Diabetes Care 1997;20(4):545–550
5. Salmeron J, Manson JE, Stampfer MJ, Colditz GA, Wing AL, Willett WC. Dietary fiber, glycemic load, and risk of non-insulin-dependent diabetes mellitus in women. JAMA 1997;277(6):472–477
6. Ludwig DS. Dietary glycemic index and the regulation of body weight. Lipids 2003;38(2):117–121
7. Bouche C, Rizkalla SW, Luo J, et al. Five-week, low-glycemic index diet decreases total fat mass and improves plasma lipid profile in moderately overweight nondiabetic men. Diabetes Care 2002;25(5):822–828
8. Spieth LE, Harnish JD, Lenders CM, et al. A low-glycemic index diet in the treatment of pediatric obesity. Arch Pediatr Adolesc Med 2000;154(9):947–951
9. Slabber M, Barnard HC, Kuyl JM, Dannhauser A, Schall R. Effects of a low-insulin-response, energy-restricted diet on weight loss and plasma insulin concentrations in hyperinsulinemic obese females. Am J Clin Nutr 1994;60(1):48–53
10. Bazzano LA, He J, Ogden LG, et al. Legume consumption and risk of coronary heart disease in US men and women: NHANES I Epidemiologic Follow-up Study. Arch Intern Med 2001;161(21):2573–2578
11. Hu FB, Rimm EB, Stampfer MJ, Ascherio A, Spiegelman D, Willett WC. Prospective study of major dietary patterns and risk of coronary heart disease in men. Am J Clin Nutr 2000;72(4):912–921
12. Fung TT, Willett WC, Stampfer MJ, Manson JE, Hu FB. Dietary patterns and the risk of coronary heart disease in women. Arch Intern Med 2001;161(15):1857–1862
13. Anderson JW, Major AW. Pulses and lipaemia, short- and long-term effect: potential in the prevention of cardiovascular disease. Br J Nutr 2002;88(Suppl 3):S263–S271
14. U.S. Food and Drug Administration. Final Rule: Food Labeling: Health Claims; Soy Protein and Coronary Heart Disease. 1999. Available at: http://www.cfsan.fda.gov/~lrd/fr991026.html. Accessed 8/1/06
15. Anderson JW, Johnstone BM, Cook-Newell ME. Meta-analysis of the effects of soy protein intake on serum lipids. N Engl J Med 1995;333(5):276–282
16. Erdman JW Jr. AHA Science Advisory: Soy protein and cardiovascular disease: a statement for healthcare professionals from the Nutrition Committee of the AHA. Circulation 2000;102(20):2555–2559
17. Sacks FM, Lichtenstein A, Van Horn L, Harris W, Kris-Etherton P, Winston M. Soy protein, isoflavones, and cardiovascular health. An American Heart Association Science Advisory for Professionals from the Nutrition Committee. Circulation 2006; Epub ahead of print.
18. Weggemans RM, Trautwein EA. Relation between soy-associated isoflavones and LDL and HDL cholesterol concentrations in humans: a meta-analysis. Eur J Clin Nutr 2003;57(8):940–946
19. Lichtenstein AH, Jalbert SM, Adlercreutz H, et al. Lipoprotein response to diets high in soy or animal protein with and without isoflavones in moderately hypercholesterolemic subjects. Arterioscler Thromb Vasc Biol 2002;22(11):1852–1858
20. Nikander E, Tiitinen A, Laitinen K, Tikkanen M, Ylikorkala O. Effects of isolated isoflavonoids on lipids, lipoproteins, insulin sensitivity, and ghrelin in postmenopausal women. J Clin Endocrinol Metab 2004;89(7):3567–3572
21. Kendall CW, Jenkins DJ. A dietary portfolio: maximal reduction of low-density lipoprotein cholesterol with diet. Curr Atheroscler Rep 2004;6(6):492–498
22. Mathers JC. Pulses and carcinogenesis: potential for the prevention of colon, breast and other cancers. Br J Nutr 2002;88(Suppl 3):S273–S279
23. World Cancer Research Fund. Food, Nutrition, and the Prevention of Cancer: A Global Perspective. Washington, DC: American Institute for Cancer Research; 1997
24. Mills PK, Beeson WL, Phillips RL, Fraser GE. Cohort study of diet, lifestyle, and prostate cancer in Adventist men. Cancer 1989;64(3):598–604
25. Schuurman AG, Goldbohm RA, Dorant E, van den Brandt PA. Vegetable and fruit consumption and prostate cancer risk: a cohort study in The Netherlands. Cancer Epidemiol Biomarkers Prev 1998;7(8):673–680
26. Kolonel LN, Hankin JH, Whittemore AS, et al. Vegetables, fruits, legumes and prostate cancer: a multi-ethnic case-control study. Cancer Epidemiol Biomarkers Prev 2000;9(8):795–804
27. Lee MM, Gomez SL, Chang JS, Wey M, Wang RT, Hsing AW. Soy and isoflavone consumption in relation to prostate cancer risk in China. Cancer Epidemiol Biomarkers Prev 2003;12(7):665–668
28. Strom SS, Yamamura Y, Duphorne CM, et al. Phytoestrogen intake and prostate cancer: a case-control study using a new database. Nutr Cancer 1999;33(1):20–25
29. Villeneuve PJ, Johnson KC, Kreiger N, Mao Y. Risk factors for prostate cancer: results from the Canadian National Enhanced Cancer Surveillance System. The Canadian Cancer Registries Epidemiology Research Group. Cancer Causes Control 1999;10(5):355–367
30. Oishi K, Okada K, Yoshida O, et al. A case-control study of prostatic cancer with reference to dietary habits. Prostate 1988;12(2):179–190
31. Sung JF, Lin RS, Pu YS, Chen YC, Chang HC, Lai MK. Risk factors for prostate carcinoma in Taiwan: a case-control study in a Chinese population. Cancer 1999;86(3):484–491
32. Jacobsen BK, Knutsen SF, Fraser GE. Does high soy milk intake reduce prostate cancer incidence? The Adventist Health Study (United States). Cancer Causes Control 1998;9(6):553–557
33. Nomura AM, Hankin JH, Lee J, Stemmermann GN. Cohort study of tofu intake and prostate cancer: no apparent association. Cancer Epidemiol Biomarkers Prev 2004;13(12):2277–2279
34. Yamamoto S, Sobue T, Kobayashi M, Sasaki S, Tsugane S. Soy, isoflavones, and breast cancer risk in Japan. J Natl Cancer Inst 2003;95(12):906–913

35. Peeters PH, Keinan-Boker L, van der Schouw YT, Grobbee DE. Phytoestrogens and breast cancer risk. Review of the epidemiological evidence. Breast Cancer Res Treat 2003;77(2):171–183

36. Shannon J, Ray R, Wu C, et al. Food and botanical groupings and risk of breast cancer: a case-control study in Shanghai, China. Cancer Epidemiol Biomarkers Prev 2005;14(1):81–90

37. Shu XO, Jin F, Dai Q, et al. Soyfood intake during adolescence and subsequent risk of breast cancer among Chinese women. Cancer Epidemiol Biomarkers Prev 2001;10(5):483–488

38. Wu AH, Wan P, Hankin J, Tseng CC, Yu MC, Pike MC. Adolescent and adult soy intake and risk of breast cancer in Asian-Americans. Carcinogenesis 2002; 23(9):1491–1496

39. U.S .Department of Health and Human Services, US Department of Agriculture. Dietary Guidelines for Americans. 2005. Available at: http://www.health-ierus.gov/dietaryguidelines/. Accessed 8/1/06

4 Nuts

In the not too distant past, nuts were considered unhealthy because of their relatively high fat content. In contrast, recent research suggests that regular nut consumption is an important part of a healthy diet.[1] Although the fat content of nuts is relatively high (14 to 19 g/oz), most of the fats in nuts are the healthier monounsaturated and polyunsaturated fats[2] (see **Table 4–1**). The term "nuts" includes almonds, Brazil nuts, cashews, hazelnuts, macadamia nuts, pecans, pistachios, walnuts, and peanuts. Despite their name, peanuts are actually legumes like peas and beans. However, they are nutritionally similar to tree nuts and have some of the same beneficial properties.

Prevention

Cardiovascular Disease

Coronary Heart Disease

In large prospective cohort studies, regular nut consumption has been consistently associated with significant reductions in the risk of coronary heart disease (CHD).[3] One of the first studies to observe a protective effect of nut consumption was the Adventist Health Study, which followed more than 30,000 Seventh Day Adventists over 12 years.[4] In general, the dietary and lifestyle habits of Seventh Day Adventists are closer to those recommended for cardiovascular disease prevention than those of average Americans. Few of those who participated in the Adventist Health Study smoked, and most consumed a diet lower in saturated fat than the average American. Even in this healthy living group, those who consumed nuts at least 5 times weekly had a risk of death from CHD that was 48% lower than those who consumed nuts less than once weekly and a risk of a nonfatal myocardial infarction (MI) that was 51% lower. Even in people over 83 years of age, those who ate nuts at least 5 times weekly had a risk of death from CHD that was 39% lower than those who consumed nuts less than once weekly.[5] The results of a smaller prospective study of more than

Table 4–1 Fat, Phytosterol, and Fiber Content of a One-Ounce Serving of Selected Nuts

Nut	Total Fat (g)	Monoun-saturated Fat (g)	Polyun-saturated Fat (g)	Phytosterols (mg)	Fiber (g)
Almonds	14.4	9.1	3.5	34.0	3.3
Brazil nuts	18.8	7.0	5.8	–	2.1
Cashews	13.3	7.2	2.4	44.8	0.9
Hazelnuts	17.2	12.9	2.2	27.2	2.8
Macadamia nuts	21.5	16.7	0.4	32.9	2.4
Peanuts	14.1	7.0	4.5	62.3	2.3
Peanut butter (2 tbs)	16.7	7.9	4.8	32.6	1.9
Pecans	20.4	11.6	6.1	28.9	2.7
Pine nuts	19.4	5.3	9.7	40.0	1.0
Pistachio nuts	12.6	6.6	3.8	60.7	2.9
Black walnuts	16.7	4.3	9.9	30.6	1.9

3000 Black men and women were similar.[6] Those who consumed nuts at least 5 times weekly had a risk of death from CHD that was 44% lower than those who consumed nuts less than once weekly.

The cardioprotective effects of nuts were not limited to Seventh Day Adventists. In a 14-year study of more than 86,000 women participating in the Nurses' Health Study, those who consumed more than 5 oz of nuts weekly had a risk of CHD that was 35% lower than those who ate less than 1 oz of nuts monthly.[7] Similar decreases were observed for the risk of death from CHD and nonfatal MI. A 17-year study of more than 21,000 male health professionals found that those who consumed nuts at least twice weekly had a risk of sudden cardiac death that was 53% lower than those who rarely or never consumed nuts, although there was no significant decrease in the risk of nonfatal MI or nonsudden CHD death.[8] The Iowa Women's Health Study, which followed more than 30,000 postmenopausal women for 12 years, is the only published prospective study that did not observe a significant inverse association between nut consumption and CHD mortality, although a slight but significant decrease in all cause mortality was observed in those who consumed nuts twice weekly.[9] Overall, the results of most prospective cohort studies suggest that regular nut consumption is associated with a substantial decrease in the risk of death related to CHD.

Serum Cholesterol

Results of controlled clinical trials indicate that at least part of the cardioprotective effect of nut consumption is derived from beneficial effects on serum total and low-density lipoprotein (LDL)-cholesterol concentrations.[3] At least 18 controlled clinical trials have found that adding nuts to a diet that is low in saturated fat results in significant reductions in serum total cholesterol and LDL-cholesterol concentrations in people with normal or elevated serum cholesterol. These effects have been observed for almonds,[10-13] hazelnuts,[14] macadamia nuts,[15,16] peanuts,[17,18] pecans,[19] pistachio nuts,[20] and walnuts.[21-26]

Cardioprotective Compounds in Nuts

Substituting dietary saturated fats with polyunsaturated and monounsaturated fats like those found in nuts can decrease serum total and LDL-cholesterol concentrations.[3] However, in some of the clinical trials, the cholesterol-lowering effect of nut consumption was greater than would be predicted from the polyunsaturated and monounsaturated fat content of the nuts, suggesting there may be other protective factors in nuts.[27] Other bioactive compounds in nuts that may contribute to their cholesterol-lowering effects include fiber (Chapter 12) and phytosterols (Chapter 19). See **Table 4–1** for the unsaturated fat, fiber, and phytosterol contents of selected nuts. Walnuts are especially rich in α-linolenic acid, an omega-3 fatty acid with several cardioprotective effects, including the prevention of cardiac arrhythmias that may lead to sudden cardiac death (Chapter 11). Other nutrients that may contribute to the cardioprotective effects of nuts include folate and potassium.[3,28] The U.S. Food and Drug Administration has acknowledged the emerging evidence for a relationship between nut consumption and cardiovascular disease risk by approving the following qualified health claim for nuts:[29] "Scientific evidence suggests but does not prove that eating 1.5 ounces per day of most nuts as part of a diet low in saturated fat and cholesterol may reduce the risk of heart disease."

Type 2 Diabetes Mellitus

Recent results from the Nurses' Health Study suggest that nut and peanut butter consumption may be inversely associated with the risk of type 2 diabetes mellitus (DM) in women.[30] In this cohort of more than 86,000 women followed over 16 years, those who consumed an ounce of nuts at least 5 times weekly had a risk of developing type 2 DM that was 27% lower than those who rarely or never consumed nuts. Similarly, those who consumed peanut butter at least 5 times weekly had a risk of developing type 2 DM that was 21% lower than those who rarely or never consumed peanut butter. Although these findings require confirmation in other studies, they provide additional evidence that nuts can be a component of a healthy diet. Compounds in nuts that could contribute to the observed decrease in type 2 DM include unsaturated fats, fiber, and magnesium.

Safety

Nut Allergies

Allergies to peanuts and tree nuts (almonds, cashews, hazelnuts, pecans, pistachios, and walnuts) are among the most common food allergies, affecting at least 1 % of the U.S. population.[31] Although all food allergies have the potential to induce severe reactions, peanuts and tree nuts are among the foods most commonly associated with anaphylaxis, a life-threatening allergic reaction.[32] People with severe peanut or tree nut allergies need to take special precautions to avoid inadvertently consuming peanuts or tree nuts by checking labels and avoiding unlabeled snacks, candies, and desserts.

Intake Recommendations

Regular nut consumption, equivalent to an ounce of nuts 5 times weekly, has been consistently associated with significant reductions in CHD risk in epidemiological studies. Consuming 1 to 2 oz of nuts daily as part of a diet that is low in saturated fat has been found to lower serum total and LDL-cholesterol in several controlled clinical trials. Since an ounce of most nuts provides at least 669 kJ (160 kcal), simply adding an ounce of nuts daily to one's habitual diet without eliminating other foods may result in weight gain. Substituting unsalted nuts for other less healthy snacks or for meat in main dishes are two ways to make nuts part of a healthy diet.

Summary

- Nuts are good sources of fiber, phytosterols, and unsaturated fat.
- The results of most prospective cohort studies suggest that regular nut consumption (equivalent to 1 oz at least 5 times weekly)

is associated with significantly lower cardiovascular disease risk.
- At least one prospective cohort study has found that regular nut consumption is associated with significantly lower risk of developing type 2 DM.
- An ounce of most nuts provides at least 669 kJ (160 kcal) of energy; therefore, substituting nuts for other less healthy snacks is a good strategy for avoiding weight gain when increasing nut intake.

References

1. Hu FB, Stampfer MJ. Nut consumption and risk of coronary heart disease: a review of epidemiologic evidence. Curr Atheroscler Rep 1999;1(3):204–209
2. Kris-Etherton PM, Yu-Poth S, Sabate J, Ratcliffe HE, Zhao G, Etherton TD. Nuts and their bioactive constituents: effects on serum lipids and other factors that affect disease risk. Am J Clin Nutr 1999;70(3 Suppl): 504S–511S
3. Kris-Etherton PM, Zhao G, Binkoski AE, Coval SM, Etherton TD. The effects of nuts on coronary heart disease risk. Nutr Rev 2001;59(4):103–111
4. Fraser GE, Sabate J, Beeson WL, Strahan TM. A possible protective effect of nut consumption on risk of coronary heart disease. The Adventist Health Study. Arch Intern Med 1992;152(7):1416–1424
5. Fraser GE, Shavlik DJ. Risk factors for all-cause and coronary heart disease mortality in the oldest-old. The Adventist Health Study. Arch Intern Med 1997; 157(19):2249–2258
6. Fraser GE, Sumbureru D, Pribis P, Neil RL, Frankson MA. Association among health habits, risk factors, and all-cause mortality in a black California population. Epidemiology 1997;8(2):168–174
7. Hu FB, Stampfer MJ, Manson JE, et al. Frequent nut consumption and risk of coronary heart disease in women: prospective cohort study. BMJ 1998; 317 (7169):1341–1345
8. Albert CM, Gaziano JM, Willett WC, Manson JE. Nut consumption and decreased risk of sudden cardiac death in the Physicians' Health Study. Arch Intern Med 2002;162(12):1382–1387
9. Ellsworth JL, Kushi LH, Folsom AR. Frequent nut intake and risk of death from coronary heart disease and all causes in postmenopausal women: the Iowa Women's Health Study. Nutr Metab Cardiovasc Dis 2001;11(6): 372–377
10. Hyson DA, Schneeman BO, Davis PA. Almonds and almond oil have similar effects on plasma lipids and LDL oxidation in healthy men and women. J Nutr 2002; 132(4):703–707
11. Jenkins DJ, Kendall CW, Marchie A, et al. Dose response of almonds on coronary heart disease risk factors: blood lipids, oxidized low-density lipoproteins, lipoprotein(a), homocysteine, and pulmonary nitric oxide: a randomized, controlled, crossover trial. Circulation 2002;106(11):1327–1332
12. Sabate J, Haddad E, Tanzman JS, Jambazian P, Rajaram S. Serum lipid response to the graduated enrichment

of a Step I diet with almonds: a randomized feeding trial. Am J Clin Nutr 2003;77(6):1379–1384

13. Spiller GA, Jenkins DA, Bosello O, Gates JE, Cragen LN, Bruce B. Nuts and plasma lipids: an almond-based diet lowers LDL-C while preserving HDL-C. J Am Coll Nutr 1998;17(3):285–290

14. Durak I, Koksal I, Kacmaz M, Buyukkocak S, Cimen BM, Ozturk HS. Hazelnut supplementation enhances plasma antioxidant potential and lowers plasma cholesterol levels. Clin Chim Acta 1999;284(1):113–115

15. Curb JD, Wergowske G, Dobbs JC, Abbott RD, Huang B. Serum lipid effects of a high-monounsaturated fat diet based on macadamia nuts. Arch Intern Med 2000;160(8):1154–1158

16. Garg ML, Blake RJ, Wills RB. Macadamia nut consumption lowers plasma total and LDL cholesterol levels in hypercholesterolemic men. J Nutr 2003;133(4):1060–1063

17. Kris-Etherton PM, Pearson TA, Wan Y, et al. High-monounsaturated fatty acid diets lower both plasma cholesterol and triacylglycerol concentrations. Am J Clin Nutr 1999;70(6):1009–1015

18. O'Byrne DJ, Knauft DA, Shireman RB. Low fat-monounsaturated rich diets containing high-oleic peanuts improve serum lipoprotein profiles. Lipids 1997;32(7):687–695

19. Morgan WA, Clayshulte BJ. Pecans lower low-density lipoprotein cholesterol in people with normal lipid levels. J Am Diet Assoc 2000;100(3):312–318

20. Edwards K, Kwaw I, Matud J, Kurtz I. Effect of pistachio nuts on serum lipid levels in patients with moderate hypercholesterolemia. J Am Coll Nutr 1999;18(3):229–232

21. Abbey M, Noakes M, Belling GB, Nestel PJ. Partial replacement of saturated fatty acids with almonds or walnuts lowers total plasma cholesterol and low-density-lipoprotein cholesterol. Am J Clin Nutr 1994;59(5):995–999

22. Almario RU, Vonghavaravat V, Wong R, Kasim-Karakas SE. Effects of walnut consumption on plasma fatty acids and lipoproteins in combined hyperlipidemia. Am J Clin Nutr 2001;74(1):72–79

23. Chisholm A, Mann J, Skeaff M, et al. A diet rich in walnuts favourably influences plasma fatty acid profile in moderately hyperlipidaemic subjects. Eur J Clin Nutr 1998;52(1):12–16

24. Morgan JM, Horton K, Reese D, Carey C, Walker K, Capuzzi DM. Effects of walnut consumption as part of a low-fat, low-cholesterol diet on serum cardiovascular risk factors. Int J Vitam Nutr Res 2002;72(5):341–347

25. Sabate J, Fraser GE, Burke K, Knutsen SF, Bennett H, Lindsted KD. Effects of walnuts on serum lipid levels and blood pressure in normal men. N Engl J Med 1993;328(9):603–607

26. Zambon D, Sabate J, Munoz S, et al. Substituting walnuts for monounsaturated fat improves the serum lipid profile of hypercholesterolemic men and women. A randomized crossover trial. Ann Intern Med 2000;132(7):538–546

27. Coulston AM. Do nuts have a place in a healthful diet? Nutr Today 2003;38(3):95–99

28. Willett WC. Eat, Drink, and Be Healthy: The Harvard Medical School Guide to Healthy Eating. New York: Simon & Schuster; 2001

29. U.S. Food and Drug Administration, Center for Food Safety and Nutrition. Summary of Qualified Health Claims Permitted. 2003. Available at: http://www.cfsan.fda.gov/~dms/qhc-sum.html#nuts. Accessed 8/1/06

30. Jiang R, Manson JE, Stampfer MJ, Liu S, Willett WC, Hu FB. Nut and peanut butter consumption and risk of type 2 diabetes in women. JAMA 2002;288(20):2554–2560

31. Sicherer SH, Munoz-Furlong A, Burks AW, Sampson HA. Prevalence of peanut and tree nut allergy in the US determined by a random digit dial telephone survey. J Allergy Clin Immunol 1999;103(4):559–562

32. Al-Muhsen S, Clarke AE, Kagan RS. Peanut allergy: an overview. CMAJ 2003;168(10):1279–1285

5 Whole Grains

Grains are the seeds of plants belonging to the grass family. Species that produce edible grains include wheat, rice, maize (corn), barley, oats, and rye.[1] An intact grain has an outer layer of bran, a carbohydrate-rich middle layer called the endosperm, and an inner germ layer. Although not always intact, whole-grain foods contain the entire grain, including the bran, the endosperm, and the germ. Whole grains are rich in potentially beneficial compounds, including vitamins, minerals, and phytochemicals, such as lignans (Chapter 17), phytosterols (Chapter 19), and fiber (Chapter 12). Most of these compounds are located in the bran or the germ of the grain, both of which are lost during the refining process, leaving only the starchy endosperm.[2] Compared with diets high in refined grains, diets rich in whole grains are associated with reduced risks of several chronic diseases. The health benefits of whole grains are not entirely explained by the individual contributions of the nutrients and phytochemicals they contain. Whole grains represent a unique package of energy, micronutrients, and phytochemicals that work synergistically to promote health and prevent disease.

Prevention

Type 2 Diabetes Mellitus

Four large prospective studies have found that higher whole-grain intakes are associated with significant reductions in the risk of developing type 2 diabetes mellitus (DM) over time.[3–6] In the studies conducted in the United States, those who consumed an average of ~3 daily servings of whole-grain foods had a risk of type 2 DM that was 21 to 30% lower than those who rarely or never consumed whole grains.[3–5] In Finland the quarter of the population with the highest whole-grain intakes had a risk of type 2 DM that was 35% lower than the quarter

with the lowest intakes.[6] Insulin resistance is a condition of decreased insulin sensitivity that increases the risk of developing type 2 DM. In observational studies, higher whole-grain intakes are associated with decreased insulin resistance[7] and increased insulin sensitivity[8] in people who do not have type 2 DM. In a controlled clinical trial that compared the effects of a diet rich in whole grains with a diet high in refined grains in overweight and obese adults, several clinical measures of insulin resistance were significantly lower after 6 weeks on the whole-grain diet compared with the refined-grain diet.[9]

The refining process makes the carbohydrate in the endosperm of the grain easier to digest. Immediately after a meal, carbohydrate from refined grains elicits a higher and more rapid elevation in blood glucose as well as greater demand for insulin.[10] Over time, elevated blood glucose levels and compensatory increases in insulin secretion may lead to the development of type 2 diabetes. The glycemic index value is a way of ranking the glucose-raising potential of carbohydrate in different foods. Foods made from whole grains generally have lower glycemic index values than do foods made from refined grains.[11] Substituting whole-grain foods for refined-grain foods decreases dietary glycemic load, which has been associated with decreased risk of type 2 DM[12,13] and improved control of blood glucose levels in people who have diabetes.[14] Thus, substituting low-glycemic index whole-grain foods for high-glycemic index refined-grain foods may substantially decrease the risk of developing type 2 diabetes. For more information on glycemic index and glycemic load, see Appendix 1.

Cardiovascular Disease

At least seven large prospective cohort studies have found that higher intakes of whole grains are associated with significant reductions in coronary heart disease (CHD) risk.[15-21] In general, those with the highest intakes of whole grains (~ 3 servings daily) had a risk of CHD that was 20 to 30% lower than those with the lowest intakes even after adjusting the risk estimates for other heart disease risk factors. Whole-grain foods consumed in these studies included dark bread, whole-grain breakfast cereals, popcorn, cooked oatmeal, brown rice, bran, barley, and other grains like bulgar and kasha. A recent study that followed more than 85,000 male physicians for 5 years found that those who consumed at least one serving of whole-grain breakfast cereal daily had a risk of death from cardiovascular disease that was 20% lower than those who rarely or never consumed whole-grain cereal.[20] Higher intakes of whole grains have also been associated with a decreased risk of ischemic stroke (a stroke caused by the obstruction of a blood vessel that supplies the brain). A study that followed more than 75,000 women participating in the Nurses' Health Study for 12 years found that women who consumed an average of almost 3 servings of whole grains daily had a risk of ischemic stroke that was more than 30% lower than women who rarely consumed whole grains.[22]

Several possible explanations can account for the cardioprotective effects associated with higher intakes of whole grains and lower intakes of refined-grain products. Compared with refined grains, whole grains are richer in nutrients associated with cardiovascular risk reduction, including folate, magnesium, and potassium. Although wheat fiber has not been found to lower serum cholesterol levels, numerous clinical studies have demonstrated that increasing oat fiber intake results in modest reductions in total and LDL-cholesterol.[1] In light of these findings, the U.S. Food and Drug Administration (FDA) approved the following health claim: "Diets low in saturated fat and cholesterol that provide 3 g or more per day of soluble fiber from oat bran, rolled oats (oatmeal), or whole oat flour may reduce the risk of heart disease."[23] Limited evidence suggests that increasing barley intake can also lower serum total and LDL cholesterol.[24] Whole grains are also sources of phytosterols (Chapter 19), compounds that decrease serum cholesterol by interfering with the intestinal

absorption of cholesterol.[25] The relatively low-glycemic index values of whole grains compared with refined grains may also play a role in decreasing the risk of heart disease. Substituting whole-grain products for refined-grain products in one's diet decreases dietary glycemic load. Recent results from large prospective studies suggest that low-glycemic load diets are associated with lower coronary heart disease risk than high-glycemic load diets.[26] For more information on glycemic index and glycemic load, see Appendix 1.

Cancer

Although the protective effects of whole grains against various types of cancer are not as well established as those against diabetes and cardiovascular disease, numerous case-control studies have found inverse associations between various measures of whole-grain intake and cancer risk.[27,28] A meta-analysis of 40 case-control studies examining 20 different types of cancer found that those with high whole-grain intakes had an overall risk of cancer that was 34% lower than those with low whole-grain intakes.[27] These studies generally used some measure of whole-grain bread intake to assess whole-grain intake, although a series of Italian case-control studies also assessed the intake of whole-grain pasta.[28] Higher intakes of whole grain were most consistently associated with decreased risk of gastrointestinal tract cancers, including cancers of the mouth, throat, stomach, colon, and rectum. A prospective cohort study that followed more than 61,000 Swedish women for 15 years found that those who consumed more than 4.5 servings of whole grain daily had a risk of colon cancer that was 35% lower than those who consumed less than 1.5 servings of whole grain daily.[29] In contrast to refined-grain products, whole grains are rich in numerous compounds that may be protective against cancer, particularly cancers of the gastrointestinal tract.[30] Higher fiber intakes are known to speed up the passage of stool through the colon allowing less time for potentially carcinogenic compounds to stay in contact with cells that line the inner surface of the colon. Lignans in whole grains are phytoestrogens, and may affect the development of hormone-dependent cancers.

Table 5–1   Examples of One Serving of Whole-Grain Food

Whole-Grain Food	Amount in One Serving
Whole-grain bread	1 slice
Whole-grain English muffin, bagel, or bun	1 half
Whole-grain cereal, ready to eat	1 oz
Oatmeal, brown rice, or whole-wheat pasta, cooked	$1/2$ cup
Whole-wheat tortilla	1 tortilla (7" diameter)
Whole-grain crackers	5–6 crackers
Popped popcorn	3 cups

Phenolic compounds in whole grains may modify signal transduction pathways that promote the development of cancer or bind potentially damaging free metal ions in the gastrointestinal tract.

Intestinal Health

Diets rich in whole grains and fiber help prevent constipation by softening and adding bulk to stool, and speeding its passage through the colon.[31] Such diets are also associated with decreased risk of diverticulosis, a condition characterized by the formation of small pouches (diverticula) in the colon. Although most people with diverticulosis experience no symptoms, ~ 15 to 20 % may develop pain or inflammation, known as diverticulitis. Diverticulitis was virtually unheard of before the practice of milling (refining) flour began in industrialized countries, and the role of a low-fiber diet in the development of diverticular disease is well-established.[32] Although high-fiber diets are recommended for people with constipation and diverticulosis, people with diverticulosis are sometimes advised to avoid eating small seeds and husks to prevent them from becoming lodged in diverticula and causing diverticulitis. However, no study has ever shown that avoiding seeds or popcorn reduces the risk of diverticulitis in an individual with diverticulosis.[32]

Intake Recommendations

Whole-grain intakes approaching 3 servings daily are associated with significant reductions in chronic disease risk in populations with relatively low whole-grain intakes. One of the objectives of the U.S. Department of Health and Human Services' prevention agenda, Healthy People 2010, is to increase the proportion of people in the United States who consume 3 servings of whole grains daily. However, most Americans consume less than one serving daily.[2] **Table 5–1** provides some examples of a serving of whole grains. The 2005 Dietary Guidelines for Americans recommend consuming 3 or more servings of whole-grain products daily.[33] In view of the potential health benefits of increasing whole-grain intake, 3 daily servings of whole-grain foods should be seen as a minimum, and whole-grain foods should be substituted for refined carbohydrates whenever possible.

Increasing Whole-Grain Intake

Finding Whole-Grain Foods

Whole-grains include amaranth, barley, brown rice, buckwheat (kasha), flaxseed, millet, oats, popcorn, quinoa, rye, spelt, triticale, whole wheat (wheat berries), and wild rice.[34] Unfortunately, it is not always clear from the label whether a product is made mostly from whole grains or refined grains. Some strategies to use when shopping for whole-grain foods include:
- Looking for products that list whole grain(s) as the first ingredient(s).
- Looking for whole-grain products that contain at least 2 g of fiber per serving; whole grains are rich in fiber.
- Looking for products that display this health claim, "Diets rich in whole grain foods and other plant foods and low in total fat, saturated fat and cholesterol may reduce the risk for heart disease and certain cancers." Products displaying this health claim must contain at least 51 % whole grain by weight.[35]
- Looking for whole-wheat pasta that lists whole-wheat flour as the first ingredient. Most pasta is made from refined semolina or durum wheat flour.

Strategies for Increasing Whole-Grain Intake

- Eat whole-grain breakfast cereals, such as wheat flakes, shredded wheat, kashi, muesli, and oatmeal. Bran cereals are not actually whole grain cereals, but their high-fiber content also makes them a good breakfast choice.
- Substitute whole-grain breads, rolls, tortillas, and crackers for those made from refined grains.
- Substitute whole-wheat pasta or pasta made from 50% whole wheat and 50% white flour for conventional pastas.
- Substitute brown rice for white rice.
- Add barley to soups and stews.
- When baking, substitute whole-wheat flour for white or unbleached flour.

Summary

- Whole-grain foods contain the entire grain, including the bran, the endosperm, and the germ.
- Epidemiological studies have found that, diets rich in whole grains are associated with reduced risks of cardiovascular disease and type 2 DM compared with diets high in refined grains.
- Although the protective effects of whole grains against cancer are not as well established as those against cardiovascular disease and type 2 DM, some epidemiological studies have found whole grain intake to be associated with decreased cancer risk.
- Diets rich in whole-grains and fiber help prevent constipation and are also associated with decreased risk of diverticulosis.
- The 2005 Dietary Guidelines for Americans recommend consuming a minimum of 3 servings of whole-grain products daily.[33]

References

1. Truswell AS. Cereal grains and coronary heart disease. Eur J Clin Nutr 2002;56(1):1–14
2. Slavin JL, Jacobs D, Marquart L, Wiemer K. The role of whole grains in disease prevention. J Am Diet Assoc 2001;101(7):780–785
3. Meyer KA, Kushi LH, Jacobs DR Jr, Slavin J, Sellers TA, Folsom AR. Carbohydrates, dietary fiber, and incident type 2 diabetes in older women. Am J Clin Nutr 2000;71(4):921–930
4. Liu S, Manson JE, Stampfer MJ, et al. A prospective study of whole-grain intake and risk of type 2 diabetes mellitus in US women. Am J Public Health 2000;90(9):1409–1415
5. Fung TT, Hu FB, Pereira MA, et al. Whole-grain intake and the risk of type 2 diabetes: a prospective study in men. Am J Clin Nutr 2002;76(3):535–540
6. Montonen J, Knekt P, Jarvinen R, Aromaa A, Reunanen A. Whole-grain and fiber intake and the incidence of type 2 diabetes. Am J Clin Nutr 2003;77(3):622–629
7. McKeown NM, Meigs JB, Liu S, Saltzman E, Wilson PW, Jacques PF. Carbohydrate nutrition, insulin resistance, and the prevalence of the metabolic syndrome in the Framingham Offspring Cohort. Diabetes Care 2004; 27(2):538–546
8. Liese AD, Roach AK, Sparks KC, Marquart L, D'Agostino RB Jr, Mayer-Davis EJ. Whole-grain intake and insulin sensitivity: the Insulin Resistance Atherosclerosis Study. Am J Clin Nutr 2003;78(5):965–971
9. Pereira MA, Jacobs DR Jr, Pins JJ, et al. Effect of whole grains on insulin sensitivity in overweight hyperinsulinemic adults. Am J Clin Nutr 2002;75(5):848–855
10. Liu S. Intake of refined carbohydrates and whole grain foods in relation to risk of type 2 diabetes mellitus and coronary heart disease. J Am Coll Nutr 2002;21(4): 298–306
11. Hallfrisch J. Facn, Behall KM. Mechanisms of the effects of grains on insulin and glucose responses. J Am Coll Nutr 2000;19(3 Suppl):320S–325S
12. Salmeron J, Ascherio A, Rimm EB, et al. Dietary fiber, glycemic load, and risk of NIDDM in men. Diabetes Care 1997;20(4):545–550
13. Salmeron J, Manson JE, Stampfer MJ, Colditz GA, Wing AL, Willett WC. Dietary fiber, glycemic load, and risk of non-insulin-dependent diabetes mellitus in women. JAMA 1997;277(6):472–477
14. Brand-Miller J, Hayne S, Petocz P, Colagiuri S. Low-glycemic index diets in the management of diabetes: a meta-analysis of randomized controlled trials. Diabetes Care 2003;26(8):2261–2267
15. Fraser GE, Sabate J, Beeson WL, Strahan TM. A possible protective effect of nut consumption on risk of coronary heart disease. The Adventist Health Study. Arch Intern Med 1992;152(7):1416–1424
16. Pietinen P, Rimm EB, Korhonen P, et al. Intake of dietary fiber and risk of coronary heart disease in a cohort of Finnish men. The Alpha-Tocopherol, Beta-Carotene Cancer Prevention Study. Circulation 1996;94(11):2720–2727
17. Jacobs DR Jr, Meyer KA, Kushi LH, Folsom AR. Whole-grain intake may reduce the risk of ischemic heart disease death in postmenopausal women: the Iowa Women's Health Study. Am J Clin Nutr 1998;68(2): 248–257
18. Liu S, Stampfer MJ, Hu FB, et al. Whole-grain consumption and risk of coronary heart disease: results from the Nurses' Health Study. Am J Clin Nutr 1999; 70(3):412–419
19. Jacobs DR Jr, Meyer HE, Solvoll K. Reduced mortality among whole grain bread eaters in men and women in the Norwegian County Study. Eur J Clin Nutr 2001; 55(2):137–143

20. Liu S, Sesso HD, Manson JE, Willett WC, Buring JE. Is intake of breakfast cereals related to total and cause-specific mortality in men? Am J Clin Nutr 2003;77(3): 594–599

21. Jensen MK, Koh-Banerjee P, Hu FB, et al. Intakes of whole grains, bran, and germ and the risk of coronary heart disease in men. Am J Clin Nutr 2004;80(6): 1492–1499

22. Liu S, Manson JE, Stampfer MJ, et al. Whole grain consumption and risk of ischemic stroke in women: a prospective study. JAMA 2000;284(12):1534–1540

23. U.S. Food and Drug Administration, HHS. Food labeling: health claims; soluble dietary fiber from certain foods and coronary heart disease. Final rule. Fed Regist. 2003;68(144):44207–44209

24. Behall KM, Scholfield DJ, Hallfrisch J. Lipids significantly reduced by diets containing barley in moderately hypercholesterolemic men. J Am Coll Nutr 2004;23(1):55–62

25. Slavin J. Why whole grains are protective: biological mechanisms. Proc Nutr Soc 2003;62(1):129–134

26. Liu S, Willett WC. Dietary glycemic load and atherothrombotic risk. Curr Atheroscler Rep 2002;4(6): 454–461

27. Jacobs DR Jr, Marquart L, Slavin J, Kushi LH. Whole-grain intake and cancer: an expanded review and meta-analysis. Nutr Cancer 1998;30(2):85–96

28. La Vecchia C, Chatenoud L, Negri E, Franceschi S. Session: Whole cereal grains, fibre and human cancer. Wholegrain cereals and cancer in Italy. Proc Nutr Soc 2003;62(1):45–49

29. Larsson SC, Giovannucci E, Bergkvist L, Wolk A. Whole grain consumption and risk of colorectal cancer: a population-based cohort of 60,000 women. Br J Cancer 2005;92(9):1803–1807

30. Slavin JL. Mechanisms for the impact of whole grain foods on cancer risk. J Am Coll Nutr 2000;19(3 Suppl): 300S–307S

31. Marlett JA, McBurney MI, Slavin JL. Position of the American Dietetic Association: health implications of dietary fiber. J Am Diet Assoc 2002;102(7):993–1000

32. Farrell RJ, Farrell JJ, Morrin MM. Diverticular disease in the elderly. Gastroenterol Clin North Am 2001;30(2): 475–496

33. U.S. Department of Health and Human Services, U.S. Department of Agriculture. Dietary Guidelines for Americans. 2005. Available at: http://www.healthierus.gov/dietaryguidelines/. Accessed 8/1/06

34. Willett WC. Eat, Drink, and Be Healthy: The Harvard Medical School Guide to Healthy Eating. New York: Simon & Schuster; 2001

35. U.S. Food and Drug Administration. Health Claim Notification for Whole Grain Foods. 1999. Available at: http://www.cfsan.fda.gov/~dms/flgrains.html. Accessed 8/1/06

6 Coffee

Coffee, an infusion of ground, roasted coffee beans, is among the most widely consumed beverages in the world. Although caffeine has received the most attention from scientists, coffee is a complex mixture of many chemicals, including carbohydrates, lipids (fats), amino acids, vitamins, minerals, alkaloids, and phenolic compounds.[1]

Some Bioactive Compounds in Coffee

Chlorogenic Acid

Chlorogenic acids are actually a family of esters formed between quinic acid and phenolic compounds known as cinnamic acids.[2] The most abundant chlorogenic acid in coffee is 5-O-caffeoylquinic acid, an ester formed between quinic acid and caffeic acid (**Fig. 6–1**). Coffee represents one of the richest dietary sources of chlorogenic acid. The chlorogenic acid content of a 200 mL (7 oz) cup of coffee has been reported to range from 70 to 350 mg, which would provide ~35 to 175 mg of caffeic acid. Although chlorogenic acid and caffeic acid have antioxidant activity in vitro,[3] it is un-clear how much antioxidant activity they contribute in vivo because they are extensively metabolized, and the metabolites often have lower antioxidant activity than the parent compounds.[4]

Caffeine

Caffeine is a purine alkaloid that occurs naturally in coffee beans (**Fig. 6–2**). At intake levels associated with coffee consumption, caffeine appears to exert most of its biological effects through antagonism of the A_1 and A_{2A} subtypes of the adenosine receptor.[5] Adenosine (**Fig. 6–3**) is an endogenous neuromodulator with mostly inhibitory effects, so the effects of adenosine antagonism by caffeine in the central nervous system are generally stimulatory. Caffeine is rapidly and almost completely absorbed in the stomach and small intestine and distributed to all tissues, including the brain. Caffeine concentrations in coffee beverages can be quite variable. A standard cup of coffee is often assumed to provide 100 mg of caffeine, but a recent analysis of 14 different specialty coffees purchased at coffee shops in the United States found that the amount of caffeine in 8 oz (~240 mL) of brewed coffee ranged from 72 to

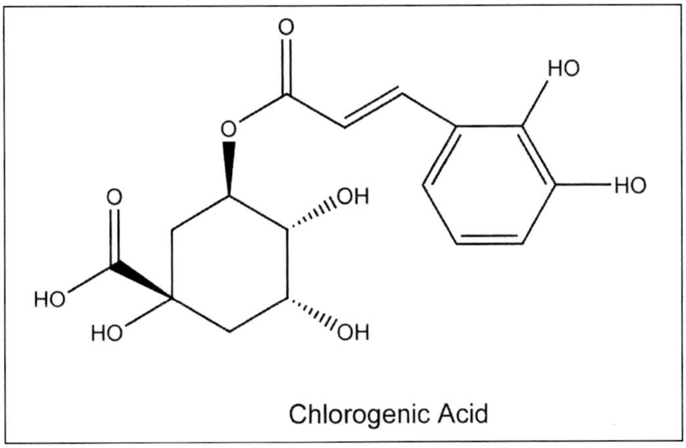

Figure 6–1 Chemical structure of 5-O-caffeoylquinic acid (chlorogenic acid).

Chlorogenic Acid

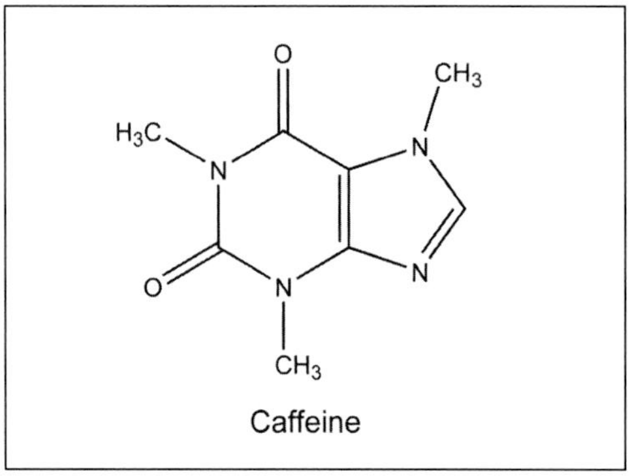

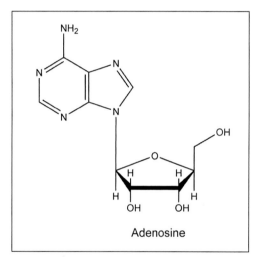

Figure 6–2 Chemical structure of caffeine.

Figure 6–3 Chemical structure of adenosine.

130 mg.[6] Caffeine in espresso coffees ranged from 58 to 76 mg in a single shot. In countries other than the United States, coffee is often stronger but the volume per cup is smaller, making 100 mg of caffeine per cup a reasonable estimate.

Diterpenes

Cafestol and kahweol are fat-soluble compounds known as diterpenes (**Fig. 6–4**), which have been found to raise serum total and low-density lipoprotein (LDL) cholesterol concentrations in humans.[7] Some cafestol and kahweol are extracted from ground coffee during brewing, but are largely removed from coffee by paper filters. Scandinavian boiled coffee, Turkish coffee, and French press (cafetiere) coffee contain relatively high levels of cafestol and kahweol (6 to 12 mg/cup), whereas filtered coffee, percolated coffee, and instant coffee contain low levels of cafestol and kahweol (0.2 to 0.6 mg/cup).[8,9] Although diterpene concentrations are relatively high in espresso coffee, the small serving size makes it an intermediate source of cafestol and kahweol (4 mg/cup). Because coffee beans are high in cafestol and kahweol, ingestion of coffee beans or grounds on a regular basis may also raise serum and LDL cholesterol.

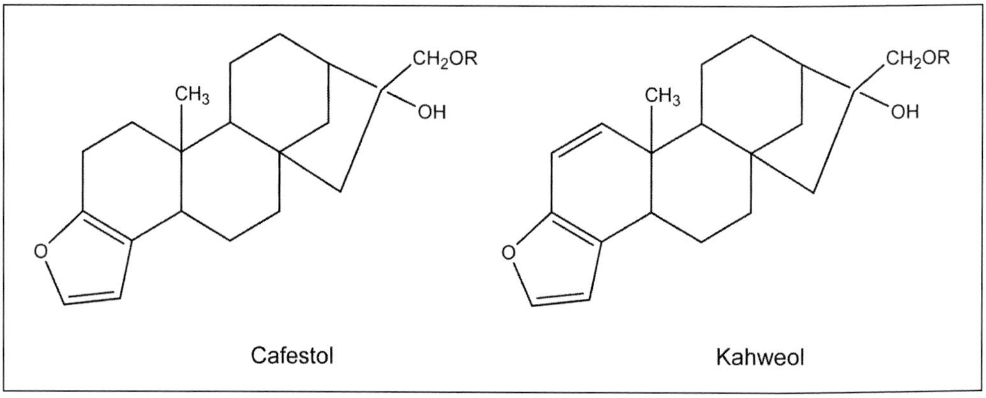

Figure 6–4 Chemical structures of cafestol and kahweol, diterpenes in coffee with cholesterol-raising effects. R = H: free diterpene; R = fatty acid: diterpene ester.

Disease Prevention

Type 2 Diabetes Mellitus

Six out of nine prospective cohort studies have found higher coffee intakes to be associated with significant reductions in the risk of type 2 diabetes mellitus (DM).[10-14] The two largest prospective cohort studies to examine the relationship between coffee consumption and type 2 DM were the Health Professionals Follow-up Study (41,934 men) and the Nurses' Health Study (84,276 women) in the United States. Men who drank at least 6 cups of coffee daily had a risk of developing type 2 DM that was 54% lower than men who did not drink coffee, and women who drank at least 6 cups of coffee daily had a risk of type 2 DM that was 29% lower than women who did not drink coffee.[12] In both cohorts, higher caffeine intakes were also associated with significant reductions in the risk of type 2 DM. Decaffeinated coffee consumption was associated with a more modest decrease in the risk of type 2 DM, suggesting that compounds other than caffeine may contribute to the reduction in risk. Recently, a systematic review of nine prospective cohort studies, including more than 193,000 men and women, found that the risk of type 2 DM was 35% lower in those who consumed at least 6 cups/d of coffee and 28% lower in those who consumed between 4 to 6 cups/d compared those who consumed less than 2 cups/d.[15] The mechanism explaining the significant reductions in the risk for type 2 DM observed in the majority of prospective studies is unclear because short-term clinical trials have found that caffeine administration impairs glucose tolerance and decreases insulin sensitivity.[16,17] Until the relationship between long-term coffee consumption and type 2 DM risk is better understood, it is premature to recommend coffee consumption as a means of preventing type 2 DM.[12,15]

Parkinson's Disease

Several large prospective cohort studies have found higher coffee and caffeine intakes to be associated with significant reductions in Parkinson's disease risk in men.[18-20] In a prospective study of 47,000 men, those who regularly consumed at least one cup of coffee daily had a risk of developing Parkinson's disease over the next 10 years that was 40% lower than men who did not drink coffee.[19] Caffeine consumption from other sources was also inversely associated with Parkinson's disease risk in a dose-dependent manner. Studies in animal models of Parkinson's disease suggest that caffeine may protect dopaminergic neurons by acting as an adenosine A_{2A}-receptor antagonist in the brain.[21] In contrast to the results of prospective studies in men, inverse associations between coffee or caffeine consumption and Parkinson's disease risk were not observed in women.[18,19] The failure of prospective studies to find inverse associations between coffee or caffeine consumption and Parkinson's disease in women may be due to the modifying effect of estrogen replacement therapy. Further analysis of a prospective study of more than 77,000 female nurses revealed that coffee consumption was inversely associated with Parkinson's disease risk in women who had never used postmenopausal estrogen, but a significant increase in Parkinson's disease risk was observed in postmenopausal estrogen users who drank at least 6 cups of coffee daily.[22] In a prospective cohort study that included more than 238,000 women, a significant inverse association between coffee consumption and Parkinson's disease mortality was also observed in women who had never used postmenopausal estrogen, but not in those who had used postmenopausal estrogen.[18] It is not known how estrogen modifies the effect of caffeine on Parkinson's disease risk.[23] Although the results of epidemiological and animal studies suggest that caffeine may reduce the risk of developing Parkinson's disease, it is premature to recommend increasing caffeine consumption to prevent Parkinson's disease, particularly in women taking estrogen.

Colorectal Cancer

In general, coffee consumption has been inversely associated with the risk of colon cancer in case-control studies, but not in prospective cohort studies.[24,25] A meta-analysis that combined the results of 12 case-control studies and 5 prospective cohort studies found that those who drank 4 or more cups of coffee daily had a risk of colorectal cancer that was 24% lower than that of nondrinkers.[25] However, coffee consumption was not associated with colorectal cancer risk when the results of only the prospective cohort studies were combined. Although case-control studies usually include more cancer cases than prospective cohort studies, they may be subject to recall bias with respect to coffee consumption and selection bias with respect to the control group. A more recent review of epidemiological studies also found evidence of an inverse association between coffee consumption and colon cancer risk from case-control studies but no evidence of such an association from prospective cohort studies.[24] No overall associations between coffee and rectal cancer emerged in this review. In contrast, the two largest prospective cohort studies to examine the relationship between coffee and colorectal cancer to date found that American men and women who regularly consumed 2 or more cups of decaffeinated coffee daily had a risk of rectal cancer that was 48% lower than those who never consumed coffee.[26] Consumption of caffeinated coffee, tea, and caffeine was not associated with either colon or rectal cancer risk. Despite promising findings in case-control studies, it is unclear whether coffee consumption decreases colon or rectal cancer risk in humans.

Cirrhosis and Hepatocellular Carcinoma

Liver injury resulting from chronic inflammation may result in cirrhosis. In cirrhosis, the formation of fibrotic scar tissue results in progressive deterioration of liver function and other complications, including liver cancer (hepatocellular carcinoma).[27] The most common causes of cirrhosis in developed countries are alcohol abuse and viral hepatitis B and C infection. Coffee consumption was inversely associated with the risk of cirrhosis in several case-control studies[28-30] and with mortality from alcoholic cirrhosis in two prospective cohort studies.[31,32] An 8-year study of more than 120,000 men and women in the United States found that the risk of death from alcoholic cirrhosis was 22% lower per cup of coffee consumed daily.[33] A 17-year study of more than 51,000 men and women in Norway found that those who consumed at least 2 cups of coffee daily had a risk of death from cirrhosis that was 40% lower than those who never consumed coffee.[32] Several case-control studies in Europe.[34,35] and two prospective cohort studies in Japan[36,37] have found significant inverse associations between coffee consumption and the risk of hepatocellular carcinoma. In the prospective cohort studies, coffee consumption was associated with significant reductions in the risk of hepatocellular carcinoma in Japanese men and women with liver disease or hepatitis C infection.[36,37] In those high-risk individuals, consumption of at least one cup of coffee daily was associated with a 50% reduction in the risk of hepatocellular carcinoma compared with those who never drank coffee.

Safety

Health Risks Associated with Coffee Consumption

Cardiovascular Disease

Coronary Heart Disease

Although limited by the potential for selection and recall bias, the results of most case-control studies suggest that people who consume 5 or more cups of coffee daily may be at increased risk of coronary heart disease.[38,39] In contrast, the majority of prospective cohort studies have not found significant associations between coffee intake and CHD risk. One exception was a prospective study in Norway, which found that high intakes of unfiltered boiled coffee were associated with increased risk of death from CHD before that population switched to filtered coffee.[40] The results of two separate meta-analyses that combined the results of more than 10 prospective cohort studies did not support an association between coffee consumption and the risk of CHD.[39,41] Similarly, most of the prospective cohort studies published since the last meta-analysis have not found significant associations between coffee consumption and CHD risk, including studies of large cohorts in the United States, Scotland, and Finland.[42-44]

Hypertension

Hypertension is a well-recognized risk factor for cardiovascular disease. It has been well-established that caffeine consumption acutely raises blood pressure, particularly in individuals with hypertension.[5] Although habitual consumption has been found to result in a degree of tolerance to the blood pressure-raising effect of caffeine, the results of several clinical trials suggest that this tolerance is not always complete even in those who consume caffeine daily.[45–47] Two meta-analyses have examined the results of randomized controlled trials of coffee consumption for more than one week on blood pressure. A meta-analysis that included 11 randomized controlled trials, in which the median duration of coffee consumption was 56 days and the median intake was 5 cups/d, found that coffee consumption significantly increased systolic and diastolic blood pressure by 2.4 and 1.2 mm Hg, respectively.[48] Recently, a meta-analysis that included 18 randomized controlled trials with a median duration of 43 days and a median intake of 725 mL/d (~3 cups/d) found that coffee consumption significantly increased systolic blood pressure by 1.2 mm Hg.[49] Although the increases in systolic blood pressure seem modest by individual standards, it has been estimated that an average systolic blood pressure reduction of 2 mm Hg in a population may result in 10% lower mortality from stroke and 7% lower mortality from CHD.[50] The available evidence from randomized controlled trials suggests that chronic coffee and caffeine consumption modestly raises systolic blood pressure, which, given the widespread consumption of caffeine and coffee, may result in increased risk of stroke and CHD in the population, particularly in those with hypertension.

Low-Density Lipoprotein Cholesterol

A meta-analysis of 14 randomized controlled trials found that the consumption of unfiltered boiled coffee dose-dependently increased serum total and LDL-cholesterol concentrations, whereas the consumption of filtered coffee resulted in very little change.[51] Overall, the consumption of boiled coffee increased serum total cholesterol by 23 mg/dL and LDL cholesterol by 14 mg/dL, while the consumption of filtered coffee raised total cholesterol by only 3 mg/dL and did not affect LDL cholesterol. The cholesterol-raising factors in unfiltered coffee have been identified as cafestol and kahweol, diterpenes that are largely removed from coffee by paper filters (see the Diterpenes section above).[7]

Homocysteine

An elevated plasma total homocysteine (tHcy) concentration is associated with increased risk of cardiovascular disease, including CHD, stroke, and peripheral vascular disease, but it is unclear whether the relationship is causal.[52] Higher coffee intakes have been associated with increased plasma tHcy concentrations in cross-sectional studies conducted in Europe, Scandinavia, and the United States.[53–57] Controlled clinical trials have confirmed the homocysteine-raising effect of coffee at intakes of ~4 cups/d.[58–60] In one clinical trial, supplementation of healthy men and women with 200 µg/d of folic acid prevented elevations in plasma tHcy induced by the consumption of 600 mL/d (2 to 3 cups/d) of filtered coffee for 4 weeks.[61]

Cardiac Arrhythmias

Clinical trials have not found coffee or caffeine intake equivalent to 5 to 6 cups/d to increase the frequency or severity of cardiac arrhythmias in healthy people or people with CHD.[62,63] A large prospective study in the United States that followed more than 128,000 people for 7 years found no association between coffee consumption and sudden cardiac death. Recently, two prospective studies in Scandinavia found no association between coffee consumption and the risk of developing atrial fibrillation, a common supraventricular arrhythmia.[64,65]

Cancer

Numerous epidemiological studies have examined relationships between coffee and caffeine intake and cancer risk in humans. In general, there is little evidence that coffee consumption increases the risk of cancer, especially when the analyses are adjusted for cigarette smoking.[66]

Pregnancy

Miscarriage

The results of epidemiological studies that have examined the relationship between maternal coffee or caffeine intake and the risk of miscarriage (spontaneous abortion) have been conflicting. Some studies have observed significant associations between high caffeine intakes, particularly from coffee, and the risk of spontaneous abortion;[67-70] however, other studies have not.[71,72] Most studies that observed significant associations between self-reported coffee or caffeine consumption and the risk of spontaneous abortion did so at intake levels of at least 300 mg/d of caffeine.[66] The only study that assessed caffeine intake by measuring serum concentrations of paraxanthine, a caffeine metabolite, found that the risk of spontaneous abortion was only elevated in women with paraxanthine concentrations that suggested caffeine intakes of at least 600 mg/d.[73] It has been proposed that an association between caffeine consumption and the risk of spontaneous abortion could be explained by the relationship between nausea and fetal viability.[74] Nausea is more common in women with viable pregnancies than nonviable pregnancies, suggesting that women with viable pregnancies are more likely to avoid or limit caffeine consumption due to nausea. However, at least one study found that the significant increase in the risk of spontaneous abortion observed in women with caffeine intakes higher than 300 mg/d was independent of nausea in pregnancy,[68] and two other studies found that caffeine consumption was associated with increased risk of spontaneous abortion in women who experienced nausea or aversion to coffee during pregnancy.[67,70] Although the topic remains controversial, the available epidemiological evidence suggests that maternal consumption of less than 300 mg/d of caffeine is unlikely to increase the risk of spontaneous abortion.

Fetal Growth

Epidemiological studies examining the effects of maternal caffeine consumption on fetal growth have assessed mean birth weight, low birth weight (less than 2500 g), and fetal growth retardation (less than the 10th percentile of birth weight for gestational age). Several studies found that maternal caffeine intakes ranging from 200 to 400 mg/d were associated with decreases in mean birth weight of ~ 100 g (3.5 oz).[75-77] However, a large prospective study found that caffeine-associated decreases in birth weight were unlikely to be clinically important in women with caffeine intakes of less than 600 mg/d.[78] The results of epidemiological studies examining the association between maternal caffeine consumption and the risk of low birth weight or fetal growth retardation have been mixed (reviewed in[66]). Moreover, some of the available epidemiological studies have been criticized for inadequately controlling for important risk factors for low birth weight and fetal growth retardation, particularly smoking.[74] Although the relationship between maternal caffeine consumption and fetal growth requires further clarification, it appears unlikely that caffeine intakes less than 300 mg/d will adversely affect fetal growth in nonsmoking women.

Birth Defects

At present, there is no convincing evidence from epidemiological studies that maternal caffeine consumption ranging from 300 to 1000 mg/d increases the risk of congenital malformations in humans.[66,79]

Lactation

The American Academy of Pediatrics categorizes caffeine as a maternal medication that is usually compatible with breastfeeding.[80] Although high maternal caffeine intakes have been reported to cause irritability and poor sleeping patterns in infants, no adverse effects have been reported with moderate maternal intake of caffeinated beverages equivalent to 2 to 3 cups of coffee daily.

Adverse Effects

Most adverse effects attributed to coffee consumption are related to caffeine. Adverse reactions to caffeine may include tachycardia (rapid heart rate), palpitations, insomnia, restlessness, nervousness, tremor, headache, abdominal pain, nausea, vomiting, diarrhea, and diuresis (increased urination).[81] Very high caffeine intakes, not usually from coffee, may induce hypokalemia (abnormally low serum potassium).[82] Sudden cessation of caffeine consumption after long-term use may result in caffeine withdrawal symptoms.[83] Commonly reported caffeine withdrawal symptoms include headaches, fatigue, drowsiness, irritability, difficulty concentrating, and depressed mood. Significant withdrawal symptoms have been observed at long-term intakes as low as 100 mg/d, although they are more common with higher intakes. Gradual withdrawal from caffeine appears less likely to result in withdrawal symptoms than abrupt withdrawal.[84]

Drug Interactions

Habitual caffeine consumption increases hepatic cytochrome P450 (CYP) 1A2 activity, which has implications for the metabolism for several medications.[85] Additionally, drugs that inhibit the activity of CYP1A2 interfere with the metabolism and elimination of caffeine, increasing the risk of adverse effects.[86]

Drugs That Alter Caffeine Metabolism

The following medications may impair the hepatic metabolism of caffeine, decreasing its elimination and potentially increasing the risk of caffeine-related side effects: cimetidine (Tagamet), disulfiram (Antabuse), estrogens, fluconazole (Diflucan), fluvoxamine (Luvox), mexiletine (Mexitil), quinolone class antibiotics, and terbinafine (Lamisil).[85]

Phenytoin (Dilantin) and cigarette smoking increase the hepatic metabolism of caffeine, resulting in increased elimination and decreased plasma caffeine concentrations.[81]

Caffeine Effects on Other Drugs

Caffeine and other methylxanthines may enhance the effects and side effects of β-adrenergic stimulating agents, such as epinephrine and albuterol.[81,85] Caffeine may inhibit the hepatic metabolism of the antipsychotic medication, clozapine, potentially elevating serum clozapine levels and increasing the risk of toxicity. Caffeine consumption can decrease the elimination of theophylline, potentially increasing serum theophylline levels. Caffeine has been found to decrease the systemic elimination of acetaminophen and to increase the bioavailability of aspirin, which may partially explain its efficacy in enhancing their analgesic effects. Caffeine may decrease serum lithium concentrations by enhancing its elimination.

Nutrient Interactions

Calcium and Osteoporosis

The results of controlled studies in humans indicate that coffee and caffeine consumption decrease the efficiency of calcium absorption resulting in a loss of ~4 to 6 mg of calcium per cup of coffee.[87,88] Most studies have found no association between caffeine consumption and change in bone mineral density (BMD) over time (reviewed in[89]). However, one study found that caffeine consumption was associated with accelerated loss of BMD only in women with calcium intakes less than 744 mg/d,[90] whereas another found that consumption of more than 300 mg/d of caffeine was associated with accelerated bone loss in elderly women.[91] Six prospective cohort studies have examined associations between caffeine (mainly from coffee) or coffee consumption and the risk of hip fracture in women. Two studies, one in Finland and one in Japan, found no association.[92,93] Another study in Norway found that women who consumed at least 9 cups of coffee daily tended to have an increased risk of hip fracture, but only 7% of women consumed this much coffee.[94] However, three prospective cohort studies in the United States found that coffee or caffeine consumption was positively associated with the risk of hip fracture in women.[95–97] In the Framingham cohort, women who consumed more than 2 cups of coffee daily had a risk of hip fracture over the next 12 years that was 69% higher than women who did not consume caffeinated beverages.[95] In the Nurses' Health Study cohort, women who consumed 4 or more cups of coffee daily had a risk of hip fracture over the next 6 years that was 3 times the risk of those who did not drink coffee.[96] A prospective cohort study of women 65 years of age and older found that a 190 mg increase in caffeine consumption increased the risk of osteoporotic fracture by ~20%.[97] Given the multifactorial etiology of osteoporosis, the impact of coffee or caffeine consumption on the risk of osteoporosis is not clear. However, currently available evidence suggests that ensuring adequate calcium and vitamin D intake and limiting coffee consumption to 3 cups/d or less may help reduce the risk of osteoporosis and osteoporotic fracture, particularly in older adults.

Nonheme Iron

Polyphenols in coffee can bind nonheme iron and inhibit its intestinal absorption.[98] Drinking 150 to 250 mL of coffee with a test meal has been found to inhibit the absorption of iron by 24 to 73%.[99,100] To maximize iron absorption from a meal or iron supplements, concomitant intake of coffee should be avoided.

Summary

- Coffee is a complex mixture of chemicals that provides significant amounts of chlorogenic acid and caffeine.
- Unfiltered coffee is a significant source of cafestol and kahweol, diterpenes that have been found to raise serum total and LDL concentrations in humans.
- The results of epidemiological studies suggest that coffee consumption is associated with decreased risk of type 2 diabetes, Parkinson's disease, and liver disease. However, it is premature to recommend coffee consumption for disease prevention based on this evidence.
- At present, there is little evidence that coffee consumption increases the risk of cancer.

- Despite evidence from clinical trials that caffeine in coffee can increase blood pressure, most prospective cohort studies have not found moderate coffee consumption to be associated with increased risk of cardiovascular disease.
- Overall, there is little evidence of health risk and some evidence of health benefits for adults consuming moderate amounts of coffee (3 to 4 cups/d providing 300 to 400 mg/d of caffeine).
- However, some people may be more vulnerable to the adverse effects of caffeine in coffee:
  - Caffeine consumption comparable to the amount in 2 to 3 cups of coffee may raise blood pressure, particularly in people with hypertension or borderline high blood pressure.
  - Until the effects of caffeine on the risk of miscarriage and fetal growth are clarified, women who are pregnant or planning to become pregnant should limit coffee intake to 3 cups/d providing no more than 300 mg/d of caffeine.
  - Ensuring adequate calcium and vitamin D intake and limiting coffee consumption to 3 cups/d (300 mg/d of caffeine) may help reduce the risk of osteoporosis and osteoporotic fracture, particularly in older adults.

References

1. Spiller MA. The chemical components of coffee. In: Spiller GA, ed. Caffeine. Boca Raton: CRC Press; 1998:97–161
2. Clifford MN. Chlorogenic acids and other cinnamates–nature occurrence and dietary burden. J Sci Food Agric 1999;79:362–372
3. Iwai K, Kishimoto N, Kakino Y, Mochida K, Fujita T. In vitro antioxidative effects and tyrosinase inhibitory activities of seven hydroxycinnamoyl derivatives in green coffee beans. J Agric Food Chem 2004;52(15): 4893–4898
4. Olthof MR, Hollman PC, Buijsman MN, van Amelsvoort JM, Katan MB. Chlorogenic acid, quercetin-3-rutinoside and black tea phenols are extensively metabolized in humans. J Nutr 2003;133(6): 1806–1814
5. James JE. Critical review of dietary caffeine and blood pressure: a relationship that should be taken more seriously. Psychosom Med 2004;66(1):63–71
6. McCusker RR, Goldberger BA, Cone EJ. Caffeine content of specialty coffees. J Anal Toxicol 2003;27(7): 520–522

7. Urgert R, Katan MB. The cholesterol-raising factor from coffee beans. Annu Rev Nutr 1997;17:305–324

8. Gross G, Jaccaud E, Huggett AC. Analysis of the content of the diterpenes cafestol and kahweol in coffee brews. Food Chem Toxicol 1997;35(6):547–554

9. Urgert R, van der Weg G, Kosmeijer-Schuil TG, van de Bovenkamp P, Hovenier R, Katan MB. Levels of the cholesterol-elevating diterpenes cafestol and kahweol in various coffee brews. J Agric Food Chem 1995; 43(8):2167–2172

10. Carlsson S, Hammar N, Grill V, Kaprio J. Coffee consumption and risk of type 2 diabetes in Finnish twins. Int J Epidemiol 2004;33(3):616–617

11. Rosengren A, Dotevall A, Wilhelmsen L, Thelle D, Johansson S. Coffee and incidence of diabetes in Swedish women: a prospective 18-year follow-up study. J Intern Med 2004;255(1):89–95

12. Salazar-Martinez E, Willett WC, Ascherio A, et al. Coffee consumption and risk for type 2 diabetes mellitus. Ann Intern Med 2004;140(1):1–8

13. Tuomilehto J, Hu G, Bidel S, Lindstrom J, Jousilahti P. Coffee consumption and risk of type 2 diabetes mellitus among middle-aged Finnish men and women. JAMA 2004;291(10):1213–1219

14. van Dam RM, Feskens EJ. Coffee consumption and risk of type 2 diabetes mellitus. Lancet 2002; 360(9344): 1477–1478

15. van Dam RM, Hu FB. Coffee consumption and risk of type 2 diabetes: a systematic review. JAMA 2005; 294(1):97–104

16. Keijzers GB, De Galan BE, Tack CJ, Smits P. Caffeine can decrease insulin sensitivity in humans. Diabetes Care 2002;25(2):364–369

17. Petrie HJ, Chown SE, Belfie LM, et al. Caffeine ingestion increases the insulin response to an oral-glucose-tolerance test in obese men before and after weight loss. Am J Clin Nutr 2004;80(1):22–28

18. Ascherio A, Weisskopf MG, O'Reilly EJ, et al. Coffee consumption, gender, and Parkinson's disease mortality in the cancer prevention study II cohort: the modifying effects of estrogen. Am J Epidemiol 2004; 160(10):977–984

19. Ascherio A, Zhang SM, Hernan MA, et al. Prospective study of caffeine consumption and risk of Parkinson's disease in men and women. Ann Neurol 2001;50(1): 56–63

20. Ross GW, Abbott RD, Petrovitch H, et al. Association of coffee and caffeine intake with the risk of Parkinson disease. JAMA 2000;283(20):2674–2679

21. Schwarzschild MA, Chen JF, Ascherio A. Caffeinated clues and the promise of adenosine A(2A) antagonists in PD. Neurology 2002;58(8):1154–1160

22. Ascherio A, Chen H, Schwarzschild MA, Zhang SM, Colditz GA, Speizer FE. Caffeine, postmenopausal estrogen, and risk of Parkinson's disease. Neurology 2003;60(5):790–795

23. Pollock BG, Wylie M, Stack JA, et al. Inhibition of caffeine metabolism by estrogen replacement therapy in postmenopausal women. J Clin Pharmacol 1999; 39(9):936–940

24. Tavani A, La Vecchia C. Coffee, decaffeinated coffee, tea and cancer of the colon and rectum: a review of epidemiological studies, 1990–2003. Cancer Causes Control 2004;15(8):743–757

25. Giovannucci E. Meta-analysis of coffee consumption and risk of colorectal cancer. Am J Epidemiol 1998;147(11):1043–1052

26. Michels KB, Willett WC, Fuchs CS, Giovannucci E. Coffee, tea, and caffeine consumption and incidence of colon and rectal cancer. J Natl Cancer Inst 2005;97(4):282–292

27. Friedman SL, Schiano TD. Cirrhosis and its sequelae. In: Goldman L, Ausiello D, eds. Cecil Textbook of Medicine. 22nd ed. St. Louis: W. B. Saunders; 2004:940–944

28. Corrao G, Lepore AR, Torchio P, et al. The effect of drinking coffee and smoking cigarettes on the risk of cirrhosis associated with alcohol consumption. A case-control study. Provincial Group for the Study of Chronic Liver Disease. Eur J Epidemiol 1994;10(6): 657–664

29. Corrao G, Zambon A, Bagnardi V, D'Amicis A, Klatsky A. Coffee, caffeine, and the risk of liver cirrhosis. Ann Epidemiol 2001;11(7):458–465

30. Gallus S, Tavani A, Negri E, La Vecchia C. Does coffee protect against liver cirrhosis? Ann Epidemiol 2002;12(3):202–205

31. Klatsky AL, Armstrong MA. Alcohol, smoking, coffee, and cirrhosis. Am J Epidemiol 1992;136(10):1248–1257

32. Tverdal A, Skurtveit S. Coffee intake and mortality from liver cirrhosis. Ann Epidemiol 2003;13(6):419–423

33. Klatsky AL, Armstrong MA, Friedman GD. Coffee, tea, and mortality. Ann Epidemiol 1993;3(4):375–381

34. Gallus S, Bertuzzi M, Tavani A, et al. Does coffee protect against hepatocellular carcinoma? Br J Cancer 2002;87(9):956–959

35. Gelatti U, Covolo L, Franceschini M, et al. Coffee consumption reduces the risk of hepatocellular carcinoma independently of its aetiology: a case-control study. J Hepatol 2005;42(4):528–534

36. Inoue M, Yoshimi I, Sobue T, Tsugane S. Influence of coffee drinking on subsequent risk of hepatocellular carcinoma: a prospective study in Japan. J Natl Cancer Inst 2005;97(4):293–300

37. Shimazu T, Tsubono Y, Kuriyama S, et al. Coffee consumption and the risk of primary liver cancer: pooled analysis of two prospective studies in Japan. Int J Cancer 2005;116(1):150–154

38. Greenland S. A meta-analysis of coffee, myocardial infarction, and coronary death. Epidemiology 1993;4(4):366–374

39. Kawachi I, Colditz GA, Stone CB. Does coffee drinking increase the risk of coronary heart disease? Results from a meta-analysis. Br Heart J 1994;72(3):269–275

40. Tverdal A, Stensvold I, Solvoll K, Foss OP, Lund-Larsen P, Bjartveit K. Coffee consumption and death from coronary heart disease in middle aged Norwegian men and women. BMJ 1990;300(6724):566–569

41. Myers MG, Basinski A. Coffee and coronary heart disease. Arch Intern Med 1992;152(9):1767–1772

42. Kleemola P, Jousilahti P, Pietinen P, Vartiainen E, Tuomilehto J. Coffee consumption and the risk of coronary heart disease and death. Arch Intern Med 2000;160(22):3393–3400

43. Willett WC, Stampfer MJ, Manson JE, et al. Coffee consumption and coronary heart disease in women. A ten-year follow-up. JAMA 1996;275(6):458–462

44. Woodward M, Tunstall-Pedoe H. Coffee and tea consumption in the Scottish Heart Health Study follow up: conflicting relations with coronary risk factors,

coronary disease, and all cause mortality. J Epidemiol Community Health 1999;53(8):481–487

45. Denaro CP, Brown CR, Jacob P III, Benowitz NL. Effects of caffeine with repeated dosing. Eur J Clin Pharmacol 1991;40(3):273–278

46. James JE. Chronic effects of habitual caffeine consumption on laboratory and ambulatory blood pressure levels. J Cardiovasc Risk 1994;1(2):159–164

47. Lovallo WR, Wilson MF, Vincent AS, Sung BH, McKey BS, Whitsett TL. Blood pressure response to caffeine shows incomplete tolerance after short-term regular consumption. Hypertension 2004;43(4):760–765

48. Jee SH, He J, Whelton PK, Suh I, Klag MJ. The effect of chronic coffee drinking on blood pressure: a meta-analysis of controlled clinical trials. Hypertension 1999;33(2):647–652

49. Noordzij M, Uiterwaal CS, Arends LR, Kok FJ, Grobbee DE, Geleijnse JM. Blood pressure response to chronic intake of coffee and caffeine: a meta-analysis of randomized controlled trials. J Hypertens 2005;23(5): 921–928

50. Lewington S, Clarke R, Qizilbash N, Peto R, Collins R. Age-specific relevance of usual blood pressure to vascular mortality: a meta-analysis of individual data for one million adults in 61 prospective studies. Lancet 2002;360(9349):1903–1913

51. Jee SH, He J, Appel LJ, Whelton PK, Suh I, Klag MJ. Coffee consumption and serum lipids: a meta-analysis of randomized controlled clinical trials. Am J Epidemiol 2001;153(4):353–362

52. Splaver A, Lamas GA, Hennekens CH. Homocysteine and cardiovascular disease: biological mechanisms, observational epidemiology, and the need for randomized trials. Am Heart J 2004;148(1):34–40

53. Husemoen LL, Thomsen TF, Fenger M, Jorgensen T. Effect of lifestyle factors on plasma total homocysteine concentrations in relation to MTHFR(C677T) genotype. Eur J Clin Nutr 2004;58(8):1142–1150

54. Mennen LI, de Courcy GP, Guilland JC, et al. Homocysteine, cardiovascular disease risk factors, and habitual diet in the French Supplementation with Antioxidant Vitamins and Minerals Study. Am J Clin Nutr 2002;76(6):1279–1289

55. de Bree A, Verschuren WM, Blom HJ, Kromhout D. Lifestyle factors and plasma homocysteine concentrations in a general population sample. Am J Epidemiol 2001;154(2):150–154

56. Stolzenberg-Solomon RZ, Miller ER III, Maguire MG, Selhub J, Appel LJ. Association of dietary protein intake and coffee consumption with serum homocysteine concentrations in an older population. Am J Clin Nutr 1999;69(3):467–475

57. Nygard O, Refsum H, Ueland PM, et al. Coffee consumption and plasma total homocysteine: The Hordaland Homocysteine Study. Am J Clin Nutr 1997;65(1):136–143

58. Christensen B, Mosdol A, Retterstol L, Landaas S, Thelle DS. Abstention from filtered coffee reduces the concentrations of plasma homocysteine and serum cholesterol–a randomized controlled trial. Am J Clin Nutr 2001;74(3):302–307

59. Urgert R, van Vliet T, Zock PL, Katan MB. Heavy coffee consumption and plasma homocysteine: a randomized controlled trial in healthy volunteers. Am J Clin Nutr 2000;72(5):1107–1110

60. Grubben MJ, Boers GH, Blom HJ, et al. Unfiltered coffee increases plasma homocysteine concentrations in healthy volunteers: a randomized trial. Am J Clin Nutr 2000;71(2):480–484

61. Strandhagen E, Landaas S, Thelle DS. Folic acid supplement decreases the homocysteine increasing effect of filtered coffee. A randomised placebo-controlled study. Eur J Clin Nutr 2003;57(11):1411–1417

62. Chelsky LB, Cutler JE, Griffith K, Kron J, McClelland JH, McAnulty JH. Caffeine and ventricular arrhythmias. An electrophysiological approach. JAMA 1990; 264(17):2236–2240

63. Myers MG. Caffeine and cardiac arrhythmias. Ann Intern Med 1991;114(2):147–150

64. Frost L, Vestergaard P. Caffeine and risk of atrial fibrillation or flutter: the Danish Diet, Cancer, and Health Study. Am J Clin Nutr 2005;81(3):578–582

65. Wilhelmsen L, Rosengren A, Lappas G. Hospitalizations for atrial fibrillation in the general male population: morbidity and risk factors. J Intern Med 2001;250(5):382–389

66. Nawrot P, Jordan S, Eastwood J, Rotstein J, Hugenholtz A, Feeley M. Effects of caffeine on human health. Food Addit Contam 2003;20(1):1–30

67. Cnattingius S, Signorello LB, Anneren G, et al. Caffeine intake and the risk of first-trimester spontaneous abortion. N Engl J Med 2000;343(25):1839–1845

68. Giannelli M, Doyle P, Roman E, Pelerin M, Hermon C. The effect of caffeine consumption and nausea on the risk of miscarriage. Paediatr Perinat Epidemiol 2003; 17(4):316–323

69. Rasch V. Cigarette, alcohol, and caffeine consumption: risk factors for spontaneous abortion. Acta Obstet Gynecol Scand 2003;82(2):182–188

70. Wen W, Shu XO, Jacobs DR Jr, Brown JE. The associations of maternal caffeine consumption and nausea with spontaneous abortion. Epidemiology 2001; 12(1):38–42

71. Fenster L, Hubbard AE, Swan SH, et al. Caffeinated beverages, decaffeinated coffee, and spontaneous abortion. Epidemiology 1997;8(5):515–523

72. Mills JL, Holmes LB, Aarons JH, et al. Moderate caffeine use and the risk of spontaneous abortion and intrauterine growth retardation. JAMA 1993;269(5): 593–597

73. Klebanoff MA, Levine RJ, DerSimonian R, Clemens JD, Wilkins DG. Maternal serum paraxanthine, a caffeine metabolite, and the risk of spontaneous abortion. N Engl J Med 1999;341(22):1639–1644

74. Leviton A, Cowan L. A review of the literature relating caffeine consumption by women to their risk of reproductive hazards. Food Chem Toxicol 2002; 40(9):1271–1310

75. Bracken MB, Triche E, Grosso L, Hellenbrand K, Belanger K, Leaderer BP. Heterogeneity in assessing self-reports of caffeine exposure: implications for studies of health effects. Epidemiology 2002; 13(2):165–171

76. Martin TR, Bracken MB. The association between low birth weight and caffeine consumption during pregnancy. Am J Epidemiol 1987;126(5):813–821

77. Peacock JL, Bland JM, Anderson HR. Effects on birthweight of alcohol and caffeine consumption in smoking women. J Epidemiol Community Health 1991; 45(2):159–163

78. Bracken MB, Triche EW, Belanger K, Hellenbrand K, Leaderer BP. Association of maternal caffeine consumption with decrements in fetal growth. Am J Epidemiol 2003;157(5):456–466

79. Christian MS, Brent RL. Teratogen update: evaluation of the reproductive and developmental risks of caffeine. Teratology 2001;64(1):51–78

80. American Academy of Pediatrics Committee on Drugs. Transfer of drugs and other chemicals into human milk. Pediatrics 2001;108(3):776–789

81. Novak K, ed. Drug Facts and Comparisons. St. Louis: Wolters Kluwer Health; 2005

82. Engebretsen KM, Harris CR. Caffeine and related nonprescription sympathomimetics. In: Ford MD, Delaney KA, Ling LJ, Erickson T, eds. Clinical Toxicology. Philadelphia: W. B. Saunders; 2001:310–315

83. Juliano LM, Griffiths RR. A critical review of caffeine withdrawal: empirical validation of symptoms and signs, incidence, severity, and associated features. Psychopharmacology (Berl) 2004;176(1):1–29

84. Dews PB, Curtis GL, Hanford KJ, O'Brien CP. The frequency of caffeine withdrawal in a population-based survey and in a controlled, blinded pilot experiment. J Clin Pharmacol 1999;39(12):1221–1232

85. Carrillo JA, Benitez J. Clinically significant pharmacokinetic interactions between dietary caffeine and medications. Clin Pharmacokinet 2000;39(2):127–153

86. Faber MS, Fuhr U. Time response of cytochrome P450 1A2 activity on cessation of heavy smoking. Clin Pharmacol Ther 2004;76(2):178–184

87. Barger-Lux MJ, Heaney RP. Caffeine and the calcium economy revisited. Osteoporos Int 1995;5(2):97–102

88. Hasling C, Sondergaard K, Charles P, Mosekilde L. Calcium metabolism in postmenopausal osteoporotic women is determined by dietary calcium and coffee intake. J Nutr 1992;122(5):1119–1126

89. Heaney RP. Effects of caffeine on bone and the calcium economy. Food Chem Toxicol 2002;40(9):1263–1270

90. Harris SS, Dawson-Hughes B. Caffeine and bone loss in healthy postmenopausal women. Am J Clin Nutr 1994;60(4):573–578

91. Rapuri PB, Gallagher JC, Kinyamu HK, Ryschon KL. Caffeine intake increases the rate of bone loss in elderly women and interacts with vitamin D receptor genotypes. Am J Clin Nutr 2001;74(5):694–700

92. Fujiwara S, Kasagi F, Yamada M, Kodama K. Risk factors for hip fracture in a Japanese cohort. J Bone Miner Res 1997;12(7):998–1004

93. Huopio J, Kroger H, Honkanen R, Saarikoski S, Alhava E. Risk factors for perimenopausal fractures: a prospective study. Osteoporos Int 2000;11(3):219–227

94. Meyer HE, Pedersen JI, Loken EB, Tverdal A. Dietary factors and the incidence of hip fracture in middle-aged Norwegians. A prospective study. Am J Epidemiol 1997;145(2):117–123

95. Kiel DP, Felson DT, Hannan MT, Anderson JJ, Wilson PW. Caffeine and the risk of hip fracture: the Framingham Study. Am J Epidemiol 1990;132(4):675–684

96. Hernandez-Avila M, Colditz GA, Stampfer MJ, Rosner B, Speizer FE, Willett WC. Caffeine, moderate alcohol intake, and risk of fractures of the hip and forearm in middle-aged women. Am J Clin Nutr 1991;54(1):157–163

97. Cummings SR, Nevitt MC, Browner WS, et al. Risk factors for hip fracture in white women. Study of Osteoporotic Fractures Research Group. N Engl J Med 1995;332(12):767–773

98. Fairweather-Tait SJ. Iron nutrition in the UK: getting the balance right. Proc Nutr Soc 2004;63(4):519–528

99. Hallberg L, Rossander L. Effect of different drinks on the absorption of non-heme iron from composite meals. Hum Nutr Appl Nutr 1982;36(2):116–123

100. Morck TA, Lynch SR, Cook JD. Inhibition of food iron absorption by coffee. Am J Clin Nutr 1983;37(3):416–420

7 Tea

Tea is an infusion of the leaves of the *Camellia sinensis* plant and is the most widely consumed beverage in the world, aside from water.[1] Herbal teas are infusions of herbs or plants other than *Camellia sinensis* and will not be discussed. Although tea contains several bioactive chemicals, including caffeine and fluoride, scientists are particularly interested in the potential health benefits of a class of compounds in tea known as flavonoids. In many cultures, tea is an important source of dietary flavonoids.

Definitions

Types of Tea

All teas are derived from the leaves of *Camellia sinensis*, but different processing methods produce different types of tea. Fresh tea leaves are rich in flavonoids known as flavanols or catechins. Tea leaves also contain polyphenol oxidase enzymes in separate compartments from catechins. When tea leaves are intentionally broken or rolled during processing, contact with polyphenol oxidase causes catechins to join together forming dimers and polymers, known as theaflavins and thearubigins, respectively. This oxidation process is known in the tea industry as "fermentation." Steaming or firing tea leaves inactivates polyphenol oxidase and stops the fermentation process.[2] Although there are thousands of tea varieties, teas may be divided into three groups based on the amount of fermentation they undergo during processing.

Unfermented Teas (White and Green Teas)

White teas are made from buds and young leaves, which are steamed or fired to inactivate polyphenol oxidase, and then dried. Thus, white tea retains the high concentrations of catechins present in fresh tea leaves. Green tea is made from more mature tea leaves than white tea and may be withered prior to steaming or firing. Although they are also rich in catechins, green teas may have different catechin profiles than white teas.[3]

Semifermented Teas (Oolong Teas)

Tea leaves destined to become oolong teas are "bruised" to allow the release of some of the polphenol oxidase present in the leaves. Oolong teas are allowed to ferment for less time than black teas before they are heated and dried. Consequently, the catechin, theaflavin, and thearubigin levels in oolong teas are generally between those of unfermented green and white teas and completely fermented black teas.[2]

Fully Fermented Teas (Black Teas)

Tea leaves destined to become black tea are rolled or broken to maximize the interaction between catechins and polyphenol oxidase. Because they are allowed to ferment completely before drying, most black teas are rich in theaflavins and thearubigins, but relatively low in catechins.[4]

Cup Sizes

The definition of a cup of tea varies in different countries or regions. In Japan, a typical cup of green tea may contain only 100 mL (3.5 oz). A traditional European teacup holds ~ 125 to 150 mL (5 oz), while a mug of tea may contain 235 mL (8 oz) or more.

Bioactive Compounds in Tea

Flavonoids

Flavanols are the most abundant class of flavonoids in tea. Flavanol monomers are also known as catechins. The principal catechins found in tea (**Fig. 7–1**) are epicatechin (EC), epigallocatechin (EGC), epicatechin gallate (ECG), and epigallocatechin gallate (EGCG).[2] When catechins are enzymatically oxidized by polyphenol oxidase during fermentation, they form polymers known as theaflavins (**Fig. 7–2**) and thearubigins. Unfermented teas are rich in catechins, whereas fermented teas are rich in theaflavins and thearubigins (see the Types of Tea section above). Tea is also a good source of another class of flavonoids, called flavonols.

Flavonols found in tea include kaempferol, quercetin, and myricitin. The flavonol content of tea is less affected by processing, and flavonols are present in comparable quantities in fermented and unfermented teas. Unlike catechins, flavonols are usually present in tea as glycosides (bound to a sugar molecule). See Chapter 13 for more information on flavonoids.

Caffeine

All teas contain caffeine, unless they are deliberately decaffeinated during processing. The caffeine content of different varieties of tea may vary considerably and is influenced by factors like brewing time, the amount of tea and water used for brewing, and whether the tea is loose or in teabags. In general, a mug of

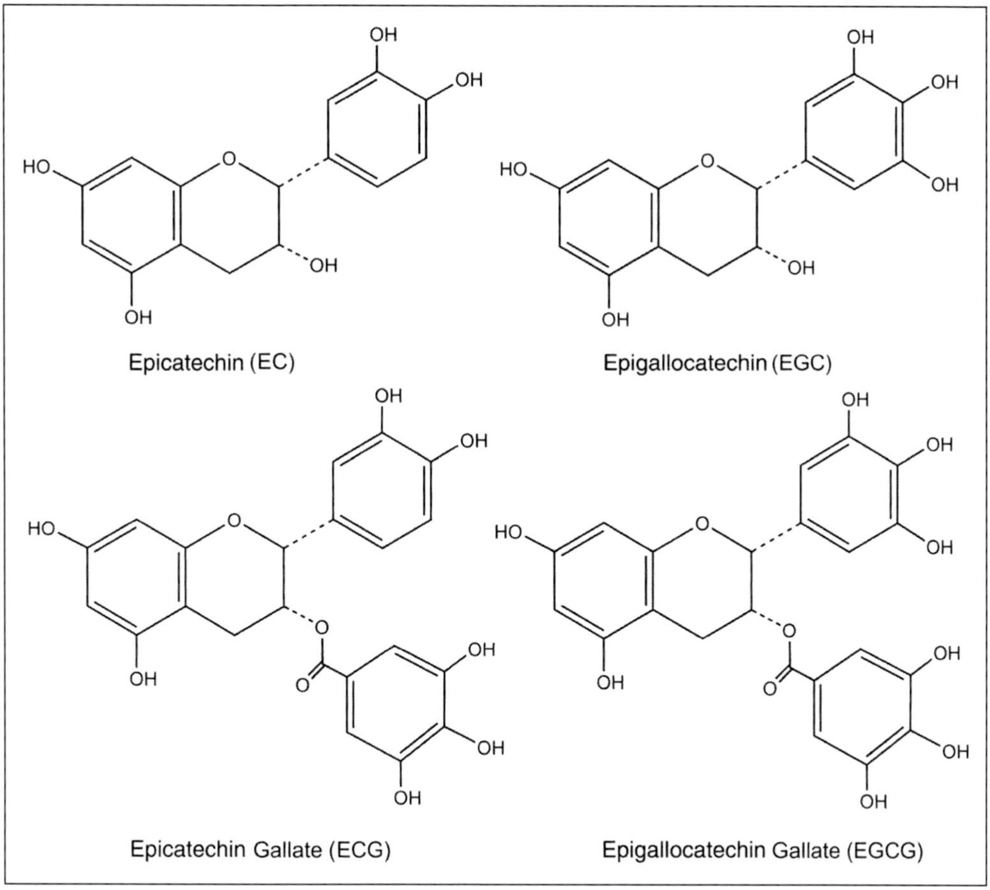

Epicatechin (EC)

Epigallocatechin (EGC)

Epicatechin Gallate (ECG)

Epigallocatechin Gallate (EGCG)

Figure 7–1   Chemical structures of principal catechins in tea.

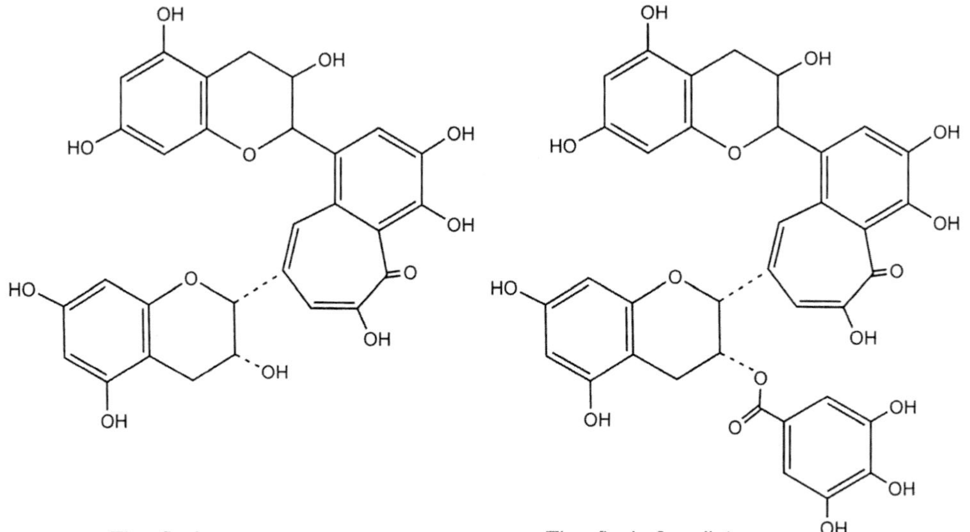

Figure 7–2   Chemical structures of some theaflavins in tea.

Table 7–1   Caffeine Content of Teas and Coffee[5,70]

Type of Tea/Coffee	Caffeine (mg/L)	Caffeine (mg/8 oz)
Green	40–211	9–50
Black	177–303	42–72
Coffee, brewed	306–553	72–130

tea contains about half as much caffeine as a mug of coffee.[4] The caffeine contents of more than 20 green and black teas prepared according to package directions are presented in **Table 7–1**.[5] The caffeine content of oolong teas is comparable to green teas.[6] There is little information on the caffeine content of white teas because they are often grouped together with green teas. Buds and young tea leaves have been found to contain higher levels of caffeine than older leaves,[7] suggesting that the caffeine content of some white teas may be slightly higher than that of green teas.[3] See Chapter 6 on Coffee for more information on caffeine.

Fluoride

Tea plants accumulate fluoride in their leaves. In general, the oldest tea leaves contain the most fluoride.[8] Most high-quality teas are made from the bud or the first four leaves—the youngest leaves on the plant. Brick tea, a lower quality tea, is made from the oldest tea leaves and is often very high in fluoride. Symptoms of fluoride excess (dental and skeletal fluorosis) have been observed in Tibetan children and adults who consume large amounts of brick tea.[9,10] Unlike brick tea, fluoride levels in green, oolong, and black teas are generally comparable to those recommended for the prevention of dental caries (cavities). Thus, daily consumption of up to 1 L of green, oolong, or black tea would be unlikely to result in fluoride intakes higher than those recommended for dental health.[11,12] The fluoride content of white tea is likely to be less than other teas; white teas are made from the buds and youngest leaves of the tea plant. The fluoride contents of 17 brands of green, oolong, and black tea are presented in **Table 7–2**.[12] These values do not include the fluoride content of the water used to make the tea.

Table 7–2   Flouride Content of Teas[12]

Type of Tea	Fluoride (mg/L)[*]	Fluoride (mg/8 oz)
Green	1.2–1.7	0.3–0.4
Oolong	0.6–1.0	0.1–0.2
Black	1.0–1.9	0.2–0.5
Brick tea	2.2–7.3	0.5–1.7

* Fluoride in 1 % w/v tea prepared by continuous infusion from 5 to 360 minutes.

Prevention

Cardiovascular Disease

Epidemiological Studies

Many epidemiological studies have examined associations between tea consumption and manifestations of cardiovascular disease, including myocardial infarction (MI) and stroke. A meta-analysis that combined the results of 10 prospective cohort studies and 7 case-control studies found that a 24-oz increase in daily tea consumption was associated with an 11% decrease in the risk of MI.[13] However, caution was urged in the interpretation of these results because of bias toward the publication of studies suggesting a protective effect. Since then, the results of several other prospective cohort studies have been mixed. A 6-year study of Dutch men and women found that those who drank at least 3 cups/d (~ 13 oz) had a significantly lower risk of MI than those who did not drink tea.[14] A 7-year study of American women found that the risk of important vascular events (MI, stroke, or death from cardiovascular disease) was significantly lower in a small number of women who drank at least 4 cups/d of black tea.[15] However, so few women fell into this group that the significance of this finding is unclear. Finally, a 15-year study of American men found no association between tea consumption and cardiovascular disease risk, but tea consumption in this population was relatively low, averaging 1 cup/d.[16] Overall, the available research suggests that consumption of at least 3 cups/d of black tea may be associated with a modest decrease in the risk of MI. Although green tea consumption may con-

fer a similar benefit,[17] there has not been enough research on green tea consumption and cardiovascular disease risk to draw any firm conclusions.

Endothelial Function

Vascular endothelial cells play an important role in maintaining cardiovascular health by producing nitric oxide, a compound that promotes arterial relaxation (vasodilation).[18] Arterial vasodilation resulting from endothelial production of nitric oxide is termed endothelium-dependent vasodilation. Two controlled clinical trials found that the daily consumption of 4 to 5 cups (900 to 1250 mL) of black tea for 4 weeks significantly improved endothelium-dependent vasodilation in patients with coronary artery disease[19] and patients with mildly elevated serum cholesterol levels[20] compared with the equivalent amount of caffeine alone or hot water. The beneficial effect of black tea consumption on vascular endothelial function could help explain the modest reduction in cardiovascular disease risk observed in some epidemiological studies.

Cancer

Animal Studies

Green and black tea have been found to have cancer preventive activity in a variety of animal models of cancer, including cancer of the skin, lung, mouth, esophagus, stomach, colon, pancreas, bladder, and prostate.[21,22] In most cases, flavonoids appear to contribute substantially to the cancer preventing effects of tea, but caffeine has also been found to have cancer preventing activity in some animal models of skin[23] and lung cancer.[24] Although beneficial effects of tea flavonoids were often attributed to their antioxidant activity, the overall contribution of tea flavonoids to plasma and tissue antioxidant activity in humans is now thought to be relatively minor.[25] Currently, scientists are focusing their attention on the potential for tea flavonoids to modulate cell signaling pathways that promote the transformation of healthy cells to cancerous cells.[26] See Chapter 13 for more information on Flavonoids.

Epidemiological Studies

Despite promising results from animal studies, it is not clear whether increasing tea consumption will help prevent cancers in humans. The results of numerous epidemiological studies of many different types of cancers do not provide any consistent evidence that green or black tea consumption is associated with significant reductions in cancer risk.[27] Tea comes into direct contact with the gastrointestinal tract; therefore, scientists have been particularly interested in the potential for increased tea consumption to prevent cancers of the stomach and colon. Although a few case-control studies suggested that higher intakes of green tea were associated with decreased stomach cancer risk, recent prospective cohort studies do not support an inverse association between green tea consumption and stomach cancer risk in Japanese men and women.[28-31] Despite promising findings in animal models of colon cancer,[32] the majority of epidemiological studies have not found tea consumption to be associated with lower colorectal cancer risk.[33,34]

There are several possible reasons for the discrepancies between findings from animal models of cancer and epidemiological studies in humans. Aside from potential species differences, it may be difficult for humans drinking tea to reach sufficient plasma and tissue levels of tea flavonoids to realize a protective effect. In general, flavonoids are rapidly metabolized and eliminated from the body, but there is considerable variation between individuals in this respect.[35] Catechol-O-methyltransferase (COMT) is one of the enzymes involved in flavonoid metabolism. There are two forms of the gene for COMT—a low activity form and a high activity form. A recent case-control study found that higher intakes of green tea were associated with lower breast cancer risk only in women who had inherited at least one copy of the low activity form of COMT, suggesting that those who are less efficient at eliminating green tea flavonoids may be more likely to benefit from their consumption.[36] Relationships between tea consumption and cancer risk are likely to be complex, and further study is needed before specific recommendations can be made regarding tea consumption and cancer prevention.

Osteoporosis

Many factors can affect the development of osteoporosis, including nutrition, physical activity, and genetic factors. Although one cross-sectional study found that black tea consumption was associated with slightly lower bone mineral density (BMD) in American women,[37] three other cross-sectional studies found that habitual tea consumption was associated with higher BMD in British[38] and Canadian women[39] and in Taiwanese men and women.[40] Hip fracture is one of the most serious consequences of osteoporosis. A large case-control study in Mediterranean countries found that low tea consumption was associated with higher risk of hip fracture in men[41] and women.[42] However, two large prospective cohort studies of women in the United States found no relationship between tea consumption and the risk of hip or wrist fracture over 4 to 6 years of follow-up.[43,44] The most recent of these studies found that higher tea intakes were associated with slightly higher BMD in postmenopausal women, but this finding did not translate into a lower risk of hip or wrist fracture.[43] Further study is required to determine whether tea consumption affects the development of osteoporosis or the risk of osteoporotic fracture in a meaningful way.

Dental Caries

Fluoride concentrations in tea are comparable to those recommended for U.S. water supplies to prevent dental caries (cavities).[45] Green, black, and oolong tea extracts have been found to inhibit the growth and acid production of cavity-producing bacteria in the test tube.[46,47] Although tea extracts have been found to prevent or decrease dental caries in animal models,[48] few published studies have examined the effect of tea consumption on dental caries in humans. A cross-sectional study of more than 6000 fourteen-year-olds in the UK found that those who drank tea had significantly fewer dental caries than nondrinkers, whether or not they added sugar to their tea.[49]

Kidney Stones

Two large prospective cohort studies in the United States found that the risk of developing symptomatic kidney stones decreased by 8% in women[50] and 14% in men[51] for each 8-oz (235 mL) mug of tea consumed daily. The implications of these findings for individuals with a previous history of calcium oxalate stone formation are unclear. High fluid intake, including tea intake, is generally considered the most effective and economical means of preventing kidney stones.[52] However, tea consumption has been found to increase urinary oxalate levels in healthy individuals,[53] and some experts continue to advise people with a history of calcium oxalate stones to limit tea consumption.[54]

Weight Loss

Weight reduction can be achieved by long-term decreases in energy intake and/or increases in energy expenditure. Several small short-term trials have reported modest 3 to 4% increases in energy expenditure after the consumption of oolong tea[55,56] or green tea extract.[57] However, none of these studies were designed to assess weight loss. A clinical trial in overweight men and women who had lost an average of 7.5% of their body weight by adhering to a very low-calorie diet for 4 weeks found that green tea capsules (573 mg/d of catechins and 104 mg/d of caffeine) were no better than placebo in preventing weight regain over the next 8 weeks.[58] At present, there is no evidence from controlled clinical trials that tea or tea extracts promote weight loss or improve weight maintenance.

Safety

Adverse Effects

Tea

Tea is generally considered to be safe, even in large amounts. However, two cases of hypokalemia (abnormally low serum potassium) in the elderly have been attributed to excessive consumption of black and oolong tea (3 to 14 L/d).[59,60] Hypokalemia is a potentially life-threatening condition that has been associated with caffeine toxicity.

Tea Extracts

Cancer patients in clinical trials of caffeinated green tea extracts who took 6 g/d in 3 to 6 divided doses have reported mild-to-moderate gastrointestinal side effects, including nausea, vomiting, abdominal pain, and diarrhea.[61,62] Central nervous system symptoms including agitation, restlessness, insomnia, tremors, dizziness, and confusion have also been reported. In one case, confusion was severe enough to require hospitalization.[61] These side effects were likely related to the caffeine in the green tea extract.[62] In a 4-week clinical trial that assessed the safety of decaffeinated green tea extracts (800 mg/d of EGCG) to healthy individuals, a few of the participants reported mild nausea, stomach upset, dizziness, or muscle pain.[63]

Pregnancy and Lactation

The safety of tea extracts or supplements for pregnant or breastfeeding women has not been established. Some organizations advise pregnant women to limit their caffeine consumption to 300 mg/d because higher caffeine intakes have been associated with increased risk of miscarriage and low birth weight in some epidemiological studies.[64] For more information on caffeine and pregnancy, see Chapter 6.

Drug Interactions

Green Tea

Excessive green tea consumption may decrease the therapeutic effects of the anticoagulant, warfarin (Coumadin). Such an effect was documented in one patient who began drinking one-half gallon to one gallon of green tea daily.[65] It is probably not necessary for people on warfarin therapy to avoid green tea entirely. However, large quantities of green tea may decrease its effectiveness.[66]

Caffeine

Several drugs can impair the metabolism of caffeine, increasing the potential for adverse effects from caffeine; high caffeine intakes may increase the risk of toxicity of some drugs.[67] See Chapter 6 for more information on caffeine-drug interactions.

Nutrient Interactions

Nonheme Iron

Flavonoids in tea can bind nonheme iron, inhibiting its intestinal absorption. Nonheme iron is the principal form of iron in plant foods, dairy products, and iron supplements. The consumption of one cup of tea with a meal has been found to decrease the absorption of nonheme iron in that meal by ~ 70 %.[68,69] To maximize iron absorption from a meal or iron supplements, tea should not be consumed at the same time.

Summary

- Tea is an infusion of the leaves of the *Camellia sinensis* plant and is not to be confused with so-called herbal teas.
- Some biologically active chemicals in tea include flavonoids, caffeine, and fluoride.
- Overall, observational studies in humans suggest that daily consumption of at least 3 cups of tea may be associated with a modest (11 %) decrease in the risk of myocardial infarction.
- Despite promising results from animal studies, it is not clear whether increasing tea consumption will help prevent cancers in humans.
- Although tea consumption has been positively associated with bone density in some studies, it is not clear whether tea consumption reduces the risk of fractures due to osteoporosis.
- Limited research suggests that tea consumption may be associated with fewer cavities and a slightly lower risk of kidney stones, but more research is needed to confirm these findings.
- At present, there is no evidence from controlled clinical trials that tea or tea extracts promote weight loss.

References

1. Graham HN. Green tea composition, consumption, and polyphenol chemistry. Prev Med 1992;21(3):334–350
2. Balentine DA, Paetau-Robinson I. Tea as a source of dietary antioxidants with a potential role in prevention of chronic diseases. In: Mazza G, Oomah BD, eds. Herbs, Botanicals, & Teas. Lancaster: Technomic Publishing Co., Inc.; 2000:265–287
3. Santana-Rios G, Orner GA, Amantana A, Provost C, Wu SY, Dashwood RH. Potent antimutagenic activity of white tea in comparison with green tea in the Salmonella assay. Mutat Res 2001;495(1–2):61–74
4. Lakenbrink C, Lapczynski S, Maiwald B, Engelhardt UH. Flavonoids and other polyphenols in consumer brews of tea and other caffeinated beverages. J Agric Food Chem 2000;48(7):2848–2852
5. Astill C, Birch MR, Dacombe C, Humphrey PG, Martin PT. Factors affecting the caffeine and polyphenol contents of black and green tea infusions. J Agric Food Chem 2001;49(11):5340–5347
6. Lin JK, Lin CL, Liang YC, Lin-Shiau SY, Juan IM. Survey of catechins, gallic acid, and methylxanthines in green, oolong, pu-erh, and black teas. J Agric Food Chem 1998;46(9):3635–3642
7. Lin YS, Tsai YJ, Tsay JS, Lin JK. Factors affecting the levels of tea polyphenols and caffeine in tea leaves. J Agric Food Chem 2003;51(7):1864–1873
8. Wong MH, Fung KF, Carr HP. Aluminium and fluoride contents of tea, with emphasis on brick tea and their health implications. Toxicol Lett 2003;137(1–2):111–120
9. Cao J, Zhao Y, Liu J, et al. Brick tea fluoride as a main source of adult fluorosis. Food Chem Toxicol 2003;41(4):535–542
10. Cao J, Bai X, Zhao Y, et al. The relationship of fluorosis and brick tea drinking in Chinese Tibetans. Environ Health Perspect 1996;104(12):1340–1343
11. Cao J, Luo SF, Liu JW, Li YH. Safety evaluation on fluoride content in black tea. Food Chem 2004;88(2):233–236
12. Fung KF, Zhang ZQ, Wong JWC, Wong MH. Fluoride contents in tea and soil from tea plantations and the release of fluoride into tea liquor during infusion. Environ Pollut 1999;104(2):197–205
13. Peters U, Poole C, Arab L. Does tea affect cardiovascular disease? A meta-analysis. Am J Epidemiol 2001;154(6):495–503
14. Geleijnse JM, Launer LJ, Van der Kuip DA, Hofman A, Witteman JC. Inverse association of tea and flavonoid intakes with incident myocardial infarction: the Rotterdam Study. Am J Clin Nutr 2002;75(5):880–886
15. Sesso HD, Gaziano JM, Liu S, Buring JE. Flavonoid intake and the risk of cardiovascular disease in women. Am J Clin Nutr 2003;77(6):1400–1408
16. Sesso HD, Paffenbarger RS Jr, Oguma Y, Lee IM. Lack of association between tea and cardiovascular disease in college alumni. Int J Epidemiol 2003;32(4):527–533
17. Nakachi K, Matsuyama S, Miyake S, Suganuma M, Imai K. Preventive effects of drinking green tea on cancer and cardiovascular disease: epidemiological evidence for multiple targeting prevention. Biofactors 2000;13(1–4):49–54
18. Vita JA. Tea consumption and cardiovascular disease: effects on endothelial function. J Nutr 2003;133(10):3293S–3297S

19. Duffy SJ, Keaney JF Jr, Holbrook M, et al. Short- and long-term black tea consumption reverses endothelial dysfunction in patients with coronary artery disease. Circulation 2001;104(2):151–156
20. Hodgson JM, Puddey IB, Burke V, Watts GF, Beilin LJ. Regular ingestion of black tea improves brachial artery vasodilator function. Clin Sci (Lond) 2002; 102(2):195–201
21. Lambert JD, Yang CS. Mechanisms of cancer prevention by tea constituents. J Nutr 2003;133(10):3262S–3267S
22. Yang CS, Maliakal P, Meng X. Inhibition of carcinogenesis by tea. Annu Rev Pharmacol Toxicol 2002;42: 25–54
23. Lu YP, Lou YR, Lin Y, et al. Inhibitory effects of orally administered green tea, black tea, and caffeine on skin carcinogenesis in mice previously treated with ultraviolet B light (high-risk mice): relationship to decreased tissue fat. Cancer Res 2001;61(13):5002–5009
24. Chung FL, Wang M, Rivenson A, et al. Inhibition of lung carcinogenesis by black tea in Fischer rats treated with a tobacco-specific carcinogen: caffeine as an important constituent. Cancer Res 1998;58(18):4096–4101
25. Williams RJ, Spencer JP, Rice-Evans C. Flavonoids: antioxidants or signalling molecules? Free Radic Biol Med 2004;36(7):838–849
26. Hou Z, Lambert JD, Chin KV, Yang CS. Effects of tea polyphenols on signal transduction pathways related to cancer chemoprevention. Mutat Res 2004;555(1–2): 3–19
27. Higdon JV, Frei B. Tea catechins and polyphenols: health effects, metabolism, and antioxidant functions. Crit Rev Food Sci Nutr 2003;43(1):89–143
28. Hoshiyama Y, Kawaguchi T, Miura Y, et al. A nested case-control study of stomach cancer in relation to green tea consumption in Japan. Br J Cancer 2004; 90(1):135–138
29. Koizumi Y, Tsubono Y, Nakaya N, et al. No association between green tea and the risk of gastric cancer: pooled analysis of two prospective studies in Japan. Cancer Epidemiol Biomarkers Prev 2003;12(5):472–473
30. Hoshiyama Y, Kawaguchi T, Miura Y, et al. A prospective study of stomach cancer death in relation to green tea consumption in Japan. Br J Cancer 2002;87(3): 309–313
31. Tsubono Y, Nishino Y, Komatsu S, et al. Green tea and the risk of gastric cancer in Japan. N Engl J Med 2001;344(9):632–636
32. Orner GA, Dashwood WM, Blum CA, Diaz GD, Li Q, Dashwood RH. Suppression of tumorigenesis in the Apc(min) mouse: down-regulation of beta-catenin signaling by a combination of tea plus sulindac. Carcinogenesis 2003;24(2):263–267
33. Arab L, Il'yasova D. The epidemiology of tea consumption and colorectal cancer incidence. J Nutr 2003; 133(10):3310S–3318S
34. Tavani A, Vecchia CL. Coffee, decaffeinated coffee, tea and cancer of the colon and rectum: a review of epidemiological studies, 1990–2003. Cancer Causes Control 2004;15(8):743–757
35. Manach C, Scalbert A, Morand C, Remesy C, Jimenez L. Polyphenols: food sources and bioavailability. Am J Clin Nutr 2004;79(5):727–747
36. Wu AH, Tseng CC, Van Den Berg D, Yu MC. Tea intake, COMT genotype, and breast cancer in Asian-American women. Cancer Res 2003;63(21):7526–7529
37. Hernandez-Avila M, Stampfer MJ, Ravnikar VA, et al. Caffeine and other predictors of bone density among pre- and perimenopausal women. Epidemiology 1993;4(2):128–134
38. Hegarty VM, May HM, Khaw KT. Tea drinking and bone mineral density in older women. Am J Clin Nutr 2000;71(4):1003–1007
39. Hoover PA, Webber CE, Beaumont LF, Blake JM. Postmenopausal bone mineral density: relationship to calcium intake, calcium absorption, residual estrogen, body composition, and physical activity. Can J Physiol Pharmacol 1996;74(8):911–917
40. Wu CH, Yang YC, Yao WJ, Lu FH, Wu JS, Chang CJ. Epidemiological evidence of increased bone mineral density in habitual tea drinkers. Arch Intern Med 2002;162(9):1001–1006
41. Kanis J, Johnell O, Gullberg B, et al. Risk factors for hip fracture in men from southern Europe: the MEDOS study. Mediterranean Osteoporosis Study. Osteoporos Int 1999;9(1):45–54
42. Johnell O, Gullberg B, Kanis JA, et al. Risk factors for hip fracture in European women: the MEDOS Study. Mediterranean Osteoporosis Study. J Bone Miner Res 1995;10(11):1802–1815
43. Chen Z, Pettinger MB, Ritenbaugh C, et al. Habitual tea consumption and risk of osteoporosis: a prospective study in the women's health initiative observational cohort. Am J Epidemiol 2003;158(8):772–781
44. Hernandez-Avila M, Colditz GA, Stampfer MJ, Rosner B, Speizer FE, Willett WC. Caffeine, moderate alcohol intake, and risk of fractures of the hip and forearm in middle-aged women. Am J Clin Nutr 1991;54(1):157–163
45. Trevisanato SI, Kim YI. Tea and health. Nutr Rev 2000;58(1):1–10
46. Rasheed A, Haider M. Antibacterial activity of Camellia sinensis extracts against dental caries. Arch Pharm Res 1998;21(3):348–352
47. Matsumoto M, Minami T, Sasaki H, Sobue S, Hamada S, Ooshima T. Inhibitory effects of oolong tea extract on caries-inducing properties of mutans streptococci. Caries Res 1999;33(6):441–445
48. Linke HA, LeGeros RZ. Black tea extract and dental caries formation in hamsters. Int J Food Sci Nutr 2003;54(1):89–95
49. Jones C, Woods K, Whittle G, Worthington H, Taylor G. Sugar, drinks, deprivation and dental caries in 14-year-old children in the north west of England in 1995. Community Dent Health 1999;16(2):68–71
50. Curhan GC, Willett WC, Speizer FE, Stampfer MJ. Beverage use and risk for kidney stones in women. Ann Intern Med 1998;128(7):534–540
51. Curhan GC, Willett WC, Rimm EB, Spiegelman D, Stampfer MJ. Prospective study of beverage use and the risk of kidney stones. Am J Epidemiol 1996; 143(3):240–247
52. Borghi L, Meschi T, Schianchi T, et al. Urine volume: stone risk factor and preventive measure. Nephron 1999;81(Suppl 1):31–37
53. Massey LK, Roman-Smith H, Sutton RA. Effect of dietary oxalate and calcium on urinary oxalate and risk of formation of calcium oxalate kidney stones. J Am Diet Assoc 1993;93(8):901–906

54. Massey LK. Tea oxalate. Nutr Rev 2000;58(3 Pt 1):88–89

55. Komatsu T, Nakamori M, Komatsu K, et al. Oolong tea increases energy metabolism in Japanese females. J Med Invest 2003;50(3–4):170–175

56. Rumpler W, Seale J, Clevidence B, et al. Oolong tea increases metabolic rate and fat oxidation in men. J Nutr 2001;131(11):2848–2852

57. Dulloo AG, Duret C, Rohrer D, et al. Efficacy of a green tea extract rich in catechin polyphenols and caffeine in increasing 24-h energy expenditure and fat oxidation in humans. Am J Clin Nutr 1999;70(6):1040–1045

58. Kovacs EM, Lejeune MP, Nijs I, Westerterp-Plantenga MS. Effects of green tea on weight maintenance after body-weight loss. Br J Nutr 2004;91(3):431–437

59. Aizaki T, Osaka M, Hara H, et al. Hypokalemia with syncope caused by habitual drinking of oolong tea. Intern Med 1999;38(3):252–256

60. Trewby PN, Rutter MD, Earl UM, Sattar MA. Teapot myositis. Lancet 1998;351(9111):1248

61. Jatoi A, Ellison N, Burch PA, et al. A phase II trial of green tea in the treatment of patients with androgen independent metastatic prostate carcinoma. Cancer 2003;97(6):1442–1446

62. Pisters KM, Newman RA, Coldman B, et al. Phase I trial of oral green tea extract in adult patients with solid tumors. J Clin Oncol 2001;19(6):1830–1838

63. Chow HH, Cai Y, Hakim IA, et al. Pharmacokinetics and safety of green tea polyphenols after multiple-dose administration of epigallocatechin gallate and polyphenon E in healthy individuals. Clin Cancer Res 2003;9(9):3312–3319

64. National Toxicology Program Center for the Evaluation of Risks to Human Reproduction. Caffeine. 2003. Available at: http://cerhr.niehs.nih.gov/genpub/topics/caffeine-ccae.html. Accessed 12/6/04

65. Taylor JR, Wilt VM. Probable antagonism of warfarin by green tea. Ann Pharmacother 1999;33(4):426–428

66. Heck AM, DeWitt BA, Lukes AL. Potential interactions between alternative therapies and warfarin. Am J Health Syst Pharm 2000;57(13):1221–1227; quiz 1228–1230.

67. Carrillo JA, Benitez J. Clinically significant pharmacokinetic interactions between dietary caffeine and medications. Clin Pharmacokinet 2000;39(2):127–153

68. Hurrell RF, Reddy M, Cook JD. Inhibition of non-haem iron absorption in man by polyphenolic-containing beverages. Br J Nutr 1999;81(4):289–295

69. Zijp IM, Korver O, Tijburg LB. Effect of tea and other dietary factors on iron absorption. Crit Rev Food Sci Nutr 2000;40(5):371–398

70. McCusker RR, Goldberger BA, Cone EJ. Caffeine content of specialty coffees. J Anal Toxicol 2003;27(7):520–522

8 Carotenoids

Carotenoids are a class of more than 600 naturally occurring pigments synthesized by plants, algae, and photosynthetic bacteria. These richly colored molecules are the sources of the yellow, orange, and red colors of many plants.[1] Fruits and vegetables provide most of the carotenoids in the human diet. Beta-carotene, α-carotene, β-cryptoxanthin, lutein, zeaxanthin, and lycopene are the most common dietary carotenoids. Beta-carotene, α-carotene, and β-cryptoxanthin are provitamin A carotenoids, meaning they can be converted by the body to retinol (**Fig. 8–1**). Lutein, zeaxanthin, and lycopene cannot be converted to retinol, so they have no vitamin A activity (**Fig. 8–2**).

Bioavailability and Metabolism

For dietary carotenoids to be absorbed intestinally, they must be released from the food matrix and incorporated into mixed micelles (mixtures of bile salts and several types of lipids).[2] Therefore, carotenoid absorption requires the presence of fat in a meal. As little as 3 to 5 g of fat in a meal appears sufficient to ensure carotenoid absorption.[3,4] Because they do not need to be released from the plant matrix, carotenoids supplements (in oil) are more efficiently absorbed than carotenoids in foods.[4] Within the cells that line the intestine (enterocytes), carotenoids are incorporated into triglyceride-rich lipoproteins called chylom-

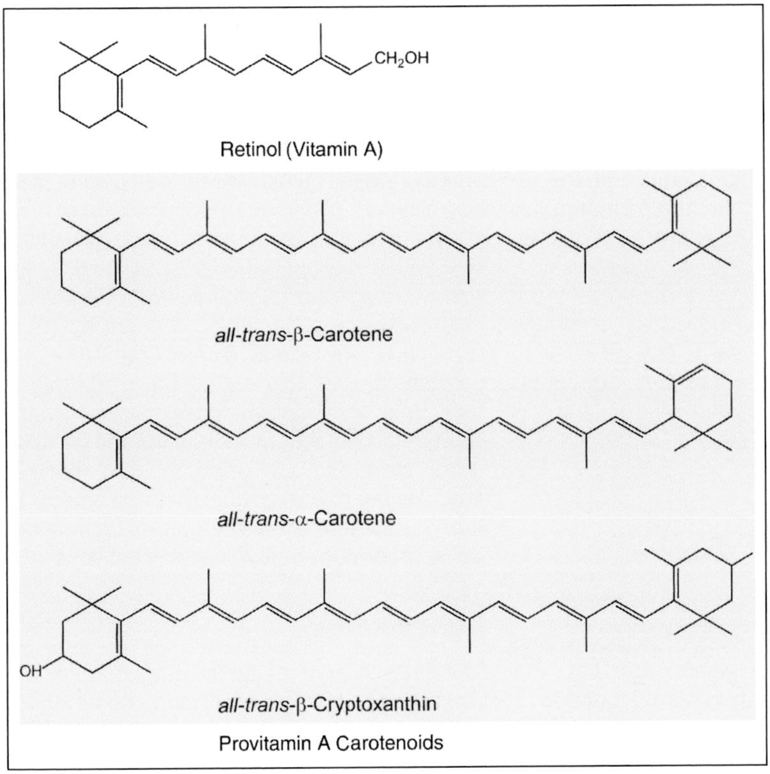

Figure 8–1 The chemical structures of retinol (vitamin A) and the provitamin A carotenoids, β-carotene, α-carotene, and β-cryptoxanthin.

Retinol (Vitamin A)

all-trans-β-Carotene

all-trans-α-Carotene

all-trans-β-Cryptoxanthin

Provitamin A Carotenoids

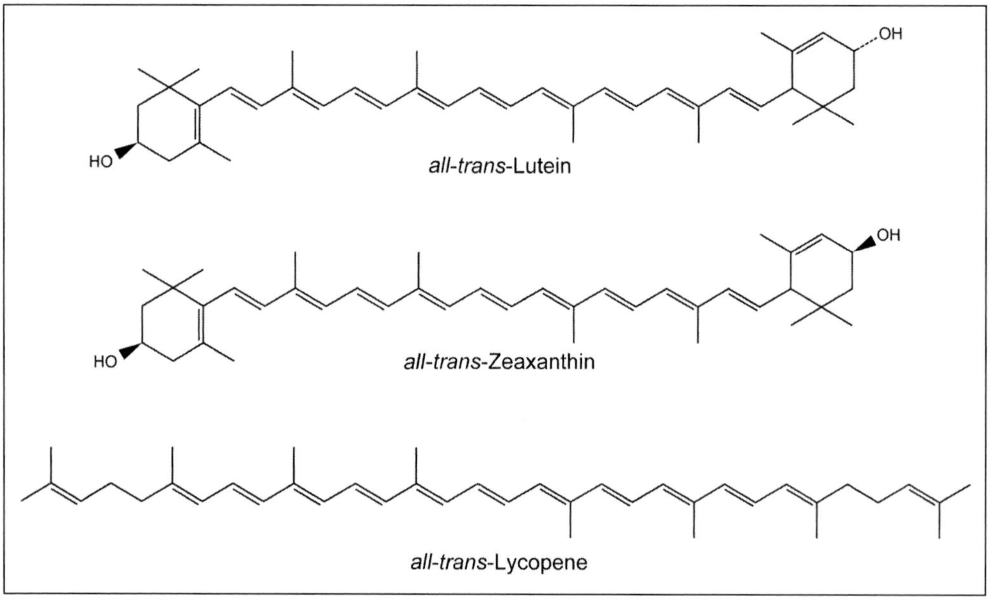

Figure 8–2   The chemical structures of lutein, zeaxanthin, and lycopene.

icrons and released into the circulation.[2] Triglycerides are depleted from circulating chylomicrons through the activity of lipo-protein lipase, resulting in the formation of chylomicron remnants. Chylomicron remnants are taken up by the liver, where carotenoids are incorporated into lipoproteins and secreted back into the circulation. In the in-testine and the liver, provitamin A carotenoids may be cleaved to produce retinal, a form of vi-tamin A. The conversion of provitamin A carotenoids to vitamin A is influenced by the vitamin A status of the individual.[5] Although the regulatory mechanism is not yet clear in humans, cleavage of provitamin A carotenoids appears to be inhibited when vitamin A stores are high.

Biological Activities

Vitamin A Activity

Vitamin A is essential for normal growth and development, immune system function, and vision. Currently, the only essential function of carotenoids recognized in humans is that of provitamin A carotenoids (β-carotene, α-carotene and β-cryptoxanthin) to serve as a source of vitamin A.[6]

Antioxidant Activity

In plants, carotenoids have the important an-tioxidant function of quenching (deactivating) singlet oxygen, an oxidant formed during pho-tosynthesis.[7] Test-tube studies indicate that ly-copene is one of the most effective quenchers of singlet oxygen among carotenoids.[8] Al-though important for plants, the relevance of singlet oxygen quenching to human health is less clear. Test-tube studies indicate that carotenoids can also inhibit the oxidation of fats (lipid peroxidation) under certain condi-tions, but their actions in humans appear to be more complex.[9] At present, it is unclear whether the biological effects of carotenoids in humans are a result of their antioxidant activ-ity or other non-antioxidant mechanisms.

Light Filtering

The long system of alternating double and single bonds common to all carotenoids allows them to absorb light in the visible range of the spectrum.[7] This feature has particular relevance to the eye, where lutein and zeaxanthin efficiently absorb blue light. Reducing the amount of blue light that reaches the structures of the eye that are critical to vision may protect them from light-induced oxidative damage.[10]

Intercellular Communication

Carotenoids can facilitate communication between neighboring cells grown in culture by stimulating the synthesis of connexin proteins.[11] Connexins form pores (gap junctions) in cell membranes, allowing cells to communicate through the exchange of small molecules. This type of intercellular communication is important for maintaining cells in a differentiated state and is often lost in cancer cells. Carotenoids facilitate intercellular communication by increasing the expression of the gene encoding a connexin protein, an effect that appears unrelated to the vitamin A or antioxidant activities of various carotenoids.[12]

Immune System Function

Because vitamin A is essential for normal immune system function, it is difficult to determine whether the effects of provitamin A carotenoids are related to their vitamin A activity or other activities of carotenoids. Although some clinical trials have found that β-carotene supplementation improves several biomarkers of immune function,[13-15] increasing intakes of lycopene and lutein—carotenoids without vitamin A activity—did not result in similar improvements in immune function biomarkers.[16-18]

Deficiency

Although consumption of provitamin A carotenoids (β-carotene, α-carotene, and β-cryptoxanthin) can prevent vitamin A deficiency, no overt deficiency symptoms have been identified in people consuming low-carotenoid diets if they consume adequate vitamin A.[6] After reviewing the published scientific research in 2000, the Food and Nutrition Board of the Institute of Medicine concluded that the existing evidence was insufficient to establish a recommended dietary allowance (RDA) or adequate intake (AI) for carotenoids. Recommendations by the National Cancer Institute, the American Cancer Society, and the American Heart Association to consume a variety of fruits and vegetables daily are aimed, in part, at increasing intakes of carotenoid-rich vegetables.

Prevention

Lung Cancer

Dietary Carotenoids

Beta-carotene was the first carotenoid to be measured in foods and human blood. The results of early observational studies suggested an inverse relationship between lung cancer risk and β-carotene intake, often assessed by measuring blood levels of β-carotene.[19,20] The development of databases for other carotenoids in foods has allowed scientists to estimate dietary intakes of total and individual dietary carotenoids more accurately. In contrast to early retrospective studies, recent prospective cohort studies have not consistently found inverse associations between β-carotene intake and lung cancer risk. Analysis of dietary carotenoid intake and lung cancer risk in two large prospective cohort studies in the United States that followed more than 120,000 men and women for at least 10 years revealed no significant association between dietary β-carotene intake and lung cancer risk.[21] However, men and women with the highest intakes of total carotenoids, β-carotene, and lycopene were at significantly lower risk of developing lung cancer than those with the lowest intakes. Dietary intakes of total carotenoids, lycopene, β-cryptoxanthin, lutein, and zeaxanthin, but not β-carotene, were associated with significant reductions in lung cancer in a 14-year study of more than 27,000 Finnish male smokers,[22] whereas only dietary intakes of β-cryptoxanthin, lutein, and zeaxanthin were inversely associated with lung cancer risk in a 6-year study of more than 58,000 Dutch men.[23] An analysis of the pooled results of six prospective cohort studies in North America and Europe also found no relationship between dietary β-carotene intake and lung cancer risk, although those with the highest β-cryptoxanthin intakes had a risk of lung cancer that was 24% lower than those with the lowest intakes.[24] Although smoking remains the strongest risk factor for lung cancer, results of recent prospective studies using accurate estimates of dietary carotenoid intake suggest that diets rich in several carotenoids—not only β-carotene—may be associated with reduced lung cancer risk.

Beta-Carotene Supplements

The effect of β-carotene supplementation on the risk of developing lung cancer has been examined in three large randomized placebo-controlled trials. In Finland, the Alpha-Tocopherol Beta-Carotene (ATBC) cancer prevention trial evaluated the effects of 20 mg/d of β-carotene and/or 50 mg/d of α-tocopherol on more than 29,000 male smokers,[25] and in the United States, the β-Carotene And Retinol Efficacy Trial (CARET) evaluated the effects of a combination of 30 mg/d of β-carotene and 25,000 IU/d of retinol (vitamin A) in more than 18,000 men and women who were smokers, former smokers, or had a history of occupational asbestos exposure.[26] Unexpectedly, the risk of lung cancer in the groups taking β-carotene supplements was increased by 16% after 6 years in the ATBC participants and increased by 28% after 4 years in the CARET participants. The Physicians' Health Study examined the effect of β-carotene supplementation (50 mg every other day) on cancer risk in more than 22,000 male physicians in the United States, of whom only 11% were current smokers.[27] In that lower risk population, β-carotene supplementation for more than 12 years was not associated with an increased risk of lung cancer. Although the reasons for the increase in lung cancer risk are not yet clear, many experts feel that the risks of high-dose β-carotene supplementation outweigh any potential benefits for cancer prevention, especially in smokers or other high-risk populations.[28,29]

Prostate Cancer

Dietary Lycopene

The results of several prospective cohort studies suggest that lycopene-rich diets are associated with significant reductions in the risk of prostate cancer, particularly more aggressive forms.[30] In a prospective study of more than 47,000 health professionals followed for 8 years, those with the highest lycopene intake had a risk of prostate cancer that was 21% lower than those with the lowest lycopene intake.[31] Those with the highest intakes of tomatoes and tomato products (accounting for 82% of total lycopene intake) had a risk of prostate cancer that was 35% lower and a risk of aggressive prostate cancer that was 53% lower than those with the lowest intakes. Similarly, a prospective study of Seventh Day Adventist men found that those who reported the highest tomato intakes were at significantly lower risk of prostate cancer,[32] and a prospective study of physicians in the United States found that those with the highest plasma lycopene levels were at significantly lower risk of developing aggressive prostate cancer.[33] However, dietary lycopene intake was not related to prostate cancer risk in a prospective study of more than 58,000 Dutch men.[34] A meta-analysis that combined the results of 10 prospective cohort studies found that an increase of one daily serving (200 g) of raw tomato was associated with a 22% reduction in the risk of prostate cancer.[35] Although there is considerable scientific interest in the potential for lycopene to help prevent prostate cancer, it is not yet clear whether the prostate cancer risk reduction observed in some epidemiological studies is related to lycopene itself, other compounds in tomatoes, or other factors associated with lycopene-rich diets.

Cardiovascular Disease

Dietary Carotenoids

Because they are very soluble in fat and insoluble in water, carotenoids circulate in lipoproteins along with cholesterol and other fats. Evidence that low-density lipoprotein (LDL) oxidation plays a role in the development of atherosclerosis led scientists to investigate the role of antioxidant compounds like carotenoids in the prevention of cardiovascular diseases.[36] The thickness of the inner layers of the carotid arteries can be measured noninvasively using ultrasound technology. This measurement of carotid intima-media thickness is considered a reliable marker of atherosclerosis.[37] Several case-control and cross-sectional studies have found higher blood levels of carotenoids to be associated with significantly lower measures of carotid artery-intima media thickness.[38-43] Higher plasma carotenoids at baseline have been associated with significant reductions in cardiovascular disease risk in some prospective studies[44-46] but not in others.[47-50] Although the results of several prospective studies indicate that people with higher intakes of carotenoid-rich fruits and vegetables are at lower risk of cardiovascular disease,[50-53] it is not yet clear whether this effect is a result of carotenoids or other factors associated with diets high in carotenoid-rich fruits and vegetables.

Beta-Carotene Supplements

In contrast to the results of epidemiological studies suggesting that high dietary intakes of carotenoid-rich fruits and vegetables may decrease cardiovascular disease risk, four randomized controlled trials found no evidence that β-carotene supplements in doses ranging from 20 to 50 mg/d were effective in preventing cardiovascular diseases.[25,27,54,55] Based on the results of these randomized controlled trials, the U.S. Preventive Health Services Task Force concluded that there was good evidence that β-carotene supplements provided no benefit in the prevention of cardiovascular disease in middle-aged and older adults.[29,56]

Although diets rich in β-carotene have generally been associated with reduced cardiovascular disease risk in observational studies, there is no evidence that β-carotene supplementation reduces cardiovascular disease risk.

Age-Related Macular Degeneration

In Western countries, degeneration of the macula, the center of the eye's retina, is the leading cause of blindness in older adults.

Dietary Lutein and Zeaxanthin

The only carotenoids found in the retina are lutein and zeaxanthin. Lutein and zeaxanthin are present in high concentrations in the macula, where they are efficient absorbers of blue light. By preventing a substantial amount of the blue light entering the eye from reaching underlying structures involved in vision, lutein and zeaxanthin may protect them from light-induced oxidative damage, which is thought to play a role in the pathology of age-related macular degeneration.[10] It is also possible, though not proven, that lutein and zeaxanthin act directly to neutralize oxidants formed in the retina. Epidemiological studies provide some evidence that higher intakes of lutein and zeaxanthin are associated with lower risk of age-related macular degeneration (AMD).[57] The relationship, however, is by no means clear-cut. Cross-sectional and retrospective case-control studies found that higher levels of lutein and zeaxanthin in the diet,[58-60] blood,[61,62] and retina[63,64] were associated with a lower incidence of AMD; nonetheless, several prospective cohort studies found no relationship between baseline dietary intakes or serum levels of lutein and zeaxanthin and the risk of developing AMD over time.[65-68] Although scientists are very interested in the potential for increased lutein and zeaxanthin intakes to reduce the risk of macular degeneration, it is premature to recommend supplements without more data from randomized controlled trials.[69] The available scientific evidence suggests that consuming at least 6 mg/d of lutein and zeaxanthin from fruits and vegetables may decrease the risk of age-related macular degeneration.[58-60]

Lutein Supplements

In a randomized controlled trial, supplementation of patients who had atrophic AMD with 10 mg/d of lutein resulted in slight improvement in visual acuity after one year compared with a placebo.[70] However, the investigators concluded that further research was needed to assess the effects of long-term lutein supplementation on atrophic AMD.

Beta-Carotene Supplements

The first randomized controlled trial designed to examine the effect of a carotenoid supplement on AMD used β-carotene in combination with vitamin C, vitamin E, and zinc because lutein and zeaxanthin were not commercially available as supplements at the time the trial began.[71] Although the combination of antioxidants and zinc lowered the risk of developing advanced macular degeneration in individuals with signs of moderate to severe macular degeneration in at least one eye, it is unlikely that the benefit was related to β-carotene because it is not present in the retina. Supplementation of male smokers in Finland with 20 mg/d of β-carotene for 6 years did not decrease the risk of AMD compared with placebo.[72]

Cataracts

Ultraviolet light and oxidants can damage proteins in the eye's lens, causing structural changes that result in the formation of opacities known as cataracts. As people age, cumulative damage to lens proteins often results in cataracts that are large enough to interfere with vision.[7]

Dietary Lutein and Zeaxanthin

The observation that lutein and zeaxanthin are the only carotenoids in the human lens has stimulated interest in the potential for increased intakes of lutein and zeaxanthin to prevent or slow the progression of cataracts.[10] Three large prospective studies found that men and women with the highest intakes of foods that are rich in lutein and zeaxanthin, particularly spinach, kale, and broccoli, were 20 to 50% less likely to require cataract extraction[73,74] or develop cataracts.[75] Additional research is required to determine whether these findings are related specifically to lutein and zeaxanthin intake or to other factors associated with diets high in lutein-rich foods.[57]

Beta-Carotene Supplements

Evidence from epidemiological studies that cataracts were less prevalent in people with high dietary intakes and blood levels of carotenoids led to the inclusion of β-carotene supplements in several large randomized controlled trials of antioxidants. The results of those trials have been somewhat conflicting. Beta-carotene supplementation (20 mg/d) for more than 6 years did not affect the prevalence of cataracts or the frequency of cataract surgery in male smokers living in Finland.[72] In contrast, a 12-year study of male physicians in the United States found that β-carotene supplementation (50 mg every other day) decreased the risk of cataracts in smokers but not in nonsmokers.[76] Two randomized controlled trials examined the effect of an antioxidant combination that included β-carotene, vitamin C, and vitamin E on the progression of cataracts. One study found no benefit after more than 6 years of supplementation;[77] the other study found a small decrease in the progression of cataracts after 3 years of supplementation.[78] Overall, the results of randomized controlled trials suggest that the benefit of β-carotene in slowing the progression of age-related cataracts does not outweigh the potential risks.

Sources

Food Sources

The most prevalent dietary carotenoids in typical Western diets are β-carotene, α-carotene, β-cryptoxanthin, lycopene, lutein, and zeaxanthin.[6] Carotenoids in foods are mainly in the *all-trans* form (**Figs. 8–1 and 8–2**), although cooking may result in the formation of other isomers. The relatively low bioavailability of carotenoids from most foods compared with supplements is partly due to the fact that they are associated with proteins in the plant matrix.[2] Chopping, homogenizing, and cooking disrupt the plant matrix, increasing the bioavailability of carotenoids.[4] The bioavailability of lycopene from tomatoes is substantially improved by heating tomatoes in oil.[79,80]

Beta-Carotene and Alpha-Carotene

Beta-carotene and α-carotene are provitamin A carotenoids; that is, they can be converted by the body to vitamin A. The vitamin A activity of β-carotene in foods is 1/12 that of retinol (preformed vitamin A). Thus, it would take 12 µg of β-carotene from foods to provide the equivalent of 1 µg of retinol. The vitamin A activity of α-carotene from foods is 1/24 that of retinol,

so it would take 24 µg of α-carotene from foods to provide the equivalent of 1 µg of retinol. Orange and yellow vegetables like carrots and winter squash are rich sources of β- and α-carotene. Spinach is also a rich source of β-carotene, although the chlorophyll in spinach leaves hides the yellow-orange pigment. Some foods that are good sources of α-carotene and β-carotene are listed in **Tables 8–1 and 8–2**, respectively.

Table 8–1   α-Carotene Content of Selected Foods

Food	Serving	α-Carotene (mg)
Pumpkin, canned	1 cup	11.7
Carrot juice, canned	1 cup (8 fl oz)	10.2
Carrots, cooked	1 cup	5.9
Carrots, raw	1 medium	2.0
Mixed vegetables, frozen cooked	1 cup	1.8
Winter squash, baked	1 cup	1.4
Plantains, raw	1 medium	0.8
Pumpkin pie	1 piece	0.7
Collards, frozen cooked	1 cup	0.2
Tomatoes, raw	1 medium	0.1
Tangerines, raw	1 medium	0.08
Peas, frozen, cooked	1 cup	0.08

Table 8–2   β-Carotene Content of Selected Foods

Food	Serving	β-Carotene (mg)
Carrot juice, canned	1 cup (8 fl oz)	22.0
Pumpkin, canned	1 cup	17.0
Sweet potato, baked	1 medium	16.8
Spinach, frozen, cooked	1 cup	13.7
Carrots, cooked	1 cup	13.0
Collards, frozen, cooked	1 cup	11.6
Kale, frozen, cooked	1 cup	11.5
Turnip greens, frozen, cooked	1 cup	10.6
Pumpkin pie	1 piece	7.4
Dandelion greens, cooked	1 cup	6.2
Winter squash, cooked	1 cup	5.7
Cantaloupe, raw	1 cup	3.2

Beta-Cryptoxanthin

Like β- and α-carotene, β-cryptoxanthin is a provitamin A carotenoid. The vitamin A activity of β-cryptoxanthin from foods is 1/24 that of retinol, so it would take 24 µg of β-cryptoxanthin from food to provide the equivalent of 1 µg of retinol. Orange and red fruits and vegetables like sweet red peppers and oranges are particularly rich sources of β-cryptoxanthin. Some foods that are good sources of β-cryptoxanthin are listed in **Table 8–3**.

Lycopene

Lycopene gives tomatoes, pink grapefruit, watermelon, and guava their red color. It has been estimated that 80% of the lycopene in the diet of the U.S. population comes from tomatoes and tomato products like tomato sauce, tomato paste, and catsup (ketchup).[81] Lycopene is not a provitamin A carotenoid, meaning the body cannot convert lycopene to vitamin A. Some foods that are good sources of lycopene are listed in **Table 8–4**.

Table 8–3　β-Cryptoxanthin Content of Selected Foods

Food	Serving	β-Cryptoxanthin (mg
Pumpkin, cooked	1 cup	3.6
Sweet red peppers, cooked	1 cup	2.8
Papayas, raw	1 medium	2.3
Sweet red peppers, raw	1 medium	0.6
Orange juice, fresh	1 cup	0.4
Tangerines, raw	1 medium	0.3
Carrots, cooked	1 cup	0.3
Watermelon, raw	1 wedge	0.2
Yellow corn, frozen, cooked	1 cup	0.2
Paprika, dried	1 tsp	0.2
Oranges, raw	1 medium	0.2
Nectarines, raw	1 medium	0.1

Table 8–4　Lycopene Content of Selected Foods

Food	Serving	Lycopene (mg)
Tomato paste, canned	1 cup	75.4
Tomato puree, canned	1 cup	54.4
Marinara sauce	1 cup	40.0
Tomato soup, canned	1 cup	25.6
Vegetable juice cocktail, canned	1 cup	23.3
Tomato juice, canned	1 cup	22.0
Watermelon, raw	1 wedge	13.0
Tomatoes, raw	1 cup	4.6
Catsup (ketchup)	1 tbs	2.6
Pink grapefruit, raw	1/2 grapefruit	1.7
Baked beans, canned	1 cup	1.3
Sweet red peppers, raw	1 cup	0.5

Table 8–5   Lutein + Zeaxanthin Content of Selected Foods

Food	Serving	Lutein + Zeaxanthin (mg)
Spinach, frozen, cooked	1 cup	29.8
Kale, frozen, cooked	1 cup	25.6
Turnip greens, frozen, cooked	1 cup	19.5
Collards, frozen, cooked	1 cup	18.5
Mustard greens, cooked	1 cup	8.3
Dandelion greens, cooked	1 cup	4.9
Summer squash, cooked	1 cup	4.0
Peas, frozen, cooked	1 cup	3.8
Winter squash, baked	1 cup	2.9
Broccoli, frozen, cooked	1 cup	2.8
Pumpkin, cooked	1 cup	2.5
Brussels sprouts, frozen, cooked	1 cup	2.4
Sweet yellow corn, boiled	1 cup	1.6

Lutein and Zeaxanthin

Although lutein and zeaxanthin are different compounds, they are both from the class of carotenoids known as xanthophylls. They are not provitamin A carotenoids. Some methods used to quantify lutein and zeaxanthin in foods do not separate the two compounds, so they are typically reported as lutein and zeaxanthin or lutein + zeaxanthin. Lutein and zeaxanthin are present in a variety of fruits and vegetables. Dark green leafy vegetables like spinach and kale are particularly rich sources of lutein and zeaxanthin. Some foods that are good sources of lutein and zeaxanthin are listed in **Table 8–5**.

Supplements

Dietary supplements providing purified carotenoids and combinations of carotenoids are commercially available in the United States without a prescription. Carotenoids are best absorbed when taken with a meal containing fat.

Beta-Carotene

Because it has vitamin A activity, β-carotene may be used to provide all or part of the vitamin A in multivitamin supplements. The vitamin A activity of β-carotene from supplements is much higher than that of β-carotene from foods. It takes only 2 μg of β-carotene from supplements to provide 1 μg of retinol (preformed vitamin A). The β-carotene content of supplements is often listed in international units (IU) rather than μg; 3000 μg (3 mg) of β-carotene provides 5000 IU of vitamin A.

Lycopene

Lycopene has no vitamin A activity. Synthetic lycopene and lycopene from natural sources (mainly tomatoes) are available as nutritional supplements.

Lutein and Zeaxanthin

Lutein and zeaxanthin have no vitamin A activity. Lutein and zeaxanthin supplements are available as free carotenoids or as esters (esterified to fatty acids). Both forms appear to have comparable bioavailability.[82] Many commercially available lutein and zeaxanthin supplements have much higher amounts of lutein than zeaxanthin.[83] Supplements containing only lutein or only zeaxanthin are also available.

Safety

Toxicity

Beta-Carotene

Although β-carotene can be converted to vitamin A, the conversion of β-carotene to vitamin A decreases when body stores of vitamin A are high. This may explain why high doses of β-carotene have never been found to cause vitamin A toxicity.[84] High doses of β-carotene (up to 180 mg/d) have been used to treat photosensitivity in erythropoietic protoporphyria without toxic effects.[6]

Lycopene, Lutein, and Zeaxanthin

No toxicities have been reported.[84]

Adverse Effects

Beta-Carotene

Increased Lung Cancer Risk

Two randomized controlled trials in smokers and former asbestos workers found that supplementation with 20 to 30 mg/d of β-carotene for 4 to 6 years was associated with significant 16 to 28% increases in the risk of lung cancer compared with placebo (see section on Lung Cancer). Although the reasons for these findings are not yet clear, many experts feel that the risks of high-dose β-carotene supplementation outweigh any potential benefits for chronic disease prevention, especially in smokers or other high-risk populations.[28,29]

Carotenodermia

High doses of β-carotene supplements (30 mg/d or more) and the consumption of large amounts of carotene-rich foods have resulted in a yellow discoloration of the skin known as carotenodermia. Carotenodermia is not associated with any underlying health problems and resolves when β-carotene supplements are discontinued or dietary carotene intake is reduced.

Lycopene

Lycopenodermia

High intakes of lycopene-rich foods or supplements may result in a deep orange discoloration of the skin known as lycopenodermia. Because lycopene is more intensely colored than the carotenes, lycopenodermia may occur at lower doses than carotenodermia.[6]

Lutein and Zeaxanthin

Adverse effects of lutein and zeaxanthin have not been reported.[83]

Safety in Pregnancy and Lactation

Beta-Carotene

Unlike vitamin A, high doses of β-carotene taken by pregnant women have not been associated with increased risk of birth defects.[6] However, the safety of high-dose β-carotene supplements in pregnancy and lactation has not been well studied. Although there is no reason to limit dietary β-carotene intake, pregnant and breastfeeding women should avoid consuming more than 3 mg/d (5,000 IU/d) of β-carotene from supplements unless prescribed under medical supervision.[83,85]

Other Carotenoids

The safety of carotenoid supplements other than β-carotene in pregnancy and lactation has not been established, so pregnant and breastfeeding women should obtain carotenoids from foods rather than supplements. There is no reason to limit the consumption of carotenoid-rich fruits and vegetables during pregnancy.[83,86]

Drug Interactions

The cholesterol-lowering agents, cholestyramine (Questran) and colestipol (Colestid), can reduce absorption of fat-soluble vitamins and carotenoids, as can mineral oil and Orlistat (Xenical), a drug used to treat obesity.[83] Colchicine, a drug used to treat gout, can cause intestinal malabsorption. However, long-term use of 1 to 2 mg/d did not affect serum β-carotene levels.[87] Increasing gastric pH through the use of proton pump inhibitors, such as omeprazole (Prilosec, Losec), lansoprazole (Prevacid), rabeprazole (Aciphex), and pantoprazole (Protonix, Pantoloc) decreased the absorption of a single dose of a β-carotene supplement, but it is not known if the absorption of dietary carotenoids is affected.[88]

Antioxidant Supplements and HMG-CoA Reductase Inhibitors

A 3-year randomized controlled trial in 160 patients with documented coronary heart disease and low-serum high-density lipoprotein (HDL) concentrations found that a combination of simvastatin (Zocor) and niacin increased HDL2 levels, inhibited the progression of coronary artery stenosis, and decreased the frequency of cardiovascular events, including MI and stroke.[89] Surprisingly, when an antioxidant combination (1000 mg of vitamin C, 800 IU of α-tocopherol, 100 μg of selenium, and 25 mg of β-carotene daily) was taken with the simvastatin-niacin combination, the protective effects were diminished. Because the antioxidants were taken together in this trial, the individual contribution of β-carotene cannot be determined. In contrast, a much larger randomized controlled trial of simvastatin and an antioxidant combination (600 mg of vitamin E, 250 mg of vitamin C, and 20 mg of β-carotene daily) in more than 20,000 men and women with coronary artery disease or diabetes found that the antioxidant combination did not diminish the cardioprotective effects of simvastatin therapy over a 5-year period,[90] suggesting that the antioxidant combination may have interfered with the HDL-raising effect of niacin in the former trial. Further research is needed to determine potential interactions between antioxidant supplements and cholesterol-lowering agents, such as niacin and HMG-CoA reductase inhibitors (statins).

Interactions with Foods

Olestra

In a controlled feeding study, consumption of 18 g/d of the fat substitute Olestra (sucrose polyester) resulted in a 27% decrease in serum carotenoid concentrations after 3 weeks.[91] Studies in free-living people before and after the introduction of Olestra-containing snacks to the marketplace found that total serum carotenoid concentrations decreased by 15% in those who reported consuming at least 2 g/d of Olestra.[92]

Plant Sterol-Containing or Stanol-Containing Foods

Some studies found that the regular use of plant sterol-containing spreads resulted in modest 10 to 20% decreases in the plasma concentrations of some carotenoids, particularly β-carotene, α-carotene, and lycopene[93,94] (see Chapter 19). However, advising people who use plant sterol- or stanol-containing margarines to consume an extra serving of carotenoid-rich fruits or vegetables daily prevented decreases in plasma carotenoid concentrations.[95,96]

Alcohol

The relationships between alcohol consumption and carotenoid metabolism are not well understood. There is some evidence that regular alcohol consumption inhibits the conversion of β-carotene to retinol.[97] Increases in lung cancer risk associated with high-dose β-carotene supplementation in two randomized controlled trials were enhanced in those with higher alcohol intakes.[26,98]

Interactions among Carotenoids

The results of metabolic studies suggest that high doses of β-carotene compete with lutein and lycopene for absorption when consumed at the same time.[99-101] However, the consumption of high-dose β-carotene supplements did not adversely affect serum carotenoid concentrations in long-term clinical trials.[102-105]

Summary

- Carotenoids are yellow, orange, and red pigments synthesized by plants. The most common dietary carotenoids are β-carotene, α-carotene, β-cryptoxanthin, lutein, zeaxanthin, and lycopene.

- Beta-carotene, α-carotene, and β-cryptoxanthin are provitamin A carotenoids, meaning they can be converted by the body to retinol (vitamin A). Lutein, zeaxanthin, and lycopene have no vitamin A activity.
- At present, it is unclear whether the biological effects of carotenoids in humans are related to their antioxidant activity or other non-antioxidant activities.
- Although the results of epidemiological studies suggest that diets high in carotenoid-rich fruits and vegetables are associated with reduced risk of cardiovascular diseases and some cancers, high dose β-carotene supplements did not reduce the risk of cardiovascular diseases or cancers in large randomized controlled trials.
- Two randomized controlled trials found that high-dose β-carotene supplements increased the risk of lung cancer in smokers and former asbestos workers.
- Several epidemiological studies found that men with high intakes of lycopene from tomatoes and tomato products were less likely to develop prostate cancer than were men with low intakes of lycopene, but it is not known whether lycopene supplements will decrease the incidence or severity of prostate cancer.
- Lutein and zeaxanthin are the only carotenoids found in the retina and lens of the eye. The results of epidemiological studies suggest that diets rich in lutein and zeaxanthin may help slow the development of age-related macular degeneration and cataracts, but it is not known whether lutein and zeaxanthin supplements will slow the development of these age-related eye diseases.
- Carotenoids are best absorbed with fat in a meal. Chopping, pureeing, and cooking carotenoid-containing vegetables in oil generally increases the bioavailability of the carotenoids they contain.

References

1. International Agency for Research on Cancer. IARC Handbooks of Cancer Prevention: Carotenoids. Lyon: International Agency for Research on Cancer; 1998
2. Yeum KJ, Russell RM. Carotenoid bioavailability and bioconversion. Annu Rev Nutr 2002;22:483–504
3. Jalal F, Nesheim MC, Agus Z, Sanjur D, Habicht JP. Serum retinol concentrations in children are affected by food sources of beta-carotene, fat intake, and anthelmintic drug treatment. Am J Clin Nutr 1998;68(3):623–629
4. van Het Hof KH, West CE, Weststrate JA, Hautvast JG. Dietary factors that affect the bioavailability of carotenoids. J Nutr 2000;130(3):503–506
5. During A, Harrison EH. Intestinal absorption and metabolism of carotenoids: insights from cell culture. Arch Biochem Biophys 2004;430(1):77–88
6. Institute of Medicine, Food and Nutrition Board. Beta-Carotene and Other Carotenoids. Dietary Reference Intakes for Vitamin C, Vitamin E, Selenium, and Carotenoids. Washington, D.C.: National Academies Press; 2000:325–400
7. Halliwell B, Gutteridge JMC. Free Radicals in Biology and Medicine. Third ed. New York, NY: Oxford University Press; 1999
8. Di Mascio P, Kaiser S, Sies H. Lycopene as the most efficient biological carotenoid singlet oxygen quencher. Arch Biochem Biophys 1989;274(2):532–538
9. Young AJ, Lowe GM. Antioxidant and prooxidant properties of carotenoids. Arch Biochem Biophys 2001;385(1):20–27
10. Krinsky NI, Landrum JT, Bone RA. Biologic mechanisms of the protective role of lutein and zeaxanthin in the eye. Annu Rev Nutr 2003;23:171–201
11. Bertram JS. Carotenoids and gene regulation. Nutr Rev 1999;57(6):182–191
12. Stahl W, Nicolai S, Briviba K, et al. Biological activities of natural and synthetic carotenoids: induction of gap junctional communication and singlet oxygen quenching. Carcinogenesis 1997;18(1):89–92
13. van Poppel G, Spanhaak S, Ockhuizen T. Effect of beta-carotene on immunological indexes in healthy male smokers. Am J Clin Nutr 1993;57(3):402–407
14. Hughes DA, Wright AJ, Finglas PM, et al. The effect of beta-carotene supplementation on the immune function of blood monocytes from healthy male nonsmokers. J Lab Clin Med 1997;129(3):309–317
15. Santos MS, Gaziano JM, Leka LS, Beharka AA, Hennekens CH, Meydani SN. Beta-carotene-induced enhancement of natural killer cell activity in elderly men: an investigation of the role of cytokines. Am J Clin Nutr 1998;68(1):164–170
16. Hughes DA, Wright AJ, Finglas PM, et al. Effects of lycopene and lutein supplementation on the expression of functionally associated surface molecules on blood monocytes from healthy male nonsmokers. J Infect Dis 2000;182(Suppl 1):S11–S15
17. Watzl B, Bub A, Blockhaus M, et al. Prolonged tomato juice consumption has no effect on cell-mediated immunity of well-nourished elderly men and women. J Nutr 2000;130(7):1719–1723
18. Corridan BM, O'Donoghue M, Hughes DA, Morrissey PA. Low-dose supplementation with lycopene or beta-carotene does not enhance cell-mediated immunity in healthy free-living elderly humans. Eur J Clin Nutr 2001;55(8):627–635
19. Peto R, Doll R, Buckley JD, Sporn MB. Can dietary beta-carotene materially reduce human cancer rates? Nature 1981;290(5803):201–208
20. Ziegler RG. A review of epidemiologic evidence that carotenoids reduce the risk of cancer. J Nutr 1989;119(1):116–122

21. Michaud DS, Feskanich D, Rimm EB, et al. Intake of specific carotenoids and risk of lung cancer in 2 prospective US cohorts. Am J Clin Nutr 2000;72(4):990–997

22. Holick CN, Michaud DS, Stolzenberg-Solomon R, et al. Dietary carotenoids, serum beta-carotene, and retinol and risk of lung cancer in the alpha-tocopherol, beta-carotene cohort study. Am J Epidemiol 2002;156(6):536–547

23. Voorrips LE, Goldbohm RA, Brants HA, et al. A prospective cohort study on antioxidant and folate intake and male lung cancer risk. Cancer Epidemiol Biomarkers Prev 2000;9(4):357–365

24. Mannisto S, Smith-Warner SA, Spiegelman D, et al. Dietary carotenoids and risk of lung cancer in a pooled analysis of seven cohort studies. Cancer Epidemiol Biomarkers Prev 2004;13(1):40–48

25. The Alpha-Tocopherol Beta Carotene Cancer Prevention Study Group. The effect of vitamin E and beta carotene on the incidence of lung cancer and other cancers in male smokers. N Engl J Med 1994;330(15):1029–1035

26. Omenn GS, Goodman GE, Thornquist MD, et al. Risk factors for lung cancer and for intervention effects in CARET, the beta-carotene and Retinol Efficacy Trial. J Natl Cancer Inst 1996;88(21):1550–1559

27. Hennekens CH, Buring JE, Manson JE, et al. Lack of effect of long-term supplementation with beta carotene on the incidence of malignant neoplasms and cardiovascular disease. N Engl J Med 1996;334(18):1145–1149

28. Vainio H, Rautalahti M. An international evaluation of the cancer preventive potential of carotenoids. Cancer Epidemiol Biomarkers Prev 1998;7(8):725–728

29. U.S. Preventive Services Task Force. Routine vitamin supplementation to prevent cancer and cardiovascular disease: recommendations and rationale. Ann Intern Med 2003;139(1):51–55

30. Giovannucci E. A review of epidemiologic studies of tomatoes, lycopene, and prostate cancer. Exp Biol Med (Maywood) 2002;227(10):852–859

31. Giovannucci E, Ascherio A, Rimm EB, Stampfer MJ, Colditz GA, Willett WC. Intake of carotenoids and retinol in relation to risk of prostate cancer. J Natl Cancer Inst 1995;87(23):1767–1776

32. Mills PK, Beeson WL, Phillips RL, Fraser GE. Cohort study of diet, lifestyle, and prostate cancer in Adventist men. Cancer 1989;64(3):598–604

33. Gann PH, Ma J, Giovannucci E, et al. Lower prostate cancer risk in men with elevated plasma lycopene levels: results of a prospective analysis. Cancer Res 1999;59(6):1225–1230

34. Schuurman AG, Goldbohm RA, Brants HA, van den Brandt PA. A prospective cohort study on intake of retinol, vitamins C and E, and carotenoids and prostate cancer risk (Netherlands). Cancer Causes Control 2002;13(6):573–582

35. Etminan M, Takkouche B, Caamano-Isorna F. The role of tomato products and lycopene in the prevention of prostate cancer: a meta-analysis of observational studies. Cancer Epidemiol Biomarkers Prev 2004;13(3):340–345

36. Kritchevsky SB. Beta-carotene, carotenoids and the prevention of coronary heart disease. J Nutr 1999;129(1):5–8

37. Bots ML, Grobbee DE. Intima media thickness as a surrogate marker for generalised atherosclerosis. Cardiovasc Drugs Ther 2002;16(4):341–351

38. Rissanen TH, Voutilainen S, Nyyssonen K, Salonen R, Kaplan GA, Salonen JT. Serum lycopene concentrations and carotid atherosclerosis: the Kuopio Ischaemic Heart Disease Risk Factor Study. Am J Clin Nutr 2003;77(1):133–138

39. Dwyer JH, Paul-Labrador MJ, Fan J, Shircore AM, Merz CN, Dwyer KM. Progression of Carotid Intima-Media Thickness and Plasma Antioxidants: The Los Angeles Atherosclerosis Study. Arterioscler Thromb Vasc Biol 2003.

40. McQuillan BM, Hung J, Beilby JP, Nidorf M, Thompson PL. Antioxidant vitamins and the risk of carotid atherosclerosis. The Perth Carotid Ultrasound Disease Assessment study (CUDAS). J Am Coll Cardiol 2001;38(7):1788–1794

41. Rissanen T, Voutilainen S, Nyyssonen K, Salonen R, Salonen JT. Low plasma lycopene concentration is associated with increased intima-media thickness of the carotid artery wall. Arterioscler Thromb Vasc Biol 2000;20(12):2677–2681

42. D'Odorico A, Martines D, Kiechl S, et al. High plasma levels of alpha- and beta-carotene are associated with a lower risk of atherosclerosis: results from the Bruneck study. Atherosclerosis 2000;153(1):231–239

43. Iribarren C, Folsom AR, Jacobs DR Jr, Gross MD, Belcher JD, Eckfeldt JH. Association of serum vitamin levels, LDL susceptibility to oxidation, and autoantibodies against MDA-LDL with carotid atherosclerosis. A case-control study. The ARIC Study Investigators. Atherosclerosis Risk in Communities. Arterioscler Thromb Vasc Biol 1997;17(6):1171–1177

44. Sesso HD, Buring JE, Norkus EP, Gaziano JM. Plasma lycopene, other carotenoids, and retinol and the risk of cardiovascular disease in women. Am J Clin Nutr 2004;79(1):47–53

45. Rissanen TH, Voutilainen S, Nyyssonen K, et al. Low serum lycopene concentration is associated with an excess incidence of acute coronary events and stroke: the Kuopio Ischaemic Heart Disease Risk Factor Study. Br J Nutr 2001;85(6):749–754

46. Street DA, Comstock GW, Salkeld RM, Schuep W, Klag MJ. Serum antioxidants and myocardial infarction. Are low levels of carotenoids and alpha-tocopherol risk factors for myocardial infarction? Circulation 1994;90(3):1154–1161

47. Sesso HD, Buring JE, Norkus EP, Gaziano JM. Plasma lycopene, other carotenoids, and retinol and the risk of cardiovascular disease in men. Am J Clin Nutr 2005;81(5):990–997

48. Hak AE, Stampfer MJ, Campos H, et al. Plasma carotenoids and tocopherols and risk of myocardial infarction in a low-risk population of US male physicians. Circulation 2003;108(7):802–807

49. Evans RW, Shaten BJ, Day BW, Kuller LH. Prospective association between lipid soluble antioxidants and coronary heart disease in men. The Multiple Risk Factor Intervention Trial. Am J Epidemiol 1998;147(2):180–186

50. Sahyoun NR, Jacques PF, Russell RM. Carotenoids, vitamins C and E, and mortality in an elderly population. Am J Epidemiol 1996;144(5):501–511

51. Rimm EB, Stampfer MJ, Ascherio A, Giovannucci E, Colditz GA, Willett WC. Vitamin E consumption and

the risk of coronary heart disease in men. N Engl J Med 1993;328(20):1450–1456

52. Gaziano JM, Manson JE, Branch LG, Colditz GA, Willett WC, Buring JE. A prospective study of consumption of carotenoids in fruits and vegetables and decreased cardiovascular mortality in the elderly. Ann Epidemiol 1995;5(4):255–260

53. Osganian SK, Stampfer MJ, Rimm E, Spiegelman D, Manson JE, Willett WC. Dietary carotenoids and risk of coronary artery disease in women. Am J Clin Nutr 2003;77(6):1390–1399

54. Greenberg ER, Baron JA, Karagas MR, et al. Mortality associated with low plasma concentration of beta carotene and the effect of oral supplementation. JAMA 1996;275(9):699–703

55. Omenn GS, Goodman GE, Thornquist MD, et al. Effects of a combination of beta carotene and vitamin A on lung cancer and cardiovascular disease. N Engl J Med 1996;334(18):1150–1155

56. Morris CD, Carson S. Routine vitamin supplementation to prevent cardiovascular disease: a summary of the evidence for the U.S. Preventive Services Task Force. Ann Intern Med 2003;139(1):56–70

57. Mares-Perlman JA, Millen AE, Ficek TL, Hankinson SE. The body of evidence to support a protective role for lutein and zeaxanthin in delaying chronic disease. Overview. J Nutr 2002;132(3):518S–524S

58. Snellen EL, Verbeek AL, Van Den Hoogen GW, Cruysberg JR, Hoyng CB. Neovascular age-related macular degeneration and its relationship to antioxidant intake. Acta Ophthalmol Scand 2002;80(4):368–371

59. Mares-Perlman JA, Fisher AI, Klein R, et al. Lutein and zeaxanthin in the diet and serum and their relation to age-related maculopathy in the third national health and nutrition examination survey. Am J Epidemiol 2001;153(5):424–432

60. Seddon JM, Ajani UA, Sperduto RD, et al. Dietary carotenoids, vitamins A, C, and E, and advanced age-related macular degeneration. Eye Disease Case-Control Study Group. JAMA 1994;272(18):1413–1420

61. Gale CR, Hall NF, Phillips DI, Martyn CN. Lutein and zeaxanthin status and risk of age-related macular degeneration. Invest Ophthalmol Vis Sci 2003;44(6):2461–2465

62. Antioxidant status and neovascular age-related macular degeneration. Eye Disease Case-Control Study Group. Arch Ophthalmol 1993;111(1):104–109

63. Bone RA, Landrum JT, Mayne ST, Gomez CM, Tibor SE, Twaroska EE. Macular pigment in donor eyes with and without AMD: a case-control study. Invest Ophthalmol Vis Sci 2001;42(1):235–240

64. Beatty S, Murray IJ, Henson DB, Carden D, Koh H, Boulton ME. Macular pigment and risk for age-related macular degeneration in subjects from a Northern European population. Invest Ophthalmol Vis Sci 2001;42(2):439–446

65. Cho E, Seddon JM, Rosner B, Willett WC, Hankinson SE. Prospective study of intake of fruits, vegetables, vitamins, and carotenoids and risk of age-related maculopathy. Arch Ophthalmol 2004;122(6):883–892

66. Flood V, Smith W, Wang JJ, Manzi F, Webb K, Mitchell P. Dietary antioxidant intake and incidence of early age-related maculopathy: the Blue Mountains Eye Study. Ophthalmology 2002;109(12):2272–2278

67. Mares-Perlman JA, Klein R, Klein BE, et al. Association of zinc and antioxidant nutrients with age-related maculopathy. Arch Ophthalmol 1996;114(8):991–997

68. Mares-Perlman JA, Brady WE, Klein R, et al. Serum antioxidants and age-related macular degeneration in a population-based case-control study. Arch Ophthalmol 1995;113(12):1518–1523

69. Mares-Perlman JA. Too soon for lutein supplements. Am J Clin Nutr 1999;70(4):431–432

70. Richer S, Stiles W, Statkute L, et al. Double-masked, placebo-controlled, randomized trial of lutein and antioxidant supplementation in the intervention of atrophic age-related macular degeneration: the Veterans LAST study (Lutein Antioxidant Supplementation Trial). Optometry 2004;75(4):216–230

71. Age-Related Eye Disease Study Research Group. A randomized, placebo-controlled, clinical trial of high-dose supplementation with vitamins C and E, beta carotene, and zinc for age-related macular degeneration and vision loss: AREDS report no. 8. Arch Ophthalmol 2001;119(10):1417–1436

72. Teikari JM, Laatikainen L, Virtamo J, et al. Six-year supplementation with alpha-tocopherol and beta-carotene and age-related maculopathy. Acta Ophthalmol Scand 1998;76(2):224–229

73. Brown L, Rimm EB, Seddon JM, et al. A prospective study of carotenoid intake and risk of cataract extraction in US men. Am J Clin Nutr 1999;70(4):517–524

74. Chasan-Taber L, Willett WC, Seddon JM, et al. A prospective study of carotenoid and vitamin A intakes and risk of cataract extraction in US women. Am J Clin Nutr 1999;70(4):509–516

75. Lyle BJ, Mares-Perlman JA, Klein BE, Klein R, Greger JL. Antioxidant intake and risk of incident age-related nuclear cataracts in the Beaver Dam Eye Study. Am J Epidemiol 1999;149(9):801–809

76. Christen WG, Manson JE, Glynn RJ, et al. A randomized trial of beta carotene and age-related cataract in US physicians. Arch Ophthalmol 2003;121(3):372–378

77. Age-Related Eye Disease Study Research Group. A randomized, placebo-controlled, clinical trial of high-dose supplementation with vitamins C and E and beta carotene for age-related cataract and vision loss: AREDS report no. 9. Arch Ophthalmol 2001;119(10):1439–1452

78. Chylack LT Jr, Brown NP, Bron A, et al. The Roche European American Cataract Trial (REACT): a randomized clinical trial to investigate the efficacy of an oral antioxidant micronutrient mixture to slow progression of age-related cataract. Ophthalmic Epidemiol 2002;9(1):49–80

79. Gartner C, Stahl W, Sies H. Lycopene is more bioavailable from tomato paste than from fresh tomatoes. Am J Clin Nutr 1997;66(1):116–122

80. Stahl W, Sies H. Uptake of lycopene and its geometrical isomers is greater from heat-processed than from unprocessed tomato juice in humans. J Nutr 1992;122(11):2161–2166

81. Clinton SK. Lycopene: chemistry, biology, and implications for human health and disease. Nutr Rev 1998;56(2 Pt 1):35–51

82. Bowen PE, Herbst-Espinosa SM, Hussain EA, Stacewicz-Sapuntzakis M. Esterification does not impair lutein bioavailability in humans. J Nutr 2002;132(12):3668–3673

83. Hendler SS, Rorvik DR, eds. PDR for Nutritional Supplements. Montvale: Medical Economics Company, Inc; 2001

84. Solomons NW. Vitamin A and carotenoids. In: Bowman BA, Russell RM, eds. Present Knowledge in Nutrition. 8th ed. Washington, D.C.: ILSI Press; 2001: 127–145

85. Beta-Carotene. Natural Medicines Comprehensive Database. 2005. Available at: http://www.naturaldatabase.com/monograph.asp?mono_id=999&brand_id=. Accessed 8/1/06

86. Lutein. Natural Medicines Comprehensive Database. 2005. Available at: http://www.naturaldatabase.com/monograph.asp?mono_id=754&brand_id=. Accessed 8/1/06

87. Ehrenfeld M, Levy M, Sharon P, Rachmilewitz D, Eliakim M. Gastrointestinal effects of long-term colchicine therapy in patients with recurrent polyserositis (familial mediterranean fever). Dig Dis Sci 1982; 27(8):723–727

88. Tang G, Serfaty-Lacrosniere C, Camilo ME, Russell RM. Gastric acidity influences the blood response to a beta-carotene dose in humans. Am J Clin Nutr 1996;64(4):622–626

89. Brown BG, Zhao XQ, Chait A, et al. Simvastatin and niacin, antioxidant vitamins, or the combination for the prevention of coronary disease. N Engl J Med 2001;345(22):1583–1592

90. Collins R, Peto R, Armitage J. The MRC/BHF Heart Protection Study: preliminary results. Int J Clin Pract 2002;56(1):53–56

91. Koonsvitsky BP, Berry DA, Jones MB, et al. Olestra affects serum concentrations of alpha-tocopherol and carotenoids but not vitamin D or vitamin K status in free-living subjects. J Nutr 1997;127(8 Suppl):1636S–1645S

92. Thornquist MD, Kristal AR, Patterson RE, et al. Olestra consumption does not predict serum concentrations of carotenoids and fat-soluble vitamins in free-living humans: early results from the sentinel site of the olestra post-marketing surveillance study. J Nutr 2000;130(7):1711–1718

93. Katan MB, Grundy SM, Jones P, Law M, Miettinen T, Paoletti R. Efficacy and safety of plant stanols and sterols in the management of blood cholesterol levels. Mayo Clin Proc 2003;78(8):965–978

94. Weststrate JA, Meijer GW. Plant sterol-enriched margarines and reduction of plasma total- and LDL-cholesterol concentrations in normocholesterolaemic and mildly hypercholesterolaemic subjects. Eur J Clin Nutr 1998;52(5):334–343

95. Ntanios FY, Duchateau GS. A healthy diet rich in carotenoids is effective in maintaining normal blood carotenoid levels during the daily use of plant sterol-enriched spreads. Int J Vitam Nutr Res 2002;72(1):32–39

96. Noakes M, Clifton P, Ntanios F, Shrapnel W, Record I, McInerney J. An increase in dietary carotenoids when consuming plant sterols or stanols is effective in maintaining plasma carotenoid concentrations. Am J Clin Nutr 2002;75(1):79–86

97. Leo MA, Lieber CS. Alcohol, vitamin A, and beta-carotene: adverse interactions, including hepatotoxicity and carcinogenicity. Am J Clin Nutr 1999;69(6):1071–1085

98. Albanes D, Heinonen OP, Taylor PR, et al. Alpha-Tocopherol and beta-carotene supplements and lung cancer incidence in the alpha-tocopherol, beta-carotene cancer prevention study: effects of baseline characteristics and study compliance. J Natl Cancer Inst 1996;88(21):1560–1570

99. van den Berg H. Carotenoid interactions. Nutr Rev 1999;57(1):1–10

100. Micozzi MS, Brown ED, Edwards BK, et al. Plasma carotenoid response to chronic intake of selected foods and beta-carotene supplements in men. Am J Clin Nutr 1992;55(6):1120–1125

101. Kostic D, White WS, Olson JA. Intestinal absorption, serum clearance, and interactions between lutein and beta-carotene when administered to human adults in separate or combined oral doses. Am J Clin Nutr 1995;62(3):604–610

102. Albanes D, Virtamo J, Taylor PR, Rautalahti M, Pietinen P, Heinonen OP. Effects of supplemental beta-carotene, cigarette smoking, and alcohol consumption on serum carotenoids in the Alpha-Tocopherol, Beta-Carotene Cancer Prevention Study. Am J Clin Nutr 1997;66(2):366–372

103. Nierenberg DW, Dain BJ, Mott LA, Baron JA, Greenberg ER. Effects of 4 y of oral supplementation with beta-carotene on serum concentrations of retinol, tocopherol, and five carotenoids. Am J Clin Nutr 1997;66(2):315–319

104. Wahlqvist ML, Wattanapenpaiboon N, Macrae FA, Lambert JR, MacLennan R, Hsu-Hage BH. Changes in serum carotenoids in subjects with colorectal adenomas after 24 mo of beta-carotene supplementation. Australian Polyp Prevention Project Investigators. Am J Clin Nutr 1994;60(6):936–943

105. Mayne ST, Cartmel B, Silva F, et al. Effect of supplemental beta-carotene on plasma concentrations of carotenoids, retinol, and alpha-tocopherol in humans. Am J Clin Nutr 1998;68(3):642–647

9 Chlorophyll and Chlorophyllin

Chlorophyll is the pigment that gives plants and algae their green color. Plants use chlorophyll to trap light needed for photosynthesis.[1] The basic structure of chlorophyll is a porphyrin ring similar to that of heme in hemoglobin, although the central atom in chlorophyll is magnesium instead of iron. The long hydrocarbon (phytol) tail attached to the porphyrin ring makes chlorophyll fat-soluble and insoluble in water. Two different types of chlorophyll (chlorophyll a and chlorophyll b) are found in plants (**Fig. 9–1**). The slight differ-

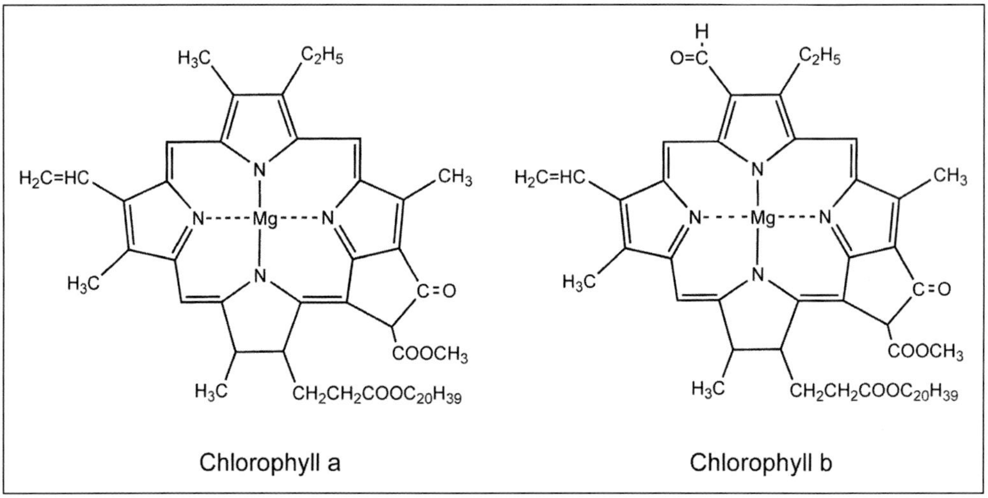

Figure 9–1 Chemical structures of natural chlorophylls, chlorophyll a and chlorophyll b.

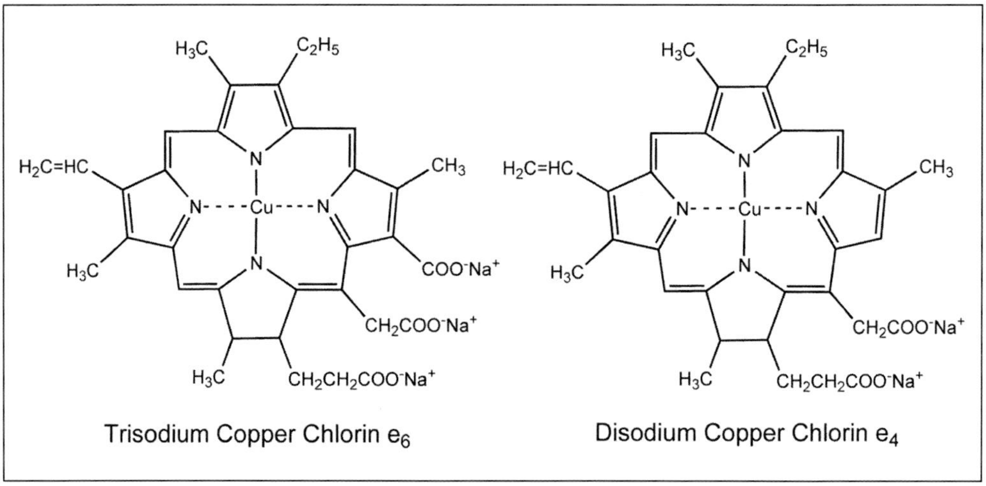

Figure 9–2 Chemical structures of some compounds found in commercial sodium copper chlorophyllin, trisodium copper chlorin e_6 and disodium copper chlorin e_4.

ence in one of the side chains allows each type of chlorophyll to absorb light at slightly different wavelengths. Chlorophyllin is a semi-synthetic mixture of sodium copper salts derived from chlorophyll.[2,3] During the synthesis of chlorophyllin, the magnesium atom at the center of the ring is replaced with copper and the phytol tail is lost. Unlike natural chlorophyll, chlorophyllin is water soluble. Although the content of different chlorophyllin mixtures may vary, two compounds commonly found in chlorophyllin mixtures are trisodium copper chlorin e_6 and disodium copper chlorin e_4 (**Fig. 9–2**).

Metabolism and Bioavailability

Little is known about the bioavailability and metabolism of chlorophyll or chlorophyllin. The lack of toxicity attributed to chlorophyllin led to the belief that it was poorly absorbed.[4] However, significant amounts of copper chlorin e_4 were measured in the plasma of people taking chlorophyllin tablets in a controlled clinical trial, indicating that is absorbed. More research is needed to understand the bioavailability and metabolism of natural chlorophylls and chlorin compounds in synthetic chlorophyllin.

Biological Activities

Complex Formation with Other Molecules

Chlorophyll and chlorophyllin are able to form tight molecular complexes with certain chemicals known or suspected to cause cancer, including polyaromatic hydrocarbons found in tobacco smoke,[5] some heterocyclic amines found in cooked meat,[6] and aflatoxin-B$_1$.[7] The tight binding of chlorophyll or chlorophyllin to these potential carcinogens may interfere with their absorption from the gastrointestinal tract and reduce the amount that reaches susceptible tissues.[8]

Antioxidant Effects

Chlorophyllin can neutralize several physically relevant oxidants in vitro,[9,10] and limited data from animal studies suggest that chlorophyllin supplementation may decrease oxidative damage induced by chemical carcinogens and radiation.[11,12]

Modification of the Metabolism and Detoxification of Carcinogens

To initiate the development of cancer, some chemicals (procarcinogens) must first be metabolized to active carcinogens that are capable of damaging DNA or other critical molecules in susceptible tissues. Enzymes in the cytochrome P450 family are required for the activation of some procarcinogens; therefore, inhibition of cytochrome P450 enzymes may decrease the risk of some types of chemically induced cancers. Studies in vitro indicate that chlorophyllin may decrease the activity of cytochrome P450 enzymes.[5,13] Phase II detoxification enzymes promote the elimination of potentially harmful toxins and carcinogens from the body. Limited data from animal studies indicate that chlorophyllin may increase the activity of the phase II enzyme quinone reductase.[14]

Prevention

Aflatoxin-Associated Hepatocellular Carcinoma

Aflatoxin-B$_1$ (AFB$_1$) is a liver carcinogen produced by certain species of fungus and found in moldy grains and legumes, such as corn, peanuts, and soybeans.[2,8] In hot, humid regions of Africa and Asia with inadequate grain storage facilities, high levels of dietary AFB$_1$ are associated with increased risk of hepatocellular carcinoma. Moreover, the combination of hepatitis B infection and high dietary AFB$_1$ exposure increases the risk of hepatocellular carcinoma still further. In the liver, AFB$_1$ is metabolized to a carcinogen capable of binding DNA and causing mutations. In animal models of AFB$_1$-induced liver cancer, administration of chlorophyllin at the same time as dietary AFB$_1$

exposure significantly reduced AFB_1-induced DNA damage in the livers of rainbow trout and rats,[15,16] and dose-dependently inhibited the development of liver cancer in trout.[17]

Because of the long time between AFB_1 exposure and the development of cancer in humans, an intervention trial might require as long as 20 years to determine whether chlorophyllin supplementation can reduce the incidence of hepatocellular carcinoma in people exposed to high levels of dietary AFB_1. However, a biomarker of AFB_1-induced DNA damage (AFB_1-N^7-guanine) can be measured in the urine, and high urinary levels of AFB_1-N^7-guanine have been associated with significantly increased risk of developing hepatocellular carcinoma.[18] To determine whether chlorophyllin could decrease AFB_1-induced DNA damage in humans, a randomized placebo-controlled intervention trial was conducted in 180 adults residing in a region of China where the risk of hepatocellular carcinoma is very high due to unavoidable dietary AFB_1 exposure and a high prevalence of chronic hepatitis B infection.[19] Participants took either 100 mg of chlorophyllin or a placebo before meals 3 times daily. After 16 weeks of treatment, urinary levels of AFB_1-N^7-guanine were 55% lower in those taking chlorophyllin than those taking the placebo, suggesting that chlorophyllin supplementation before meals can substantially decrease AFB_1-induced DNA damage. Although a reduction in hepatocellular carcinoma has not yet been demonstrated in humans taking chlorophyllin, scientists are hopeful that chlorophyllin supplementation will provide some protection to high-risk populations with unavoidable dietary AFB_1 exposure.[8] It is not known whether chlorophyllin will be useful in the prevention of cancers in people who are not exposed to significant levels of dietary AFB_1, as is the case for most people living in the United States. Many questions remain to be answered regarding the exact mechanisms of cancer prevention by chlorophyllin, the implications for the prevention of other types of cancer, and the potential for natural chlorophylls in the diet to provide cancer protection.

Treatment

Internal Deodorant

Observations in the 1940s and 1950s that topical chlorophyllin had deodorizing effects on foul-smelling wounds led clinicians to administer chlorophyllin orally to patients with colostomies and ileostomies to control fecal odor.[20] Although early case reports indicated that chlorophyllin doses of 100 to 200 mg/d were effective in reducing fecal odor in ostomy patients,[21,22] at least one placebo-controlled trial found that 75 mg of oral chlorophyllin 3 times a day was no more effective than placebo in decreasing fecal odor assessed by colostomy patients.[23] Several case reports have been published indicating that oral chlorophyllin (100 to 300 mg/d) decreased subjective assessments of urinary and fecal odor in incontinent patients.[20,24] Trimethylaminuria is a hereditary disorder characterized by the excretion of trimethylamine, a compound with a "fishy" or foul odor. A recent study in a small number of Japanese patients with trimethylaminuria found that oral chlorophyllin (60 mg 3 times a day) for 3 weeks significantly decreased urinary trimethylamine concentrations.[25]

Wound Healing

Research in the 1940s indicating that chlorophyllin solutions slowed the growth of certain anaerobic bacteria in the test tube and accelerated the healing of experimental wounds in animals led to the use of topical chlorophyllin solutions and ointments in the treatment of persistent open wounds in humans.[26] During the late 1940s and 1950s, a series of largely uncontrolled studies in patients with slow-healing wounds, such as vascular ulcers and pressure (decubitus) ulcers, reported that the application of topical chlorophyllin promoted healing more effectively than other commonly used treatments.[27,28] In the late 1950s, chlorophyllin was added to papain and urea-containing ointments used for the chemical debridement of wounds to reduce local inflammation, promote healing, and control odor.[20] Chlorophyllin-containing papain/urea ointments are still available in the United States by prescription.[29]

Sources

Food Sources

Chlorophylls are the most abundant pigments in plants. Dark green leafy vegetables like spinach are rich sources of natural chlorophylls. The chlorophyll contents of selected vegetables are presented in **Table 9–1**.[30]

Supplements

Chlorophyll

Green algae, such as chlorella, are often marketed as supplemental sources of chlorophyll. Natural chlorophyll is not as stable as chlorophyllin and is much more expensive; therefore, most over-the-counter chlorophyll supplements actually contain chlorophyllin.

Chlorophyllin

Oral preparations of sodium copper chlorophyllin (also called chlorophyllin copper complex) are available in supplements and as an over-the-counter drug (Derifil) used to reduce odor from colostomies or ileostomies or to reduce fecal odor due to incontinence.[31] Sodium copper chlorophyllin may also be used as a color additive in foods, drugs, and cosmetics.[32] Oral doses of 100 to 300 mg/d in 3 divided doses have been used to control fecal and urinary odor (see Treatment section above).

Safety

Natural chlorophylls are not known to be toxic, and no toxic effects have been attributed to chlorophyllin despite more than 50 years of clinical use in humans.[8,20,26] When taken orally, chlorophyllin may cause green discoloration of urine or feces or yellow or black discoloration of the tongue.[33] There have also been occasional reports of diarrhea related to oral chlorophyllin use. When applied topically to wounds, chlorophyllin has been reported to cause mild burning or itching in some cases.[34] Oral chlorophyllin may result in false-positive results on guaiac card tests for occult blood.[35] The safety of chlorophyll or chlorophyllin supplements has not been tested in pregnant

Table 9–1 Chlorophyll Content of Selected Raw Vegetables[30]

Food	Serving	Chlorophyll (mg)
Spinach	1 cup	23.7
Parsley	1/2 cup	19.0
Cress, garden	1 cup	15.6
Green beans	1 cup	8.3
Arugula (rocket)	1 cup	8.2
Leeks	1 cup	7.7
Endive	1 cup	5.2
Sugar peas	1 cup	4.8
Chinese cabbage	1 cup	4.1

or lactating women; therefore, they should be avoided during pregnancy and lactation.

Summary

- Chlorophyll a and chlorophyll b are natural, fat-soluble chlorophylls found in plants.
- Chlorophyllin is a semi-synthetic mixture of water-soluble sodium copper salts derived from chlorophyll.
- Chlorophyllin has been used orally as an internal deodorant and topically in the treatment of slow-healing wounds for more than 50 years without any serious side effects.
- Chlorophylls and chlorophyllin form tight molecular complexes with some chemicals known or suspected to cause cancer, and in doing so, may block their carcinogenic effects. No carefully controlled studies have been undertaken to determine whether a similar mechanism might limit uptake of required nutrients or minerals.
- Supplementation with chlorophyllin before meals substantially decreased a urinary biomarker of aflatoxin-induced DNA damage in a Chinese population at high risk of liver cancer due to unavoidable dietary aflatoxin exposure.
- Scientists are hopeful that chlorophyllin supplementation will be helpful in decreasing the risk of liver cancer in high-risk populations with unavoidable dietary afla-

toxin exposure. However, it is not yet known whether chlorophyllin or natural chlorophylls will be useful in the prevention of cancers in people who are not exposed to significant levels of dietary aflatoxin.

References

1. Matthews CK, van Holde KE. Biochemistry. 2nd ed. Menlo Park: The Benjamin/Cummings Publishing Company; 1996
2. Sudakin DL. Dietary aflatoxin exposure and chemoprevention of cancer: a clinical review. J Toxicol Clin Toxicol 2003;41(2):195–204
3. Dashwood RH. The importance of using pure chemicals in (anti) mutagenicity studies: chlorophyllin as a case in point. Mutat Res 1997;381(2):283–286
4. Egner PA, Stansbury KH, Snyder EP, Rogers ME, Hintz PA, Kensler TW. Identification and characterization of chlorin e(4) ethyl ester in sera of individuals participating in the chlorophyllin chemoprevention trial. Chem Res Toxicol 2000;13(9):900–906
5. Tachino N, Guo D, Dashwood WM, Yamane S, Larsen R, Dashwood R. Mechanisms of the in vitro antimutagenic action of chlorophyllin against benzo[a]pyrene: studies of enzyme inhibition, molecular complex formation and degradation of the ultimate carcinogen. Mutat Res 1994;308(2):191–203
6. Dashwood R, Yamane S, Larsen R. Study of the forces of stabilizing complexes between chlorophylls and heterocyclic amine mutagens. Environ Mol Mutagen 1996;27(3):211–218
7. Breinholt V, Schimerlik M, Dashwood R, Bailey G. Mechanisms of chlorophyllin anticarcinogenesis against aflatoxin B1: complex formation with the carcinogen. Chem Res Toxicol 1995;8(4):506–514
8. Egner PA, Munoz A, Kensler TW. Chemoprevention with chlorophyllin in individuals exposed to dietary aflatoxin. Mutat Res 2003;523–524:209–216
9. Kumar SS, Devasagayam TP, Bhushan B, Verma NC. Scavenging of reactive oxygen species by chlorophyllin: an ESR study. Free Radic Res 2001;35(5):563–574
10. Kamat JP, Boloor KK, Devasagayam TP. Chlorophyllin as an effective antioxidant against membrane damage in vitro and ex vivo. Biochim Biophys Acta 2000;1487(2–3):113–127
11. Park KK, Park JH, Jung YJ, Chung WY. Inhibitory effects of chlorophyllin, hemin and tetrakis(4-benzoic acid)porphyrin on oxidative DNA damage and mouse skin inflammation induced by 12-O-tetradecanoylphorbol-13-acetate as a possible anti-tumor promoting mechanism. Mutat Res 2003;542(1–2):89–97
12. Kumar SS, Shankar B, Sainis KB. Effect of chlorophyllin against oxidative stress in splenic lymphocytes in vitro and in vivo. Biochim Biophys Acta 2004;1672(2):100–111
13. Yun CH, Jeong HG, Jhoun JW, Guengerich FP. Nonspecific inhibition of cytochrome P450 activities by chlorophyllin in human and rat liver microsomes. Carcinogenesis 1995;16(6):1437–1440
14. Dingley KH, Ubick EA, Chiarappa-Zucca ML, et al. Effect of dietary constituents with chemopreventive potential on adduct formation of a low dose of the heterocyclic amines PhIP and IQ and phase II hepatic enzymes. Nutr Cancer 2003;46(2):212–221
15. Dashwood RH, Breinholt V, Bailey GS. Chemopreventive properties of chlorophyllin: inhibition of aflatoxin B1 (AFB1)-DNA binding in vivo and anti-mutagenic activity against AFB1 and two heterocyclic amines in the Salmonella mutagenicity assay. Carcinogenesis 1991;12(5):939–942
16. Kensler TW, Groopman JD, Roebuck BD. Use of aflatoxin adducts as intermediate endpoints to assess the efficacy of chemopreventive interventions in animals and man. Mutat Res 1998;402(1–2):165–172
17. Breinholt V, Hendricks J, Pereira C, Arbogast D, Bailey G. Dietary chlorophyllin is a potent inhibitor of aflatoxin B1 hepatocarcinogenesis in rainbow trout. Cancer Res 1995;55(1):57–62
18. Qian GS, Ross RK, Yu MC, et al. A follow-up study of urinary markers of aflatoxin exposure and liver cancer risk in Shanghai, People's Republic of China. Cancer Epidemiol Biomarkers Prev 1994;3(1):3–10
19. Egner PA, Wang JB, Zhu YR, et al. Chlorophyllin intervention reduces aflatoxin-DNA adducts in individuals at high risk for liver cancer. Proc Natl Acad Sci USA 2001;98(25):14601–14606
20. Chernomorsky SA, Segelman AB. Biological activities of chlorophyll derivatives. N J Med 1988;85(8):669–673
21. Siegel LH. The control of ileostomy and colostomy odors. Gastroenterology 1960;38:634–636
22. Weingarten M, Payson B. Deodorization of colostomies with chlorophyll. Rev Gastroenterol 1951;18(8):602–604
23. Christiansen SB, Byel SR, Stromsted H, Stenderup JK, Eickhoff JH. [Can chlorophyll reduce fecal odor in colostomy patients?] Ugeskr Laeger 1989;151(27):1753–1754. Danish
24. Young RW, Beregi JS Jr. Use of chlorophyllin in the care of geriatric patients. J Am Geriatr Soc 1980;28(1):46–47
25. Yamazaki H, Fujieda M, Togashi M, et al. Effects of the dietary supplements, activated charcoal and copper chlorophyllin, on urinary excretion of trimethylamine in Japanese trimethylaminuria patients. Life Sci 2004;74(22):2739–2747
26. Kephart JC. Chlorophyll derivatives – their chemistry, commercial preparation and uses. Econ Bot 1955;9:3–38
27. Bowers WF. Chlorophyll in wound healing and suppurative disease. Am J Surg 1947;73:37–50
28. Carpenter EB. Clinical experiences with chlorophyll preparations. Am J Surg 1949;77:167–171
29. 2004 Physicians' Desk Reference. 58th ed. Stamford: Thomson Health Care, Inc.; 2003
30. Bohn T, Walczyk S, Leisibach S, Hurrell RF. Chlorophyll-bound magnesium in commonly consumed vegetables and fruits: relevance to magnesium nutrition. J Food Sci 2004;69(9):S347–S350
31. Food and Drug Administration. Code of Federal Regulations: Miscellaneous Internal Drug Products for Over the Counter Use. 2002. Available at: http://www.fda.gov/cder/otcmonographs/Internaleodorant/internaleodorant(357I).html.

32. Food and Drug Administration. Code of Federal Regulations: Listing of Color Additives Exempt from Certification. 2002. Available at: http://vm.cfsan.fda.gov/~lrd/cf732125.html.

33. Hendler SS, Rorvik DR, eds. PDR for Nutritional Supplements. Montvale: Medical Economics Company, Inc; 2001

34. Smith LW. The present status of topical chlorophyll therapy. N Y State J Med 1955;55(14):2041–2050

35. Gogel HK, Tandberg D, Strickland RG. Substances that interfere with guaiac card tests: implications for gastric aspirate testing. Am J Emerg Med 1989;7(5):474–480

10 Curcumin

Turmeric is a spice derived from the rhizomes of *Curcuma longa*, which is a member of the ginger family (*Zingiberaceae*).[1] Rhizomes are horizontal underground stems that send out shoots as well as roots. The bright yellow color of turmeric comes mainly from polyphenolic pigments, known as curcuminoids (**Fig. 10–1**). Curcumin is the principal curcuminoid found in turmeric and is generally considered its most active constituent.[2] Other curcuminoids found in turmeric include demethoxycurcumin and bisdemethoxycurcumin. In addition to its use as a spice and a pigment, turmeric has been used in India for medicinal purposes for centuries. Evidence that curcumin may have anti-inflammatory and anti-cancer activities has renewed scientific interest in its potential to prevent and treat disease.

Metabolism and Bioavailability

Clinical trials in humans indicate that the systemic bioavailability of orally administered curcumin is relatively low.[2] Curcumin is readily conjugated in the intestine and liver to form curcumin glucuronides and curcumin sulfates or reduced to hexahydrocurcumin (**Fig. 10–2**).[3]

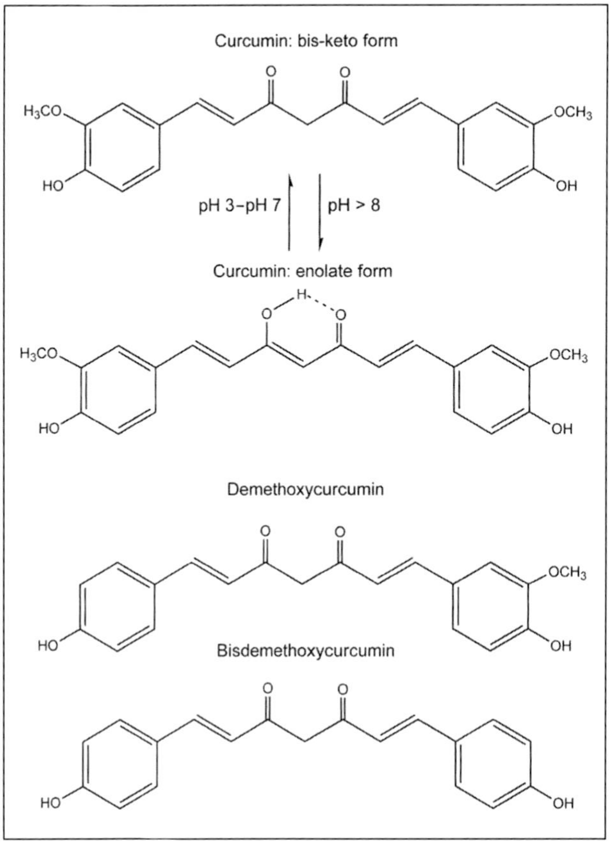

Curcumin: bis-keto form

pH 3–pH 7   pH > 8

Curcumin: enolate form

Demethoxycurcumin

Bisdemethoxycurcumin

Figure 10–1 Chemical structures of the curcuminoids, curcumin, demethoxycurcumin, and bisdemethoxycurcumin. Curcumin exists in equilibrium between its bis-keto and enolate form.[2] The bis-keto form predominates at acidic and neutral pH, whereas the enolate form predominates at pH greater than 8.

Curcumin metabolites may not have the same biological activity as the parent compound. In one study, conjugated or reduced metabolites of curcumin were less-effective inhibitors of inflammatory enzyme expression in cultured human colon cells than curcumin itself.[4] In a clinical trial conducted in Taiwan, serum curcumin concentrations peaked 1 to 2 hours after an oral dose, and peak serum concentrations were 0.5, 0.6, and 1.8 µmol/L at doses of 4, 6, and 8 g/d, respectively.[5] Curcumin could not be detected in serum at lower doses than 4 g/d. More recently, a clinical trial conducted in the UK found that plasma curcumin, curcumin sulfate, and curcumin glucuronide concentrations were in the range of 10 nmol/L (0.01 µmol/L) one hour after a 3.6 g dose of oral curcumin.[6] Curcumin and its metabolites could not be detected in plasma at doses lower than 3.6 g/d. Curcumin and its glucuronidated and sulfated metabolites were also measured in urine at a dose of 3.6 g/d. There is some evidence that orally administered curcumin accumulates in gastrointestinal tissues. When colorectal cancer patients took 3.6 g/d of curcumin orally for 7 days prior to surgery, curcumin was detected in malignant and normal colorectal tissue.[7] In contrast, curcumin was not detected in the liver tissue of patients with liver metastases of colorectal cancer after the same dose of oral curcumin,[8] suggesting that oral curcumin administration may not effectively deliver curcumin to tissues outside the gastrointestinal tract.

Biological Activities

Antioxidant Activity

Curcumin is an effective scavenger of reactive oxygen species and reactive nitrogen species in

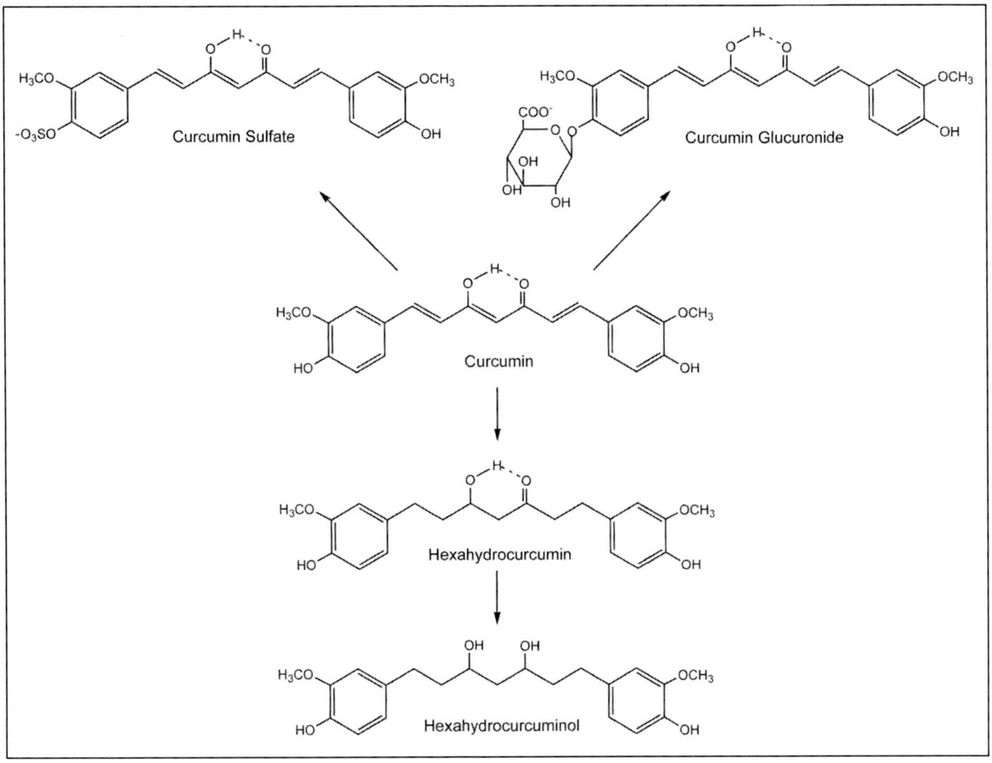

Figure 10–2 Chemical structures of curcumin metabolites, including O-conjugation products, curcumin glucuronide and curcumin sulfate, as well as curcumin bioreduction products, hexahydrocurcumin and hexahydrocurcuminol.[3]

the test tube (in vitro).[9,10] However, it is not clear whether curcumin acts directly as an antioxidant in vivo. Due to its limited oral bioavailability in humans (see the Metabolism and Bioavailability section above), plasma and tissue curcumin concentrations are likely to be much lower than that of other fat-soluble antioxidants, such as α-tocopherol. However, the finding that 7 days of oral curcumin supplementation (3.6 g/d) decreased the number of oxidative DNA adducts in malignant colorectal tissue suggests that curcumin taken orally may reach sufficient concentrations in the gastrointestinal tract to inhibit oxidative DNA damage.[7] In addition to direct antioxidant activity, curcumin may function indirectly as an antioxidant by inhibiting the activity of inflammatory enzymes or by enhancing the synthesis of glutathione, an important intracellular antioxidant (see below).

Anti-inflammatory Activity

The metabolism of arachidonic acid in cell membranes plays an important role in the inflammatory response by generating potent chemical messengers known as eicosanoids.[11] Membrane phospholipids are hydrolyzed by phospholipase A_2 (PLA$_2$), releasing arachidonic acid, which may be metabolized by cyclooxygenases (COX) to form prostaglandins and thromboxanes, or lipoxygenases (LOX) to form leukotrienes. Curcumin has been found to inhibit PLA$_2$, COX-2, and 5-LOX activity in cultured cells.[12] Although curcumin inhibited the catalytic activity of 5-LOX directly, it inhibited PLA$_2$ by preventing its phosphorylation and COX-2 mainly by inhibiting its transcription. Nuclear factor-κB (NF-κB) is a transcription factor that binds DNA and enhances the transcription of the COX-2 gene and other pro-inflammatory genes, such as inducible nitric oxide synthase (iNOS). In inflammatory cells, such as macrophages, iNOS catalyzes the synthesis of nitric oxide, which can react with superoxide to form peroxynitrite, a reactive nitrogen species that can damage proteins and DNA. Curcumin has been found to inhibit NF-κB-dependent gene transcription,[13] and to inhibit the induction of COX-2 and iNOS in cell culture and animal studies.[14,15]

Glutathione Synthesis

Glutathione is an important intracellular antioxidant that plays a critical role in cellular adaptation to stress.[16] Stress-related increases in cellular glutathione levels result from increased expression of glutamate cysteine ligase (GCL), the rate-limiting enzyme in glutathione synthesis. Studies in cell culture suggest that curcumin can increase cellular glutathione levels by enhancing the transcription of the genes for GCL.[17]

Effects on Biotransformation Enzymes Involved in Carcinogen Metabolism

Biotransformation enzymes play important roles in the metabolism and elimination of a variety of biologically active compounds, including drugs and carcinogens. In general, phase I biotransformation enzymes, including those of the cytochrome P450 (CYP) family, catalyze reactions that increase the reactivity of hydrophobic (fat-soluble) compounds, preparing them for reactions catalyzed by phase II biotransformation enzymes. Reactions catalyzed by phase II enzymes generally increase water solubility and promote the elimination of these compounds.[18] Although increasing biotransformation enzyme activity may enhance the elimination of potential carcinogens, some carcinogen precursors (procarcinogens) are metabolized to active carcinogens by phase I enzymes.[19] CYP1A1 is involved in the metabolic activation of several chemical carcinogens. Curcumin has been found to inhibit increases in CYP1A1 activity induced by procarcinogens in cell culture and animal studies.[20–23] Increasing phase II biotransformation enzyme activity is generally thought to enhance the elimination of potential carcinogens. Several studies in animals have found that dietary curcumin increased the activity of phase II enzymes, such as glutathione S-transferases (GSTs).[22,24,25] However, curcumin intakes ranging from 0.45 to 3.6 g/d for up to 4 months did not increase leukocyte GST activity in humans.[6]

Induction of Cell-Cycle Arrest and Apoptosis

After a cell divides, it passes through a sequence of stages collectively known as the cell cycle before it can divide again. Following DNA damage, the cell cycle can be transiently arrested to allow for DNA repair or activation of pathways leading to cell death (apoptosis) if the damage cannot be repaired.[26] Defective cell-cycle regulation may result in the propagation of mutations that contribute to the development of cancer. Curcumin has been found to induce cell-cycle arrest and apoptosis in a variety of cancer cell lines grown in culture.[2,27] The mechanisms by which curcumin induces apoptosis are varied but may include inhibitory effects on several cell signaling pathways. However, not all studies have found that curcumin induces apoptosis in cancer cells. Curcumin inhibited apoptosis induced by the tumor suppressor protein p53 in cultured human colon cancer cells,[28,29] and one study found that curcumin inhibited apoptosis induced by several chemotherapeutic agents in cultured breast cancer cells at concentrations of 1 to 10 µmol/L.[30]

Inhibition of Tumor Invasion and Angiogenesis

Cancerous cells invade normal tissue aided by enzymes called matrix metalloproteinases. Curcumin has been found to inhibit the activity of several matrix metalloproteinases in cell culture studies.[31-33] Invasive tumors must also develop new blood vessels to fuel their rapid growth by a process known as angiogenesis. Curcumin has been found to inhibit angiogenesis in cultured vascular endothelial cells[34] and in an animal model.[35]

It is important to keep in mind that many of the biological activities discussed above were observed in cells cultured in the presence of curcumin at higher concentrations than are likely to be achieved in humans consuming curcumin orally (see the Metabolism and Bioavailability section at the beginning of this chapter).

Prevention

Cancer

The ability of curcumin to induce apoptosis in cultured cancer cells by several different mechanisms has generated scientific interest in the potential for curcumin to prevent some types of cancer.[2] Oral curcumin administration has been found to inhibit the development of chemically induced cancer in animal models of oral,[36,37] stomach,[38,39] liver,[40] and colon cancers.[41-43] ApcMin/+ mice have a mutation in the Apc (adenomatous polyposis coli) gene similar to that in humans with familial adenomatous polyposis, a genetic condition that is characterized by the development of numerous colorectal adenomas (polyps) and a high risk for colorectal cancer. Oral curcumin administration has been found to inhibit the development of intestinal adenomas in ApcMin/+ mice.[44,45] In contrast, oral curcumin administration has not consistently been found to inhibit the development of mammary (breast) cancer in animal models.[41,46,47]

Although the results of animal studies are promising, particularly with respect to colorectal cancer, there is presently little evidence that high intakes of curcumin or turmeric are associated with decreased cancer risk in humans. A phase I clinical trial in Taiwan examined the effects of oral curcumin supplementation up to 8 g/d for 3 months in patients with precancerous lesions of the mouth (oral leukoplakia), cervix (high grade cervical intraepithelial neoplasia), skin (squamous carcinoma in situ), or stomach (intestinal metaplasia).[5] Histologic improvement on biopsy was observed in 2 out of 7 patients with oral leukoplakia, 1 out of 4 patients with cervical intraepithelial neoplasia, 2 out of 6 patients with squamous carcinoma in situ, and 1 out of 6 patients with intestinal metaplasia. However, cancer developed in 1 out of 7 patients with oral leukoplakia and 1 out of 4 patients with cervical intraepithelial neoplasia by the end of the treatment period. This study was designed mainly to examine the bioavailability and safety of oral curcumin, and interpretation of its results is limited by the lack of a control group for comparison. Because of the promising findings in animal studies, several controlled clinical trials in humans designed to evaluate the effect of oral curcumin supplementation on precancerous colorectal lesions, such as adenomas, are under way.[48]

Alzheimer's Disease

In Alzheimer's disease, a peptide called amyloid β (Aβ) forms aggregates (oligomers), which accumulate in the brain and form deposits known as amyloid plaques.[49] Inflammation and oxidative damage are also associated with the progression of Alzheimer's disease.[50] Curcumin has been found to inhibit Aβ oligomer formation in vitro.[51] When injected peripherally, curcumin was found to cross the blood–brain barrier in an animal model of Alzheimer's disease.[51] Dietary curcumin has been found to decrease biomarkers of inflammation and oxidative damage and to decrease amyloid plaque burden in the brain and Aβ-induced memory deficits in animal models of Alzheimer's disease.[51–53] It is not known whether curcumin taken orally can cross the blood–brain barrier or inhibit the progression of Alzheimer's disease in humans. Because of the promising findings in animal models, several clinical trials of oral curcumin supplementation in patients with early Alzheimer's disease are under way.[48]

Treatment

Cancer

The ability of curcumin to induce apoptosis in a variety of cancer cell lines in culture and its low toxicity have led to scientific interest in its potential for cancer therapy as well as cancer prevention.[54] To date, most of the controlled clinical trials of curcumin supplementation in cancer patients have been phase I trials. Phase I trials are clinical trials in small groups of people, aimed at determining bioavailability, optimal dose, safety, and early evidence of the efficacy of a new therapy.[55] A phase I clinical trial in patients with advanced colorectal cancer found that doses up to 3.6 g/d for 4 months were well tolerated, although the systemic availability of oral curcumin was low.[6] When colorectal cancer patients with liver

metastases took 3.6 g/d of curcumin orally for 7 days, trace levels of curcumin metabolites were measured in liver tissue, but curcumin itself was not detected.[8] In contrast, curcumin was measured in normal and malignant colorectal tissue after patients with advanced colorectal cancer took 3.6 g/d of curcumin orally for 7 days.[7] These findings suggest that oral curcumin is more likely to be effective as a therapeutic agent in cancers of the gastrointestinal tract than other tissues. Phase II trials are clinical trials designed to investigate the effectiveness of a new therapy in larger numbers of people and to further evaluate short-term side effects and safety of the new therapy. Phase II clinical trials of curcumin in patients with advanced pancreatic cancer are currently under way,[48] and phase II trials of curcumin for colorectal cancer have been recommended.[2]

Inflammatory Diseases

Although the anti-inflammatory activity of curcumin has been demonstrated in cell culture and animal studies, few controlled clinical trials have examined the efficacy of curcumin in the treatment of inflammatory conditions. A preliminary intervention trial that compared curcumin with a nonsteroidal anti-inflammatory drug (NSAID) in 18 rheumatoid arthritis patients found that improvements in morning stiffness, walking time, and joint swelling after 2 weeks of curcumin supplementation (1200 mg/d) were comparable to those experienced after 2 weeks of phenylbutazone therapy (300 mg/d).[56] A placebo-controlled trial in 40 men who had surgery to repair an inguinal hernia or hydrocele found that 5 days of oral curcumin supplementation (1200 mg/d) was more effective than placebo in reducing postsurgical edema, tenderness, and pain, and was comparable to phenylbutazone therapy (300 mg/d).[57] Two uncontrolled studies found that oral curcumin (1125 mg/d) for 12 weeks or longer improved the inflammatory ophthalmological conditions, anterior uveitis and idiopathic inflammatory orbital pseudotumor.[58,59] However, without a control group, it is difficult to draw conclusions regarding the antiinflammatory effects of curcumin in these conditions. Larger randomized controlled trials are needed to determine whether oral curcumin supplementation is effective in the treatment of inflammatory diseases, such as rheumatoid arthritis.

Cystic Fibrosis

Cystic fibrosis is a hereditary disease caused by mutations in the cystic fibrosis transmembrane conductance regulator (CFTCR) gene.[60] CFTCR is a transmembrane protein that acts as a chloride channel and plays a critical role in ion and fluid transport. In the lungs, CFTCR mutations ultimately result in increased mucus concentration and decreased clearance, which leads to progressive lung disease. The most common CFTCR mutation contributing to the development of cystic fibrosis is the ΔF508 mutation, which results in CFTCR protein misfolding and degradation before the protein can be targeted to the cell membrane. However, the mutated protein retains some ability to function as a chloride channel if it can be inserted in the cell membrane. In 2004, a study in mice with the ΔF508 mutation found that oral curcumin administration corrected abnormal ion transport and improved the survival of these mice.[61] However, unlike humans, mice with the ΔF508 mutation experience only the digestive complications of cystic fibrosis without the lung complications, and treatment benefits in the mouse model are not always realized in humans.[60] Another group of scientists was unable to duplicate the beneficial effects of curcumin in the same mouse model given the same dose of curcumin.[62] It is unclear whether curcumin supplementation will be of benefit to humans with cystic fibrosis. The Cystic Fibrosis Foundation is funding a phase I clinical trial to determine the safety of curcumin supplementation in cystic fibrosis patients.[63] Until the safety and efficacy of curcumin in individuals with cystic fibrosis has been evaluated in clinical trials, the Cystic Fibrosis Foundation does not recommend the use of curcumin as a therapy for cystic fibrosis.[64]

Sources

Food Sources

Tumeric is the dried ground rhizome of *Curcuma longa Linn.*[65] It is used as a spice in Indian, Southeast Asian, and Middle Eastern cuisines. Curcuminoids make up ~2 to 9% of turmeric.[66] Curcumin is the most abundant curcuminoid in turmeric, providing ~75% of the total curcuminoids; demethoxycurcumin provides 10 to 20% and bisdemethoxycurcumin generally provides less than 5%. Curry powder contains turmeric along with other spices, but the amount of curcumin in curry powders is variable and often relatively low.[67] Curcumin extracts are also used as food-coloring agents.[68]

Supplements

Curcumin extracts are available as dietary supplements without a prescription in the United States. The labels of several of these extracts state that they are standardized to contain 95% curcuminoids, although such claims are not strictly regulated by the U.S. Food and Drug Administration (FDA). Some curcumin preparations also contain piperine, which may increase the bioavailability of curcumin by inhibiting its metabolism. However, piperine may also affect the metabolism of drugs (see the Drug Interactions section below). Optimal doses of curcumin for cancer chemoprevention or therapeutic uses have not been established. It is unclear whether doses less than 3.6 g/d are biologically active in humans (see the Metabolism and Bioavailability section above).

Safety

Adverse Effects

In the United States, turmeric is generally recognized as a safe (GRAS) food additive by the FDA.[68] Serious adverse effects have not been reported in humans taking high doses of curcumin. In a phase I trial in Taiwan, curcumin supplementation up to 8 g/d for 3 months was reported to be well-tolerated in patients with precancerous conditions or noninvasive cancer.[5] In another clinical trial in the UK, curcumin supplementation ranging from 0.45 to 3.6 g/d for 4 months was generally well-tolerated by people with advanced colorectal cancer, although two participants experienced diarrhea and another reported nausea.[6] Increases in serum alkaline phosphatase and lactate dehydrogenase were also observed in several participants, but it was not clear whether these increases were related to curcumin supplementation or cancer progression.[2] Curcumin supplementation of 20 to 40 mg has been reported to increase gall bladder contractions in healthy people.[69,70] In light of this finding, people with gall bladder disease are often advised to avoid curcumin supplements.

Pregnancy and Lactation

Although there is no evidence that dietary consumption of turmeric as a spice adversely affects pregnancy or lactation, the safety of curcumin supplements in pregnancy and lactation has not been established.

Drug Interactions

Curcumin has been found to inhibit platelet aggregation in vitro,[71,72] suggesting a potential for curcumin supplementation to increase the risk of bleeding in people taking anticoagulant or antiplatelet medications, such as aspirin, clopidogrel (Plavix), dalteparin (Fragmin), enoxaparin (Lovenox), heparin, ticlopidine (Ticlid), and warfarin (Coumadin). In cultured breast cancer cells, curcumin inhibited apoptosis induced by the chemotherapeutic agents, campothecin, mechlorethamine, and doxorubicin at concentrations of 1 to 10 μmol/L.[30] In an animal model of breast cancer, dietary curcumin inhibited cyclophosphamide-induced tumor regression. Although it is not known whether oral curcumin administration will result in breast tissue concentrations that are high enough to inhibit cancer chemotherapeutic agents in humans,[8] it may be advisable for women undergoing chemotherapy for breast cancer to avoid curcumin supplements.[30] Some curcumin supplements also contain piperine for the purpose of increasing the bioavailability of curcumin. However, piperine may also increase the bioavailability and slow the elimination of several drugs, including phenytoin (Dilantin), propranolol (Inderal), and theophylline.[73,74]

Summary

- Turmeric is a spice derived from the rhizomes of *Curcuma longa*, a member of the ginger family.
- Curcuminoids are polyphenolic compounds that give turmeric its yellow color.
- Curcumin is the principal curcuminoid in turmeric.
- The results of phase I clinical trials in colorectal cancer patients suggest that biologically active levels of curcumin can be achieved in the gastrointestinal tract through oral curcumin supplementation and provide support for further clinical evaluation in people at risk for gastrointestinal cancers.
- Because of promising findings in animal models of Alzheimer's disease, clinical trials of curcumin supplementation in patients with early Alzheimer's disease are under way.
- Until the safety and efficacy of curcumin in individuals with cystic fibrosis has been evaluated in clinical trials, the Cystic Fibrosis Foundation does not recommend the use of curcumin as a therapy for cystic fibrosis.
- Although a few preliminary trials suggest that curcumin may have anti-inflammatory activity in humans, larger randomized controlled trials are needed to determine whether oral curcumin supplementation is effective in the treatment of inflammatory diseases.

References

1. Aggarwal BB, Kumar A, Aggarwal MS, Shishodia S. Curcumin derived from turmeric (*Curcuma longa*): a spice for all seasons. In: Preuss H, ed. Phytopharmaceuticals in Cancer Chemoprevention. Boca Raton: CRC Press; 2005:349–387
2. Sharma RA, Gescher AJ, Steward WP. Curcumin: the story so far. Eur J Cancer 2005;41(13):1955–1968
3. Ireson CR, Jones DJ, Orr S, et al. Metabolism of the cancer chemopreventive agent curcumin in human and rat intestine. Cancer Epidemiol Biomarkers Prev 2002;11(1):105–111

4. Ireson C, Orr S, Jones DJ, et al. Characterization of metabolites of the chemopreventive agent curcumin in human and rat hepatocytes and in the rat in vivo, and evaluation of their ability to inhibit phorbol ester-induced prostaglandin E2 production. Cancer Res 2001;61(3):1058–1064

5. Cheng AL, Hsu CH, Lin JK, et al. Phase I clinical trial of curcumin, a chemopreventive agent, in patients with high-risk or pre-malignant lesions. Anticancer Res 2001;21(4B):2895–2900

6. Sharma RA, Euden SA, Platton SL, et al. Phase I clinical trial of oral curcumin: biomarkers of systemic activity and compliance. Clin Cancer Res 2004;10(20):6847–6854

7. Garcea G, Berry DP, Jones DJ, et al. Consumption of the putative chemopreventive agent curcumin by cancer patients: assessment of curcumin levels in the colorectum and their pharmacodynamic consequences. Cancer Epidemiol Biomarkers Prev 2005;14(1):120–125

8. Garcea G, Jones DJ, Singh R, et al. Detection of curcumin and its metabolites in hepatic tissue and portal blood of patients following oral administration. Br J Cancer 2004;90(5):1011–1015

9. Sreejayan N, Rao MN. Nitric oxide scavenging by curcuminoids. J Pharm Pharmacol 1997;49(1):105–107

10. Sreejayan N, Rao MN. Free radical scavenging activity of curcuminoids. Arzneimittelforschung 1996;46(2):169–171

11. Steele VE, Hawk ET, Viner JL, Lubet RA. Mechanisms and applications of non-steroidal anti-inflammatory drugs in the chemoprevention of cancer. Mutat Res 2003;523-524:137–144

12. Hong J, Bose M, Ju J, et al. Modulation of arachidonic acid metabolism by curcumin and related beta-diketone derivatives: effects on cytosolic phospholipase A(2), cyclooxygenases and 5-lipoxygenase. Carcinogenesis 2004;25(9):1671–1679

13. Plummer SM, Holloway KA, Manson MM, et al. Inhibition of cyclo-oxygenase 2 expression in colon cells by the chemopreventive agent curcumin involves inhibition of NF-kappaB activation via the NIK/IKK signalling complex. Oncogene 1999;18(44):6013–6020

14. Brouet I, Ohshima H. Curcumin, an anti-tumour promoter and anti-inflammatory agent, inhibits induction of nitric oxide synthase in activated macrophages. Biochem Biophys Res Commun 1995;206(2):533–540

15. Nanji AA, Jokelainen K, Tipoe GL, Rahemtulla A, Thomas P, Dannenberg AJ. Curcumin prevents alcohol-induced liver disease in rats by inhibiting the expression of NF-kappa B-dependent genes. Am J Physiol Gastrointest Liver Physiol 2003;284(2):G321–G327

16. Dickinson DA, Levonen AL, Moellering DR, et al. Human glutamate cysteine ligase gene regulation through the electrophile response element. Free Radic Biol Med 2004;37(8):1152–1159

17. Dickinson DA, Iles KE, Zhang H, Blank V, Forman HJ. Curcumin alters EpRE and AP-1 binding complexes and elevates glutamate-cysteine ligase gene expression. FASEB J 2003;17(3):473–475

18. Lampe JW, Peterson S. Brassica, biotransformation and cancer risk: genetic polymorphisms alter the preventive effects of cruciferous vegetables. J Nutr 2002;132(10):2991–2994

19. Baird WM, Hooven LA, Mahadevan B. Carcinogenic polycyclic aromatic hydrocarbon-DNA adducts and mechanism of action. Environ Mol Mutagen 2005;45(2-3):106–114

20. Ciolino HP, Daschner PJ, Wang TT, Yeh GC. Effect of curcumin on the aryl hydrocarbon receptor and cytochrome P450 1A1 in MCF-7 human breast carcinoma cells. Biochem Pharmacol 1998;56(2):197–206

21. Rinaldi AL, Morse MA, Fields HW, et al. Curcumin activates the aryl hydrocarbon receptor yet significantly inhibits (-)-benzo(a)pyrene-7R-trans-7,8-dihydrodiol bioactivation in oral squamous cell carcinoma cells and oral mucosa. Cancer Res 2002;62(19):5451–5456

22. Singh SV, Hu X, Srivastava SK, et al. Mechanism of inhibition of benzo[a]pyrene-induced forestomach cancer in mice by dietary curcumin. Carcinogenesis 1998;19(8):1357–1360

23. Thapliyal R, Maru GB. Inhibition of cytochrome P450 isozymes by curcumins in vitro and in vivo. Food Chem Toxicol 2001;39(6):541–547

24. Iqbal M, Sharma SD, Okazaki Y, Fujisawa M, Okada S. Dietary supplementation of curcumin enhances antioxidant and phase II metabolizing enzymes in ddY male mice: possible role in protection against chemical carcinogenesis and toxicity. Pharmacol Toxicol 2003;92(1):33–38

25. Susan M, Rao MN. Induction of glutathione S-transferase activity by curcumin in mice. Arzneimittelforschung 1992;42(7):962–964

26. Stewart ZA, Westfall MD, Pietenpol JA. Cell-cycle dysregulation and anticancer therapy. Trends Pharmacol Sci 2003;24(3):139–145

27. Duvoix A, Blasius R, Delhalle S, et al. Chemopreventive and therapeutic effects of curcumin. Cancer Lett 2005;223(2):181–190

28. Moos PJ, Edes K, Mullally JE, Fitzpatrick FA. Curcumin impairs tumor suppressor p53 function in colon cancer cells. Carcinogenesis 2004;25(9):1611–1617

29. Tsvetkov P, Asher G, Reiss V, Shaul Y, Sachs L, Lotem J. Inhibition of NAD(P)H: quinone oxidoreductase 1 activity and induction of p53 degradation by the natural phenolic compound curcumin. Proc Natl Acad Sci U S A 2005;102(15):5535–5540

30. Somasundaram S, Edmund NA, Moore DT, Small GW, Shi YY, Orlowski RZ. Dietary curcumin inhibits chemotherapy-induced apoptosis in models of human breast cancer. Cancer Res 2002;62(13):3868–3875

31. Banerji A, Chakrabarti J, Mitra A, Chatterjee A. Effect of curcumin on gelatinase A (MMP-2) activity in B16F10 melanoma cells. Cancer Lett 2004;211(2):235–242

32. Ohashi Y, Tsuchiya Y, Koizumi K, Sakurai H, Saiki I. Prevention of intrahepatic metastasis by curcumin in an orthotopic implantation model. Oncology 2003;65(3):250–258

33. Menon LG, Kuttan R, Kuttan G. Anti-metastatic activity of curcumin and catechin. Cancer Lett 1999;141(1–2):159–165

34. Thaloor D, Singh AK, Sidhu GS, Prasad PV, Kleinman HK, Maheshwari RK. Inhibition of angiogenic differentiation of human umbilical vein endothelial cells by curcumin. Cell Growth Differ 1998;9(4):305–312

35. Arbiser JL, Klauber N, Rohan R, et al. Curcumin is an in vivo inhibitor of angiogenesis. Mol Med 1998;4(6):376–383

36. Krishnaswamy K, Goud VK, Sesikeran B, Mukundan MA, Krishna TP. Retardation of experimental tumori-

genesis and reduction in DNA adducts by turmeric and curcumin. Nutr Cancer 1998;30(2):163–166

37. Li N, Chen X, Liao J, et al. Inhibition of 7,12-dimethyl-benz[a]anthracene (DMBA)-induced oral carcino-genesis in hamsters by tea and curcumin. Carcino-genesis 2002;23(8):1307–1313

38. Ikezaki S, Nishikawa A, Furukawa F, et al. Chemo-preventive effects of curcumin on glandular stomach carcinogenesis induced by N-methyl-N'-nitro-N-nitrosoguanidine and sodium chloride in rats. Anti-cancer Res 2001;21(5):3407–3411

39. Huang MT, Lou YR, Ma W, Newmark HL, Reuhl KR, Conney AH. Inhibitory effects of dietary curcumin on forestomach, duodenal, and colon carcinogenesis in mice. Cancer Res 1994;54(22):5841–5847

40. Chuang SE, Kuo ML, Hsu CH, et al. Curcumin-contain-ing diet inhibits diethylnitrosamine-induced murine hepatocarcinogenesis. Carcinogenesis 2000;21(2):331–335

41. Pereira MA, Grubbs CJ, Barnes LH, et al. Effects of the phytochemicals, curcumin and quercetin, upon azoxymethane-induced colon cancer and 7,12-dim-ethylbenz[a]anthracene-induced mammary cancer in rats. Carcinogenesis 1996;17(6):1305–1311

42. Rao CV, Rivenson A, Simi B, Reddy BS. Chemopreven-tion of colon carcinogenesis by dietary curcumin, a naturally occurring plant phenolic compound. Cancer Res 1995;55(2):259–266

43. Kawamori T, Lubet R, Steele VE, et al. Chemopreven-tive effect of curcumin, a naturally occurring anti-in-flammatory agent, during the promotion/progression stages of colon cancer. Cancer Res 1999;59(3):597–601

44. Mahmoud NN, Carothers AM, Grunberger D, et al. Plant phenolics decrease intestinal tumors in an ani-mal model of familial adenomatous polyposis. Car-cinogenesis 2000;21(5):921–927

45. Perkins S, Verschoyle RD, Hill K, et al. Chemopreven-tive efficacy and pharmacokinetics of curcumin in the min/+ mouse, a model of familial adenomatous poly-posis. Cancer Epidemiol Biomarkers Prev 2002;11(6):535–540

46. Singletary K, MacDonald C, Iovinelli M, Fisher C, Wal-lig M. Effect of the beta-diketones diferuloylmethane (curcumin) and dibenzoylmethane on rat mammary DNA adducts and tumors induced by 7,12-dimethyl-benz[a]anthracene. Carcinogenesis 1998;19(6):1039–1043

47. Huang MT, Lou YR, Xie JG, et al. Effect of dietary cur-cumin and dibenzoylmethane on formation of 7,12-dimethylbenz[a]anthracene-induced mammary tu-mors and lymphomas/leukemias in Sencar mice. Car-cinogenesis 1998;19(9):1697–1700

48. National Institutes of Health. Clinical Trials.gov. 2005. Available at: http://clinicaltrials.gov/. Accessed 7/26/06

49. Gandy S. The role of cerebral amyloid beta accumula-tion in common forms of Alzheimer disease. J Clin In-vest 2005;115(5):1121–1129

50. Cole GM, Morihara T, Lim GP, Yang F, Begum A, Fraut-schy SA. NSAID and antioxidant prevention of Alzheimer's disease: lessons from in vitro and animal models. Ann N Y Acad Sci 2004;1035:68–84

51. Yang F, Lim GP, Begum AN, et al. Curcumin inhibits for-mation of amyloid beta oligomers and fibrils, binds plaques, and reduces amyloid in vivo. J Biol Chem 2005;280(7):5892–5901

52. Frautschy SA, Hu W, Kim P, et al. Phenolic anti-inflam-matory antioxidant reversal of Abeta-induced cogni-tive deficits and neuropathology. Neurobiol Aging 2001;22(6):993–1005

53. Lim GP, Chu T, Yang F, Beech W, Frautschy SA, Cole GM. The curry spice curcumin reduces oxidative damage and amyloid pathology in an Alzheimer transgenic mouse. J Neurosci 2001;21(21):8370–8377

54. Karunagaran D, Rashmi R, Kumar TR. Induction of apoptosis by curcumin and its implications for cancer therapy. Curr Cancer Drug Targets 2005;5(2):117–129

55. National Institutes of Health. An introduction to clini-cal trials. 2005. Available at: http://clinicaltrials.gov/ct/info/whatis. Accessed 7/26/06

56. Deodhar SD, Sethi R, Srimal RC. Preliminary study on antirheumatic activity of curcumin (diferuloyl meth-ane). Indian J Med Res 1980;71:632–634

57. Satoskar RR, Shah SJ, Shenoy SG. Evaluation of anti-in-flammatory property of curcumin (diferuloyl meth-ane) in patients with postoperative inflammation. Int J Clin Pharmacol Ther Toxicol 1986;24(12):651–654

58. Lal B, Kapoor AK, Agrawal PK, Asthana OP, Srimal RC. Role of curcumin in idiopathic inflammatory orbital pseudotumours. Phytother Res 2000;14(6):443–447

59. Lal B, Kapoor AK, Asthana OP, et al. Efficacy of cur-cumin in the management of chronic anterior uveitis. Phytother Res 1999;13(4):318–322

60. Mall M, Kunzelmann K. Correction of the CF defect by curcumin: hypes and disappointments. Bioessays 2005;27(1):9–13

61. Egan ME, Pearson M, Weiner SA, et al. Curcumin, a major constituent of turmeric, corrects cystic fibrosis defects. Science 2004;304(5670):600–602

62. Song Y, Sonawane ND, Salinas D, et al. Evidence against the rescue of defective DeltaF508-CFTR cellu-lar processing by curcumin in cell culture and mouse models. J Biol Chem 2004;279(39):40629–40633

63. Cystic Fibrosis Foundation. Cystic Fibrosis Foundation to Fund Clinical Trial of Potential Curcumin Therapy. 2004. Available at: http://www.cff.org/research/cf_research_inhe_news/index.cfm?ID=2635&bln ShowBack=False&idContentType=1213.

64. Cystic Fibrosis Foundation. Curcumin: information for patients and families. 2004. Available at: http://www.cff.org/images/customcontent/CurcuminQAFinal.pdf.

65. Joe B, Vijaykumar M, Lokesh BR. Biological properties of curcumin-cellular and molecular mechanisms of action. Crit Rev Food Sci Nutr 2004;44(2):97–111

66. Lechtenberg M, Quandt B, Nahrstedt A. Quantitative determination of curcuminoids in Curcuma rhizomes and rapid differentiation of Curcuma domestica Val. and Curcuma xanthorrhiza Roxb. by capillary electro-phoresis. Phytochem Anal 2004;15(3):152–158

67. Heath DD, Khwaja F, Rock CL. Curcumin content of turmeric and curry powders. 2004;18(4):A125–A125

68. U.S. Food and Drug Administration. Food additives. 1991. Available at: http://www.cfsan.fda.gov/~lrd/foodaddi.html

69. Rasyid A, Lelo A. The effect of curcumin and placebo on human gall-bladder function: an ultrasound study. Aliment Pharmacol Ther 1999;13(2):245–249

70. Rasyid A, Rahman AR, Jaalam K, Lelo A. Effect of differ-ent curcumin dosages on human gall bladder. Asia Pac J Clin Nutr 2002;11(4):314–318

71. Shah BH, Nawaz Z, Pertani SA, et al. Inhibitory effect of curcumin, a food spice from turmeric, on platelet-ac-tivating factor- and arachidonic acid-mediated plate-

let aggregation through inhibition of thromboxane formation and Ca2+ signaling. Biochem Pharmacol 1999;58(7):1167–1172

72. Srivastava KC, Bordia A, Verma SK. Curcumin, a major component of food spice turmeric (Curcuma longa) inhibits aggregation and alters eicosanoid metabolism in human blood platelets. Prostaglandins Leukot Essent Fatty Acids 1995;52(4):223–227

73. Bano G, Raina RK, Zutshi U, Bedi KL, Johri RK, Sharma SC. Effect of piperine on bioavailability and pharmacokinetics of propranolol and theophylline in healthy volunteers. Eur J Clin Pharmacol 1991;41(6):615–617

74. Velpandian T, Jasuja R, Bhardwaj RK, Jaiswal J, Gupta SK. Piperine in food: interference in the pharmacokinetics of phenytoin. Eur J Drug Metab Pharmacokinet 2001;26(4):241–247

11 Essential Fatty Acids (Omega-3 and Omega-6)

Omega-3 and omega-6 fatty acids are polyunsaturated fatty acids (PUFA), which means they contain more than one *cis* double bond.[1] In all omega-3 fatty acids, the first double bond is located between the third and fourth carbon atom counting from the methyl end of the fatty acid (n-3). Similarly, the first double bond in all omega-6 fatty acids is located between the sixth and seventh carbon atom from the methyl end of the fatty acid (n-6). Scientific abbreviations for fatty acids tell the reader something about their structure. One scientific abbreviation for α-linolenic acid (ALA) is 18:3n-3. The first part (18:3) tells the reader that ALA is an 18-carbon fatty acid with 3 double bonds; the second part (n-3) tells the reader that the first double bond is in the n-3 position, which defines it as an omega-3 fatty acid.

Although humans and other mammals can synthesize saturated and some monounsaturated fatty acids from carbon groups in carbohydrate and protein, they lack the enzymes necessary to insert a *cis* double bond at the n-6 or the n-3 position of a fatty acid.[1] Consequently, omega-6 and omega-3 fatty acids are essential nutrients. The parent fatty acid of the omega-6 series is linoleic acid (LA; 18:2n-6), and the parent fatty acid of the omega-3 series is ALA (**Fig. 11–1**). Humans can synthesize long-chain (≥ 20 carbons) omega-6 fatty acids, such as dihomo-γ-linolenic acid (DGLA;

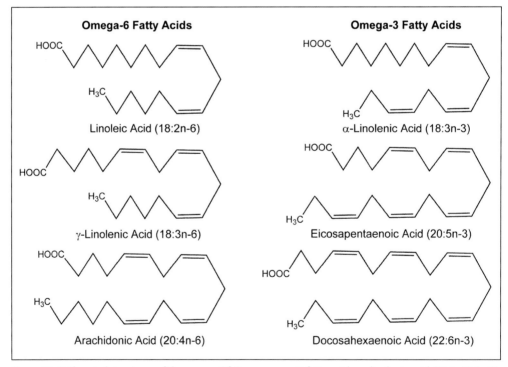

Figure 11–1 Chemical structures of the omega-6 fatty acids, linoleic acid (LA, 18:2n-6), γ-linolenic acid (GLA, 18:3n-6), and arachidonic acid (AA, 20:4n-6), and the omega-3 fatty acids, α-linolenic acid (ALA, 18:3n-3), eicosapentaenoic acid (EPA, 20:5n-3), and docosahexaenoic acid (DHA, 22:6n-3).

20:3n-6) and arachidonic acid (AA; 20:4n-6) from LA and long-chain omega-3 fatty acids, such as eicosapentaenoic acid (EPA; 20:5n-3) and docosahexaenoic acid (DHA; 22:6n-3) from ALA (see the Metabolism and Bioavailability section below). It has been estimated that the ratio of omega-6 to omega-3 fatty acids in the diet of early humans was 1:1,[2] but the ratio in the typical Western diet is now almost 10:1 due to increased use of vegetable oils rich in LA and declining fish consumption.[3] A large body of scientific research suggests that increasing the relative abundance of dietary omega-3 fatty acids may have several health benefits.

Metabolism and Bioavailability

Prior to absorption in the small intestine, fatty acids must be hydrolyzed from dietary fats (triglycerides, phospholipids, and cholesterol) by pancreatic enzymes.[4] Bile salts must also be present in the small intestine to allow for the incorporation of fatty acids and other fat digestion products into mixed micelles. Fat absorption from mixed micelles occurs throughout the small intestine and is 85 to 95% efficient under normal conditions. Humans can synthesize longer omega-6 and omega-3 fatty acids from the essential fatty acids LA and ALA, respectively, through a series of desaturation (addition of a double bond) and elongation (addition of two carbon atoms) reactions (**Fig. 11–2**).[5] LA

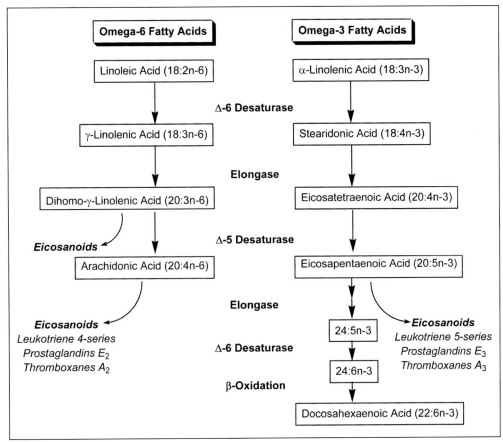

Figure 11–2 Synthesis of long-chain omega-6 and omega-3 polyunsaturated fatty acids from the parent fatty acids, linoleic acid (LA, 18:2n-6) and α-linolenic acid (ALA, 18:3n-3), in humans.

and ALA compete for the same elongase and desaturase enzymes in the synthesis of longer polyunsaturated fatty acids, such as AA and EPA. Although ALA is the preferred substrate of the Δ6 desaturase enzyme, the excess of dietary LA compared with ALA results in greater net formation of AA (20:4n-6) than EPA (20:5n-3).[6] The capacity for conversion of ALA to DHA is higher in women than in men. Studies of ALA metabolism indicate that ~ 8 % of dietary ALA is converted to EPA and 0 to 4 % is converted to DHA in healthy young men.[7] In healthy young women, ~ 21 % of dietary ALA is converted to EPA and 9 % is converted to DHA.[8] The better conversion efficiency of young women compared with men appears to be related to the effects of estrogen.[6,9] Although ALA is considered the essential omega-3 fatty acid because it cannot be synthesized by humans, evidence that human conversion of EPA and, particularly, DHA is relatively inefficient suggests that EPA and DHA may also be essential under some conditions.[10,11]

Biological Activities

Membrane Structure and Function

Omega-6 and omega-3 PUFA are important structural components of cell membranes. When incorporated into phospholipids, they affect cell membrane properties such as fluidity, flexibility, permeability, and the activity of membrane-bound enzymes.[12] DHA is selectively incorporated into retinal cell membranes and postsynaptic neuronal cell membranes, suggesting it plays important roles in vision and nervous system function.

Vision

DHA is found in very high concentrations in the cell membranes of the retina, which conserves and recycles DHA even when omega-3 fatty acid intake is low.[13] Animal studies indicate that DHA is required for the normal development and function of the retina. Moreover, these studies suggest that there is a critical period during retinal development when inadequate DHA will result in permanent abnormalities in retinal function. Recent research indicates that DHA plays an important role in the regeneration of the visual pigment rhodopsin, which plays a critical role in the visual transduction system that converts light to vision.[14]

Nervous System

The phospholipids of brain gray matter contain high proportions of DHA and AA, suggesting they are important to central nervous system function.[15] Brain DHA content may be particularly important because animal studies have shown that depletion of DHA in the brain can result in learning deficits. It is not clear how DHA affects brain function, but changes in neuronal cell membrane DHA content could alter the function of ion channels or membrane associated receptors, as well as the availability of neurotransmitters.[16]

Eicosanoid Synthesis

Eicosanoids are potent chemical messengers derived from 20-carbon PUFA that play critical roles in immune and inflammatory responses. During an inflammatory response, DGLA, AA, and EPA in cell membranes can be metabolized by enzymes known as cyclooxygenases and lipoxygenases to form prostaglandins and leukotrienes, respectively (**Fig. 11–2**). In those who consume typical Western diets the amount of AA in cell membranes is much greater than the amount of EPA, resulting in the formation of more eicosanoids derived from AA than EPA. However, increasing omega-3 fatty acid intake increases the EPA content of cell membranes, resulting in higher proportions of eicosanoids derived from EPA. Physiological responses to AA-derived eicosanoids differ from responses to EPA-derived eicosanoids. In general, eicosanoids derived from EPA are less potent inducers of inflammation, blood vessel constriction, and coagulation than eicosanoids derived from AA.[3,17]

Regulation of Gene Expression

The results of cell culture and animal studies indicate that omega-6 and omega-3 fatty acids can modulate the expression of several genes, including those involved with fatty acid metabolism and inflammation.[17,18] Although the mechanisms require further clarification, omega-6 and omega-3 fatty acids may regulate gene expression by interacting with specific transcription factors, including peroxisome proliferator-activated receptors (PPARs), liver X receptors (LXRs), and hepatic nuclear factor (HNF)-4α.[19]

Deficiency

Essential Fatty Acid Deficiency

Clinical signs of essential fatty acid deficiency include a dry scaly rash, decreased growth in infants and children, increased susceptibility to infection, and poor wound healing.[20] Omega-3, omega-6, and omega-9 fatty acids compete for the same desaturase enzymes. The desaturase enzymes show preference for the different series of fatty acids in the following order: omega-3 > omega-6 > omega-9. Consequently, synthesis of the omega-9 fatty acid eicosatrienoic acid (20:3n-9) increases only when dietary intakes of omega-3 and omega-6 fatty acids are very low.[21] A plasma eicosatrienoic acid:arachidonic acid (triene:tetraene) ratio greater than 0.2 is generally considered indicative of essential fatty acid deficiency.[20,22] In patients who were given total parenteral nutrition containing fat-free glucose amino acid mixtures, biochemical signs of essential fatty acid deficiency developed in as short a time as 7 to 10 days.[23] In these cases, the continuous glucose infusion resulted in high circulating insulin levels, which inhibited the release of essential fatty acids stored in adipose tissue. When glucose-free amino acid solutions were used, parenteral nutrition up to 14 days did not result in biochemical signs of essential fatty acid deficiency. Essential fatty acid deficiency has also been found to occur in patients with chronic fat malabsorption[24] and cystic fibrosis.[25] It has been proposed that essential fatty acid deficiency may play a role in the pathology of protein energy malnutrition.[21]

Omega-3 Fatty Acid Deficiency

At least one case of isolated omega-3 fatty deficiency has been reported. A young girl who received intravenous lipid emulsions with very little ALA developed visual problems and sensory neuropathy, which resolved when she was switched to an emulsion containing more ALA.[26] Plasma DHA concentrations decrease when omega-3 fatty acid intake is insufficient, but no cutoff values have been established. Isolated omega-3 fatty acid deficiency does not result in increased plasma triene:tetraene ratios.[1]

Prevention

Visual and Neurological Development

The last trimester of pregnancy is a critical period for the accumulation of DHA in the brain and retina; hence, preterm infants are thought to be particularly vulnerable to adverse effects of insufficient DHA on visual and neurological development.[27] Human milk contains DHA in addition to ALA and EPA, but until recently, ALA was the only omega-3 fatty acid present in conventional infant formulas. Although preterm infants can synthesize DHA from ALA, they generally cannot synthesize enough to prevent declines in plasma and cellular DHA concentrations without additional dietary intake. Therefore, it was proposed that preterm infant formulas be supplemented with enough DHA to bring plasma and cellular DHA levels of formula-fed infants up to those of breast-fed infants.[28] Although formulas enriched with DHA raise plasma and red blood cell DHA concentrations in preterm and term infants, the results of randomized controlled trials examining measures of visual acuity and neurological development in infants fed formulas with and without added DHA have been mixed.[29-31] Although several controlled trials found that healthy preterm infants fed formulas with DHA added showed subtle but significant improvements in visual acuity at 2 and 4 months of age compared with those fed DHA-free formulas,[32] most randomized controlled trials found no differences in visual acuity between healthy preterm infants fed formulas with or without DHA added.[30] Similarly, most randomized controlled trials that assessed general measures of infant development at 12 and 24 months of age found no difference between preterm infants fed formula with or without DHA added.[33,34] Infant formulas enriched with DHA are also commercially available for term infants, but the results of randomized controlled trials of these formulas on visual acuity and development in term infants have also been mixed.[29,35–37] Although DHA appears to be important for visual and neurological development, it is not yet clear whether feeding infants formula enriched with DHA enhances visual acuity or neurological development in preterm or term infants.[38]

Pregnancy

Although infant requirements for DHA have been the subject of a great deal of research, there has been relatively little investigation of maternal requirements for omega-3 fatty acids, despite the fact that the mother is the sole source of omega-3 fatty acids for the fetus and exclusively breast-fed infant.[39] The results of randomized controlled trials during pregnancy suggest that omega-3 fatty acid supplementation does not decrease the incidence of gestational diabetes, pregnancy-induced hypertension, or preeclampsia,[40–42] but may result in modest increases in length of gestation, especially in women with low omega-3 fatty acid consumption. In European women with high-risk pregnancies, fish oil supplementation that provided 2.7 g/d of EPA + DHA during the last trimester of pregnancy lowered the risk of premature delivery from 33 to 21%.[43] In healthy Danish women, fish oil supplementation that provided 2.7 g/d of EPA + DHA increased the length of gestation by an average of 4 days.[41] In a recent study, consumption of only 0.13 g/d of DHA from enriched eggs during the last trimester of pregnancy increased the length of gestation by an average of 6 days in a low-income population in the United States.[40] In Norway, children born to mothers who were supplemented with cod liver oil (2 g/d of EPA + DHA) during pregnancy and the first 3 months of lactation scored higher on mental processing tests at 4 years of age when compared

with the children whose mothers were not supplemented with cod liver oil.[44] However, only 14% of the original study participants were available for testing when the children were 4 years of age. Although promising, these findings need to be replicated in other studies before it can be concluded that EPA and DHA supplementation during pregnancy has beneficial effects on long-term cognitive development in children.

Cardiovascular Disease

Omega-6 Fatty Acids: Linoleic Acid

Linoleic acid is the most abundant dietary polyunsaturated fatty acid (PUFA). The results of prospective cohort studies examining the relationships between PUFA intake and the risk of coronary heart disease (CHD) have been somewhat inconsistent.[45] Some, but not all, prospective cohort studies have found that higher PUFA and LA intakes are associated with significant reductions in CHD risk.[46–48] The largest prospective cohort study to examine the effects of dietary fat intake on CHD risk is the Nurses' Health Study, which followed more than 78,000 women for 20 years. In that cohort, those with the highest intakes of total PUFA (7.4% of energy) and LA had a risk of CHD that was 25% lower than those with the lowest intakes of total PUFA (5% of energy) and LA.[47] Although saturated fatty acid (SFA) intake was not associated with CHD risk, the ratio of PUFA:SFA intake was inversely associated with CHD risk. In controlled feeding trials, replacing dietary SFA with PUFA consistently lowers serum and total low-density lipoprotein (LDL) cholesterol concentrations.[49] In fact, LA has been shown to be the most potent fatty acid for lowering serum total and LDL cholesterol when substituted for dietary SFA.[50] Several dietary intervention trials have compared the effects of diets high in SFA (18 to 19% of energy) with diets low in SFA (8 to 9% of energy) and high in PUFA (14 to 21% of energy) on morbidity and mortality from CHD.[45] Although most of the increase in dietary PUFA was provided by LA, ALA intakes were also increased in these trials.[49] Several dietary intervention trials in men found that replacing dietary SFA with PUFA reduced morbidity or mortality from

CHD.[51-54] However, two similar dietary intervention trials in women did not result in significant reductions in morbidity or mortality from CHD.[55,56]

Omega-3 Fatty Acids: Alpha-Linolenic Acid

Several prospective cohort studies have examined the relationship between dietary ALA intake and CHD risk. In a cohort of more than 45,000 American men followed for 14 years, each 1-g/d increase in dietary ALA intake was associated with a 16% reduction in the risk of CHD.[57] Moreover, in those who ate little or no seafood, each 1-g/d increase in dietary ALA intake was associated with a 47% reduction in the risk of CHD. In a cohort of more than 76,000 American women followed for 10 years, those with the highest ALA intakes (~ 1.4 g/d) had a risk of fatal CHD that was 45% lower than women with the lowest intakes (~ 0.7 g/d).[58] Interestingly, oil and vinegar salad dressing was an important source of dietary ALA in this population. Women who consumed oil and vinegar salad dressing 5 to 6 times weekly had a risk of fatal CHD that was 54% lower than those who rarely consumed it, even after adjusting the analysis for vegetable intake. In a smaller cohort of more than 6000 American men, those with the highest intakes of ALA had a risk of death from CHD over the next 10 years that was 40% lower than those with the lowest intakes.[59] In contrast, two studies in Europe found no association between dietary ALA intake and CHD risk.[60,61] Although not as consistent as the evidence supporting higher intakes of long-chain omega-3 fatty acids from seafood, the results of most prospective studies suggest that higher dietary ALA intakes (2 to 3 g/d) are associated with significant reductions in CHD risk, especially in populations with low levels of fish consumption.[62] Unlike LA, the cardioprotective effects of higher ALA intakes do not appear to be related to changes in serum lipid profiles. However, several controlled clinical trials found that increasing ALA intake decreased serum concentrations of C-reactive protein (CRP), a marker of inflammation that is strongly associated with the risk of cardiovascular events, such as myocardial infarction (MI) and stroke.[63-65]

Long-Chain Omega-3 Fatty Acids: Eicosapentaenoic Acid and Docosahexaenoic Acid

Evidence is accumulating that increasing intakes of long-chain omega-3 fatty acids (EPA and DHA) can decrease the risk of cardiovascular disease by (1) preventing arrhythmias that can lead to sudden cardiac death, (2) decreasing the risk of thrombosis that can lead to myocardial infarction (MI) or stroke, (3) decreasing serum triglyceride levels, (4) slowing the growth of atherosclerotic plaque, (5) improving vascular endothelial function, (6) lowering blood pressure slightly, and (7) decreasing inflammation.[66]

Coronary Heart Disease

Several prospective cohort studies have found that men who eat fish at least once weekly have lower mortality from CHD than men who do not eat fish.[67-69] One such study followed 1822 men for 30 years and found that mortality from CHD was 38% lower in men who consumed an average of at least 35 g (1.2 oz) of fish daily than in men who did not eat fish, whereas mortality from MI was 67% lower.[70] The cardioprotective effects of fish consumption may not be confined to those consuming a typical Western diet. A study in Shanghai, China, that followed more than 18,000 men for 10 years found that men who consumed more than 200 g (~ 7 oz) of fish or shellfish weekly had a risk of fatal MI that was 59% lower than men who consumed less than 50 g (~ 2 oz) weekly.[71] Less information is available regarding the effects of higher omega-3 fatty acid and fish intakes in women. In the Nurses' Health Study, which followed more than 84,000 women for 16 years, CHD mortality was 29 to 34% lower in women who ate fish at least once a week compared with women who ate fish less than once a month.[72]

Sudden Cardiac Death

Sudden cardiac death is the result of a fatal ventricular arrhythmia, which usually occurs in people with coronary artery disease. Studies in cell culture indicate that long-chain omega-3 fatty acids decrease the excitability of cardiac myocytes by modulating ion channel conductance.[73] The results of epidemiological studies suggest that regular fish consumption is inversely associated with the risk of sudden cardiac death. In a large prospective cohort study that followed more than 20,000 men for 11 years, those who ate fish at least once a week had a risk of sudden cardiac death that was 52% lower than those who ate fish less than once a month.[74] Plasma levels of EPA and DHA were also inversely related to the risk of sudden cardiac death, supporting the idea that omega-3 fatty acids are at least partially responsible for the beneficial effect of fish consumption on sudden cardiac death.[75] A prospective study that followed more than 45,000 men for 14 years found that the risk of sudden cardiac death was ~40 to 50% lower in those who consumed an average of at least 250 mg/d of dietary EPA + DHA, the equivalent of 1 to 2 oily fish meals weekly, than those who consumed less than 250 mg/d.[57] Dietary EPA + DHA intake was not related to the risk of nonfatal MI or total CHD events, suggesting the antiarrhythmic effects of long-chain omega-3 fatty acids may be important at usual dietary intake levels

Stroke

Ischemic strokes are the result of insufficient blood flow to an area of the brain, which may occur when an artery supplying the brain becomes occluded by a clot. Hemorrhagic strokes occur when a blood vessel ruptures and bleeds into the brain. In the United States, 70 to 80% of strokes are ischemic strokes.[76] Some prospective studies that have examined the relationship between fish or omega-3 fatty acid intake and total stroke incidence have found increased fish intake to be beneficial,[77,78] whereas others found no beneficial effect.[79,80] Two large prospective studies found that increased fish and omega-3 fatty acid intakes were associated with significantly lower risks of ischemic stroke, but not hemorrhagic stroke. In a study that followed more than 79,000 women for 14 years, those who ate fish at least twice weekly had a risk of thrombotic (ischemic) stroke that was 52% lower than those who ate fish less than once monthly.[81] Similarly, in a study that followed more than

43,000 men for 12 years, those who ate fish at least once monthly had a risk of ischemic stroke that was 43% lower than men who ate fish less than once monthly.[82] Although the effects of long-chain omega-3 fatty acid intake on the incidence of stroke have not been studied as thoroughly as that of CHD, available evidence suggests that increased fish intake may decrease the risk of ischemic stroke, but not hemorrhagic stroke.

Serum Triglycerides

A meta-analysis of 17 prospective studies found hypertriglyceridemia to be an independent risk factor for cardiovascular disease.[83] Numerous controlled clinical trials in humans have demonstrated that increasing intakes of EPA and DHA significantly lowers serum triglyceride concentrations.[84] The triglyceride-lowering effects of EPA and DHA increase with dose, but clinically meaningful reductions in serum triglyceride concentrations have been demonstrated at doses of 2 g/d of EPA + DHA.[3] In its recommendations regarding omega-3 fatty acids and cardiovascular disease (see Intake Recommendations below), the American Heart Association indicates that an EPA + DHA supplement may be useful in patients with hypertriglyceridemia (serum triglycerides ≥ 200 mg/dL).[66]

Summary: Omega-3 and Omega-6 PUFA and Cardiovascular Disease Prevention

The results of epidemiological studies and randomized controlled trials suggest that replacing dietary SFA with omega-6 and omega-3 PUFA lowers LDL cholesterol and decreases cardiovascular disease risk. Additionally, the results of epidemiological studies provide strong evidence that increasing dietary omega-3 fatty intake is associated with significant reductions in cardiovascular disease risk through mechanisms other than lowering LDL cholesterol. In particular, increasing EPA and DHA intake from seafood has been associated with significant reductions in sudden cardiac death, suggesting that long-chain omega-3 fatty acids have antiarrhythmic effects at intake levels equivalent to the amount in 2 small servings of oily fish per week.

Treatment

Coronary Heart Disease

Dietary Intervention Trials

Total mortality and fatal MI decreased by 29% in male MI survivors advised to increase their weekly intake of oily fish to 200 to 400 g (7 to 14 oz), which was estimated to provide an additional 500 to 800 mg/d of marine-derived omega-3 fatty acids.[85] In another dietary intervention trial, patients who survived a first MI were randomly assigned to usual care or advised to adopt a Mediterranean diet that was higher in omega-3 fatty acids (especially ALA) and lower in omega-6 fatty acids than the standard Western diet. After almost 4 years, those on the Mediterranean diet had a risk of cardiac death and nonfatal MI that was 38% lower than the group that was assigned to usual care.[86] Although higher plasma ALA levels were associated with better outcomes, the benefit of the Mediterranean diet cannot be attributed entirely to increased ALA intakes because intakes of monounsaturated fatty acids and fruits and vegetables also increased.

Supplementation Trials

In the largest randomized controlled trial of supplemental omega-3 fatty acids to date, CHD patients who received supplements providing 850 mg/d of EPA + DHA for 3.5 years had a risk of sudden death that was 45% lower than those who did not take supplements and a risk of death from all causes that was 20% lower.[87] Interestingly, it took only 3 months of supplementation to demonstrate a significant decrease in total mortality and 4 months to demonstrate a significant decrease in sudden death.[88] In another supplementation trial, patients admitted to the hospital with an acute MI were randomized to receive capsules containing fish oil (1.8 g/d of EPA + DHA), mustard oil (2.9 g/d of ALA), or a placebo.[89] After a year, total cardiac events, including nonfatal MI, were significantly lower in the groups that received fish oil or mustard oil compared with the groups that received a placebo. In contrast, acute MI patients did not realize any additional benefit from supplementation with 3.5 g/d of EPA + DHA compared with corn oil in a region of Norway where fish intakes are relatively high.[90] The results of a meta-analysis that pooled the findings of 11 randomized controlled trials of dietary or supplementary omega-3 fatty acids indicated that increased omega-3 fatty acid intakes significantly decreased overall mortality, mortality due to MI and sudden cardiac death in patients with CHD.[91]

Two randomized controlled trials have examined the effect of fish oil supplementation on the progression of coronary artery atherosclerosis measured by coronary angiography. Although a study of 59 patients with coronary artery disease found no benefit after 2 years of supplementation with fish oil providing 6 g/d of EPA +DHA compared with olive oil,[92] a larger trial of 223 patients found that supplementation with 3.3 g/d of EPA + DHA for 3 months and 1.65 g/d for an additional 21 months resulted in a modest decrease in the progression of coronary atherosclerosis compared with a placebo.[93] Numerous randomized controlled trials have examined the effect of fish oil supplementation on coronary artery restenosis after percutaneous transluminal coronary angioplasty (PTCA). A meta-analysis that combined the results of 12 randomized controlled trials found that fish oil supplementation resulted in a 14% reduction of coronary restenosis, but this reduction did not quite reach statistical significance.[94] Supplemental fish oil doses in the coronary artery restenosis trials ranged from 2.6 to 6.0 g/d.

Summary

The results of randomized controlled trials in individuals with documented CHD suggest a beneficial effect of dietary and supplemental omega-3 fatty acids. Based on the results of these trials, the American Heart Association recommends that individuals with documented CHD consume ∼1 g/d of EPA + DHA (see the Intake Recommendations section below).[3]

Diabetes Mellitus

Cardiovascular diseases are the leading causes of death in individuals with diabetes mellitus (DM). Hypertriglyceridemia is a common lipid abnormality in individuals with type 2 DM, and several randomized controlled trials have found that fish oil supplementation significantly lowers serum triglyceride levels in diabetic individuals.[95] Although early uncontrolled studies raised concerns that fish oil supplementation adversely affected glycemic control,[96,97] randomized controlled trials have not generally found adverse effects of fish oil supplementation on long-term glycemic control.[98] A systematic review that pooled the results of 18 randomized controlled trials including more than 800 diabetic patients found that fish oil supplementation significantly lowered serum triglycerides, especially in those with hypertriglyceridemia.[95] A meta-analysis that combined the results of 18 randomized controlled trials in individuals with type 2 DM or metabolic syndrome found that fish oil supplementation decreased serum triglycerides by 31 mg/dL compared with placebo, but had no effect on serum cholesterol, fasting glucose, or hemoglobin A1c concentrations.[98] Although few controlled trials have examined the effect of fish oil supplementation on cardiovascular disease outcomes in diabetics, a prospective study that followed 5103 women diagnosed with type 2 DM, but free of cardiovascular disease or cancer at the start of the study, found that higher fish intakes were associated with significantly decreased risks of CHD over a 16-year follow-up period.[99] Thus, increasing EPA and DHA intakes may be beneficial to diabetic individuals, especially those with elevated serum triglycerides.[100] Moreover, there is little evidence that daily EPA + DHA intakes of less than 3 g/d adversely affect long-term glycemic control in diabetics.[95,101] The American Diabetes Association recommends that diabetic individuals increase omega-3 fatty acid consumption by consuming two to three 3-oz servings of fish weekly.[102]

Inflammatory Diseases

Rheumatoid Arthritis

Two meta-analyses of randomized controlled trials in rheumatoid arthritis patients found that fish oil supplementation significantly decreased the number of tender joints on physical examination.[98,103] In general, clinical benefits were observed at a minimum dose of 3 g/d of EPA + DHA and were not apparent until at least 12 weeks of supplementation.[104] Neither meta-analysis found that fish oil supplementation had a significant effect on erythrocyte sedimentation rate (ESR), a measure of inflammation. Six out of seven studies that examined the effect of long-chain omega-3 fatty acid supplementation on nonsteroidal anti-inflammatory drug (NSAID) or corticosteroid use in rheumatoid arthritis patients demonstrated a reduced requirement for anti-inflammatory medication.[98]

Inflammatory Bowel Disease

Clinical trials of long-chain omega-3 fatty acid supplementation have demonstrated beneficial effects less consistently in patients with inflammatory bowel disease than in patients with rheumatoid arthritis. Although two randomized controlled trials of fish oil supplementation in Crohn's disease patients reported no benefit,[105,106] a significantly higher proportion of Crohn's disease patients supplemented with 2.7 g/d of EPA + DHA remained in remission over a 12-month period than those given a placebo.[107] Three randomized controlled trials of EPA + DHA supplementation (4.2 to 5.4 g/d for 3 to 12 months) in ulcerative colitis patients reported significant improvement in at least one outcome measure, including weight gain, decreased corticosteroid use, improved disease activity scores, and improved histology scores.[108–110] In contrast, supplementation of ulcerative colitis patients in remission with 5.1 g/d of EPA + DHA did not significantly alter the incidence of relapse over a 2-year period.[111]

Asthma

Inflammatory eicosanoids (leukotrienes) derived from AA (20:4n-6) are thought to play an important role in the pathology of asthma.[17] Increasing omega-3 fatty acid intake has been found to decrease the formation of AA-derived leukotrienes; therefore, several clinical trials have examined the effects of long-chain omega-3 fatty acid supplementation on asthma. Although there is some evidence that omega-3 fatty acid supplementation can decrease the production of inflammatory mediators in asthmatic patients,[112,113] evidence that omega-3 fatty acid supplementation decreases the clinical severity of asthma in controlled trials has been inconsistent.[114] Two recent systematic reviews of randomized controlled trials of long-chain omega-3 fatty acid supplementation in asthmatic adults and children found no consistent effects on clinical outcome measures, including pulmonary function tests, asthmatic symptoms, medication use, or bronchial hyperreactivity.[115,116]

Immunoglobulin A Nephropathy

Immunoglobulin A (IgA) nephropathy is a kidney disorder that results from the deposition of IgA in the glomeruli of the kidney. The cause of IgA nephropathy is not clear, but progressive renal failure may eventually develop in 15 to 40% of patients.[117] Because glomerular IgA deposition results in increased production of inflammatory mediators, omega-3 fatty acid supplementation could potentially modulate the inflammatory response and preserve renal function. In a multicenter randomized controlled trial, supplementation of IgA nephropathy patients with fish oil (1.8 g/d of EPA + 1.2 g/d of DHA) for 2 years significantly slowed declines in renal function.[118] Over the 2-year treatment period, 33% of the placebo group experienced a 50% increase in serum creatinine (evidence of declining renal function) compared with only 6% in the fish oil supplemented group. These results were sustained over an average of 6 years of follow-up,[119] but were not improved with higher doses of fish oil.[120] In contrast, several smaller studies failed to find a significant benefit of fish oil supplementation in IgA nephropathy patients.[121-123] Interestingly, fish oil treatment (3 g/d of EPA + DHA) for 6 months did not decrease the urinary excretion of inflammatory mediators in IgA nephropathy patients.[124] Two meta-analyses of randomized controlled trials of fish oil supplementation did not find evidence of a statistically significant benefit in IgA nephropathy patients overall.[125,126] Due to the inconsistent results of available randomized controlled trials, it is not clear whether fish oil supplementation will prevent the progression of IgA nephropathy in children or adults.[98]

Major Depression and Bipolar Disorder

Data from ecological studies across different countries suggest an inverse association between seafood consumption and national rates of major depression[127] and bipolar disorder.[128] Several small studies have found omega-3 fatty acid concentrations to be lower in the plasma[129,130] and adipose tissue[131] of individuals suffering from depression compared with controls. Although it is not known how increased omega-3 fatty acid intake affects the incidence of depression, modulation of neuronal signaling pathways and eicosanoid production have been proposed as possible mechanisms.[132] The results of randomized controlled trials of supplementation with long-chain omega-3 fatty acids on depression have been mixed. Adding fish oil supplements (8 g/d) to existing therapy in people who were being treated for depression was not significantly more effective than adding the same amount of olive oil for 12 weeks.[133] Supplementation with 2 g/d of DHA for 6 weeks was not significantly more effective than a placebo in the treatment of major depression.[134] However, a small randomized controlled trial in Chinese patients diagnosed with major depression found that supplementation with 6.6 g/d of EPA + DHA for 8 weeks improved scores on the Hamilton Rating Scale for Depression compared with placebo.[135] Another small randomized controlled trial in 30 women diagnosed with borderline personality disorder found that the 20 women randomized to treatment with 1 g/d of ethyl-EPA for 8 weeks experienced less severe depressive symptoms than the 10 women randomized to treatment with a placebo.[136] Unipolar depression and bipolar disorder are considered distinct psychiatric conditions, although major depression occurs in both. A randomized controlled trial that assessed the effects of high doses of EPA (6.2 g/d) + DHA (3.4 g/d) in patients with bipolar disorder found that those supplemented with EPA + DHA had a significantly longer period of remission than those on an olive oil placebo over a 4-month period.[137] Patients who took the EPA + DHA supplements also experienced less depression than those who took the placebo. Although the results of a few small controlled trials are somewhat optimistic, larger and long-term randomized controlled trials are required to determine the efficacy of long-chain omega-3 fatty acid supplementation on major depression.

Schizophrenia

Findings of decreased omega-3 fatty acid levels in the red blood cells[138] and brains[139] of a limited number of schizophrenic patients and the results of uncontrolled supplementation studies[140] have created interest in the use of long-chain omega-3 fatty acid supplements as an adjunct to conventional antipsychotic therapy regimens for schizophrenia. A pilot study in 45 schizophrenic patients found that the addition of 2 g/d of EPA to standard antipsychotic therapy was superior to the addition of a 2 g/d of DHA or a placebo in decreasing residual symptoms.[141] When EPA supplementation was used as the sole treatment for schizophrenic patients experiencing a relapse, 8 out of 14 patients supplemented with 2 g/d of EPA required antipsychotic medication by the end of the 12-week study period compared with 12 out of 12 of those on the placebo.[141] Results of randomized controlled trials using ethyl-EPA as an adjunct to standard antipsychotic therapy in schizophrenic patients have been somewhat contradictory. In one trial, the addition of 3 g/d of ethyl-EPA to standard antipsychotic treatment for 12 weeks improved symptom scores and decreased dyskinesia scores;[142] in a larger trial, supplementation with the same dose of ethyl-EPA was not different from placebo in improving symptoms, mood, or cognition.[143] In a placebo-controlled trial comparing the addition of 1, 2, or 4 g/d of ethyl-EPA to different medication regimens, ethyl-EPA supplementation improved symptoms of schizophrenic patients on the antipsychotic medication clozapine, but not other medications.[144] Although limited evidence suggests that EPA supplementation may be a useful adjunct to antipsychotic therapy in schizophrenic patients, larger long-term studies addressing clinically relevant outcomes are needed.[145]

Sources

Food Sources

Omega-6 Fatty Acids

Linoleic Acid

Food sources of LA include vegetable oils, such as soybean, safflower, and corn oils; nuts; seeds, and some vegetables. Dietary surveys in the United States indicate that the average adult intake of LA ranges from 12 to 17 g/d for men and 9 to 11 g/d for women.[1] Some foods that are rich in LA are listed in **Table 11–1**.[146]

Arachidonic Acid

Animals, but not plants, can convert LA to AA. Therefore, AA is present in the diet in small amounts in meat, poultry, and eggs.

Omega-3 Fatty Acids

Alpha-Linolenic Acid

Flaxseeds, walnuts, and their oils are among the richest dietary sources of ALA. Canola oil is also an excellent source of ALA. Dietary surveys in the United States indicate that average adult intakes for ALA range from 1.2 to 1.6 g/d for men and from 0.9 to 1.1 g/d for women.[1] Some foods that are rich in ALA are listed in the **Table 11–2**.[146]

Eicosapentaenoic Acid and Docosahexaenoic Acid

Oily fish are the major dietary source of EPA and DHA. Dietary surveys in the United States indicate that average adult intakes of EPA range from 0.04 to 0.07 g/d and average adult intakes of DHA range from 0.05 to 0.09 g/d.[1] Omega-3 fatty acid-enriched eggs are also available in the United States. Some foods that are rich in EPA and DHA are listed in **Table 11–3**.[3]

Biosynthesis

Humans can synthesize AA from LA and EPA and DHA from ALA through a series of desaturation and elongation reactions (see the Metabolism and Bioavailability section on page 79).

Supplements

Omega-6 Fatty Acids

Borage seed oil, evening primrose oil, and black currant seed oil are rich in γ-linolenic acid (GLA) and are often marketed as GLA or essential fatty acid (EFA) supplements.[147]

Omega-3 Fatty Acids

Flaxseed oil (also known as flax oil or linseed oil) is available as an ALA supplement. Several fish oils are marketed as omega-3 fatty acid supplements. Ethyl esters of EPA and DHA (ethyl-EPA and ethyl-DHA) are concentrated sources of long-chain omega-3 fatty acids. Because EPA and DHA content will vary in fish oil and ethyl ester preparations, it is necessary to read the label to determine the EPA and DHA content of a particular supplement. DHA supplements derived from algal and fungal sources are also available. All omega-3 fatty acid supplements are absorbed more efficiently with meals. Dividing one's daily dose into two or three smaller doses throughout the day will decrease the risk of gastrointestinal side effects (see the Safety section below). Cod liver oil is a rich source of EPA and DHA, but some cod liver oil preparations may contain excessive amounts of preformed vitamin A (retinol).[147]

Table 11–1   Some Food Sources of Linoleic Acid (18:2n-6)[146]

Food	Serving	Linoleic Acid (g)
Safflower oil	1 tbs	10.1
Sunflower seeds, oil roasted	1 oz	9.7
Pine nuts	1 oz	9.4
Sunflower oil	1 tbs	8.9
Corn oil	1 tbs	7.2
Soybean oil	1 tbs	6.9
Pecans, oil roasted	1 oz	6.4
Brazil nuts	1 oz	5.8
Sesame oil	1 tbs	5.6

Table 11–2   Some Food Sources of α-Linolenic Acid (18:3n-3)[146]

Food	Serving	α-Linolenic Acid (g)
Flaxseed (linseed) oil	1 tbs	8.5
Walnuts, English	1 oz	2.6
Flaxseeds	1 tbs	2.2
Walnut oil	1 tbs	1.4
Canola oil	1 tbs	1.2
Mustard oil	1 tbs	0.8
Soybean oil	1 tbs	0.9
Walnuts, Black	1 oz	0.6
Tofu, firm	1/2 cup	0.7

Table 11–3   Some Food Sources of Eicosapentaenoic Acid (EPA; 20:5n-3) and Docosahexaenoic Acid (DHA; 22:6n-3)[3]

Food	Serving	EPA (g)	DHA (g)	Amount providing 1 g of EPA + DHA
Herring, Pacific	3 oz*	1.06	0.75	1.5 oz
Salmon, Chinook	3 oz	0.86	0.62	2 oz
Salmon, Atlantic	3 oz	0.28	0.95	2.5 oz
Oysters, Pacific	3 oz	0.75	0.43	2.5 oz
Salmon, sockeye	3 oz	0.45	0.60	3 oz
Trout, rainbow	3 oz	0.40	0.44	3.5 oz
Tuna, canned, white	3 oz	0.20	0.54	4 oz
Crab, Dungeness	3 oz	0.24	0.10	9 oz
Tuna, canned, light	3 oz	0.04	0.19	12 oz

* A 3-oz serving of fish is about the size of a deck of cards.

Infant Formula

In 2001, the FDA began permitting the addition of DHA and AA to infant formula in the United States.[148] Presently, manufacturers are not required to list the amounts of DHA and AA added to infant formula on the label. However, most infant formula manufacturers provide this information. The amounts added to formulas range from 8 to 17 mg DHA/100 calories (5 fl oz) and from 16 to 34 mg AA/100 calories. For example, an infant drinking 20 fl oz of DHA-enriched formula daily would receive 32 to 68 mg/d of DHA and 64 to 136 mg/d of AA.

Safety

Adverse Effects

Gamma-Linolenic Acid (18:3n-6)

Supplemental γ-linolenic acid is generally well-tolerated, and serious adverse side effects have not been observed at doses up to 2.8 g/d for 12 months.[149] High doses of borage seed oil, evening primrose oil, or black currant seed oil may cause gastrointestinal upset, loose stools, or diarrhea.[147] Because of case reports that supplementation with evening primrose oil induced seizure activity in people with undiagnosed temporal lobe epilepsy,[150] people with a history of seizures or seizure disorder are generally advised to avoid evening primrose oil and other γ-linolenic acid-rich oils.[147]

Alpha-Linolenic Acid (18:3n-3)

Although flaxseed oil is generally well tolerated, high doses may cause loose stools or diarrhea.[151] Allergic and anaphylactic reactions have been reported with flaxseed and flaxseed oil ingestion.[152]

Eicosapentaenoic Acid (20:5n-3) and Docosahexaenoic Acid (22:6n-3)

Serious adverse reactions have not been reported in those using fish oil or other EPA and DHA supplements. The most common adverse effect of fish oil or EPA and DHA supplements is a fishy aftertaste. Belching and heartburn have also been reported. High doses may cause nausea and loose stools.

Potential for Excessive Bleeding

The potential for high omega-3 fatty acid intakes, especially EPA and DHA, to prolong bleeding times has been well studied and may play a role in the cardioprotective effects of omega-3 fatty acids. Although excessively long bleeding times and increased incidence of hemorrhagic stroke have been observed in Greenland Eskimos with very high intakes of EPA + DHA (6.5 g/d), it is not known whether high intakes of EPA and DHA are the only factor responsible for these observations.[1] The FDA has ruled that intakes up to 3 g/d of long-chain omega-3 fatty acids (EPA and DHA) are generally recognized as safe (GRAS) for inclusion in the diet, and available evidence suggests that intakes less than 3 g/d are unlikely to result in clinically significant bleeding.[3] Although the Institute of Medicine did not establish a tolerable upper level of intake (UL) for omega-3 fatty acids, caution was advised with the use of supplemental EPA and DHA, especially in those who are at increased risk of excessive bleeding (see the Drug Interactions section below).[1]

Potential for Immune System Suppression

Although the suppression of inflammatory responses resulting from increased omega-3 fatty acid intakes may benefit individuals with inflammatory or autoimmune diseases, anti-inflammatory doses of omega-3 fatty acids could decrease the potential of the immune system to destroy pathogens.[153] Studies comparing measures of immune cell function outside the body (ex vivo) at baseline and after supplementing people with omega-3 fatty acids, mainly EPA and DHA, have demonstrated immunosuppressive effects at doses as low as 0.9 g/d for EPA and 0.6 g/d for DHA.[1] Although it is not clear if these findings translate to impaired immune responses in vivo, caution should be observed when considering omega-3 fatty acid supplementation in individuals with compromised immune systems.

Infant Formula

In early studies of DHA-enriched infant formula, EPA- and DHA-rich fish oil was used as a source of DHA. However, some preterm infants receiving fish oil-enriched formula had decreased plasma AA concentrations, which were associated with decreased growth.[154] This effect was attributed to the potential for high concentrations of EPA to interfere with the synthesis of AA, which is essential for normal growth. Consequently, EPA was removed and AA was added to DHA-enriched formula. Infant formulas currently available in the United States contain only AA and DHA derived from algal or fungal sources, rather than fish oil. Randomized controlled trials have not found any adverse effects on growth in infants fed formulas enriched with AA and DHA for up to one year.[29,30]

Pregnancy and Lactation

The safety of supplemental omega-3 and omega-6 fatty acids, including borage seed oil, evening primrose oil, black currant seed oil, and flaxseed oil has not been established in pregnant or lactating women.[147] Studies of fish oil supplementation during pregnancy and lactation have not reported any serious adverse effects (see the Contaminants in Fish and Contaminants in Supplements sections below).

Contaminants in Fish

Some species of fish may contain significant levels of methylmercury, polychlorinated biphenyls (PCBs), or other environmental contaminants. In general, larger predatory fish, such as swordfish, tend to contain the highest levels of these contaminants. Removing the skin, fat, and internal organs of the fish prior to cooking and allowing the fat to drain from the fish while it cooks will decrease exposure to several fat-soluble pollutants, such as PCBs.[155] However, methylmercury is found throughout the muscle of fish, so these cooking precautions will not reduce exposure to methylmercury. Organic mercury compounds are toxic, and excessive exposure can cause brain and kidney damage. Unborn children, infants, and young children are especially vulnerable to the toxic effects of mercury on the brain. To limit their exposure to methylmercury, the U.S. Department of Health and Human Services (DHHS) and Environmental Protection Agency (EPA) have made the following joint recommendations for women who may become pregnant, pregnant women, and breastfeeding women[156]:

1. Do not eat shark, swordfish, king mackerel, and tile fish (also known as golden bass or golden snapper) because they contain high methylmercury levels.
2. Eat up to 12 oz (two average meals) per week of a variety of fish that are lower in mercury.
   a. The five most commonly consumed fish that are low in mercury include canned light tuna, shrimp, salmon, catfish, and pollock.
   b. Limit the consumption of canned white (albacore) tuna and tuna steak to 6 oz (one average meal) per week.
3. Check local advisories regarding the safety of fish caught by friends or family in local lakes, rivers, and coastal areas.

When feeding fish to young children, the DHHS and EPA advise following the above guidelines but serving smaller portions, such as 3 oz, for an average meal.

Contaminants in Supplements

Although concerns have been raised regarding the potential for omega-3 fatty acid supplements derived from fish oil to contain methylmercury, PCBs, and dioxins, several independent laboratory analyses in the United States have found commercially available omega-3 fatty acid supplements to be free of methylmercury, PCBs, and dioxins.[157-159] The absence of methylmercury in omega-3 fatty acid supplements can be explained by the fact that mercury accumulates in the muscle, rather than the fat of fish.[3] In general, fish body oils contain lower levels of PCBs and other fat-soluble contaminants than fish liver oils. Additionally, fish oils that have been more highly refined and deodorized contain lower levels of PCBs.[160] Pyrrolizidine alkaloids, potentially hepatotoxic, and carcinogenic compounds are found in various parts of the borage plant. People who take borage oil supplements should use products that are certified free of pyrrolizidine alkaloids.[147]

Drug Interactions

γ-Linolenic acid supplements, such as evening primrose oil or borage seed oil, may increase the risk of seizures in people on phenothiazines, such as chlorpromazine.[150] High doses of black currant seed oil, borage seed oil, evening primrose oil, flaxseed oil, and fish oil may inhibit platelet aggregation, and should be used with caution in people on anticoagulant medications. In particular, people taking fish oil or long-chain omega-3 fatty acid (EPA and DHA) supplements in combination with anticoagulant drugs, including aspirin, copidogrel (Plavix), dalteparin (Fragmin), dipyridamole (Persantine), enoxaparin (Lovenox), heparin, ticlopidine (Ticlid), and warfarin (Coumadin), should have their coagulation status monitored using a standardized prothrombin time assay (INR). One small study found that 3 g/d or 6 g/d of fish oil did not affect INR values in 10 patients on warfarin over a 4-week period[161] However, a recent case report described an individual who required a reduction of her warfarin dose when she doubled her fish oil dose from 1 g/d to 2 g/d.[162]

Nutrient Interactions

Vitamin E

Outside the body, PUFA become rancid (oxidized) more easily than SFA. Fat-soluble antioxidants, such as vitamin E, play an important role in preventing the oxidation of PUFA. Inside the body, results of animal studies and limited data in humans suggest that the amount of vitamin E required to prevent lipid peroxidation increases with the amount of polyunsaturated fat consumed.[163] One widely used recommendation for vitamin E intake is 0.6 mg of α-tocopherol per g of dietary PUFA. This recommendation was based on a small study in men and the ratio of α-tocopherol to LA in the diet of the U.S. population and has not been verified in studies that are more comprehensive. Although EPA and DHA are easily oxi-

dized outside the body, it is presently unclear whether EPA and DHA are more susceptible to oxidative damage within the body.[164] High vitamin E intakes have not been found to decrease biomarkers of oxidative damage when EPA and DHA intakes are increased,[165,166] but some experts believe that an increase in PUFA intake, particularly omega-3 PUFA intake, should be accompanied by an increase in vitamin E intake.[1]

Intake Recommendations

U.S. Institute of Medicine

In 2002, the Food and Nutrition Board of the U.S. Institute of Medicine established adequate intake (AI) levels for omega-6 and omega-3 fatty acids, which are listed in **Tables 11–4 and 11–5**, respectively.[1] The acceptable macronutrient distribution ranges established by the Food and Nutrition Board are 5 to 10 % of energy for omega-6 fatty acids and 0.6 to 1.2 % of energy for omega-3 fatty acids.

International Recommendations

The European Commission recommends an omega-6 fatty acid intake of 4 to 8 % of energy and an omega-3 fatty acid intake of 2 g/d of ALA and 200 mg/d of long-chain omega-3 fatty acids (EPA and DHA).[167] The World Health Organization recommends an omega-6 fatty acid intake of 5 to 8 % of energy and an omega-3 fatty acid intake of 1 to 2 % of energy.[168] However, the Japan Society for Lipid Nutrition has recommended that LA intake be reduced to 3 to 4 % of energy in Japanese people whose omega-3 fatty acid intakes average 2.6 g/d, including ~ 1 g/d of EPA + DHA.[169]

American Heart Association

The American Heart Association recommends that people without documented CHD eat a variety of fish (preferably oily) at least twice weekly, in addition to consuming oils and foods rich in ALA.[3] People with documented CHD are advised to consume ~ 1 g/d of EPA + DHA, preferably from oily fish, or to consider EPA + DHA supplements in consultation with a

Table 11–4   Adequate Intake Levels for Omega-6 Fatty Acids[1]

Life Stage	Age	Source	Males (g/d)	Females (g/d)
Infants	0–6 mo	Omega-6 PUFA*	4.4	4.4
Infants	7–12 mo	Omega-6 PUFA*	4.6	4.6
Children	1–3 y	LA	7	7
Children	4–8 y	LA	10	10
Children	9–13 y	LA	12	10
Adolescents	14–18 y	LA	16	11
Adults	19–50 y	LA	17	12
Adults	51 y or older	LA	14	11
Pregnancy	All ages	LA	–	13
Lactation	All ages	LA	–	13

*   The various omega-6 fatty polyunsaturated fatty acids (PUFA) present in human milk can contribute to the adequate intake for infants.
Abbreviations: LA, linoleic acid.

Table 11–5   Adequate Intake Levels for Omega-3 Fatty Acids[1]

Life Stage	Age	Source	Males (g/d)	Females (g/d)
Infants	0–6 mo	ALA, EPA, DHA	0.5	0.5
Infants	7–12 mo	ALA, EPA, DHA	0.5	0.5
Children	1–3 y	ALA	0.7	0.7
Children	4–8 y	ALA	0.9	0.9
Children	9–13 y	ALA	1.2	1.0
Adolescents	14–18 y	ALA	1.6	1.1
Adults	19 y and older	ALA	1.6	1.1
Pregnancy	All ages	ALA	-	1.4
Lactation	All ages	ALA	-	1.3

Abbreviations: ALA, α-linolenic acid; DHA, docosahexaenoic acid; EPA, eicosapentaenoic acid.

physician. Patients who need to lower serum triglycerides may take 2 to 4 g/d of EPA + DHA supplements under a physician's care.

Summary

- α-Linolenic acid (ALA), an omega-3 fatty acid, and linoleic acid (LA), an omega-6 fatty acid, are considered essential fatty acids because they cannot be synthesized by humans.
- The long-chain omega-6 fatty acid, arachidonic acid (AA), can be synthesized from LA.
- The long-chain omega-3 fatty acids, eicosapentaenoic acid (EPA) and docosahexaenoic acid (DHA), can be synthesized from ALA, but EPA and DHA synthesis may be insufficient under certain conditions.
- Typical Western diets tend to be much higher in omega-6 fatty acids than omega-3 fatty acids.
- DHA appears to be important for visual and neurological development; however, it is not yet clear whether feeding infants formula enriched with DHA and AA enhances visual acuity or neurological development in preterm or term infants.

- A large body of scientific research suggests that higher dietary omega-3 fatty acid intakes are associated with reductions in cardiovascular disease risk, prompting the American Heart Association to recommend that all adults eat fish, particularly oily fish, at least twice weekly.
- The results of randomized controlled trials indicate that increasing omega-3 fatty acid intake can decrease the risk of MI and sudden cardiac death in individuals with CHD.
- Increasing EPA and DHA intake may be beneficial to individuals with diabetes, especially those with elevated serum triglycerides.
- Randomized controlled trials have found that fish oil supplementation decreases joint tenderness and reduces the requirement for anti_inflammatory medication in rheumatoid arthritis patients.
- Although limited preliminary data suggests that omega-3 fatty acid supplementation may be beneficial in the therapy of depression, bipolar disorder, and schizophrenia, larger controlled clinical trials are needed to determine their efficacy.

References

1. Institute of Medicine. Dietary Reference Intakes for Energy, Carbohydrate, Fiber, Fat, Fatty Acids, Cholesterol, Protein, and Amino Acids. Washington, D.C.: National Academies Press; 2002
2. Simopoulos AP, Leaf A, Salem N Jr. Workshop statement on the essentiality of and recommended dietary intakes for omega-6 and omega-3 fatty acids. Prostaglandins Leukot Essent Fatty Acids 2000; 63(3):119–121
3. Kris-Etherton PM, Harris WS, Appel LJ. Fish consumption, fish oil, omega-3 fatty acids, and cardiovascular disease. Circulation 2002;106(21):2747–2757
4. Lichtenstein AH, Jones PJ. Lipids: absorption and transport. In: Bowman BA, Russel RM, eds. Present Knowledge in Nutrition. 8th ed. Washington, D.C.: ILSI Press; 2001:93–103
5. Nakamura MT, Nara TY. Structure, function, and dietary regulation of delta6, delta5, and delta9 desaturases. Annu Rev Nutr 2004;24:345–376
6. Burdge G. Alpha-linolenic acid metabolism in men and women: nutritional and biological implications. Curr Opin Clin Nutr Metab Care 2004;7(2): 137–144
7. Burdge GC, Jones AE, Wootton SA. Eicosapentaenoic and docosapentaenoic acids are the principal products of alpha-linolenic acid metabolism in young men. Br J Nutr 2002;88(4):355–364
8. Burdge GC, Wootton SA. Conversion of alpha-linolenic acid to eicosapentaenoic, docosapentaenoic and docosahexaenoic acids in young women. Br J Nutr 2002;88(4):411–420
9. Giltay EJ, Gooren LJ, Toorians AW, Katan MB, Zock PL. Docosahexaenoic acid concentrations are higher in women than in men because of estrogenic effects. Am J Clin Nutr 2004;80(5):1167–1174
10. Cunnane SC. Problems with essential fatty acids: time for a new paradigm? Prog Lipid Res 2003; 42(6):544–568
11. Muskiet FA, Fokkema MR, Schaafsma A, Boersma ER, Crawford MA. Is docosahexaenoic acid (DHA) essential? Lessons from DHA status regulation, our ancient diet, epidemiology and randomized controlled trials. J Nutr 2004;134(1):183–186
12. Stillwell W, Wassall SR. Docosahexaenoic acid: membrane properties of a unique fatty acid. Chem Phys Lipids 2003;126(1):1–27
13. Jeffrey BG, Weisingerb HS, Neuringer M, Mitcheli DC. The role of docosahexaenoic acid in retinal function. Lipids 2001;36(9):859–871
14. SanGiovanni JP, Chew EY. The role of omega-3 long-chain polyunsaturated fatty acids in health and disease of the retina. Prog Retin Eye Res 2005;24(1): 87–138
15. Innis SM. Perinatal biochemistry and physiology of long-chain polyunsaturated fatty acids. J Pediatr 2003;143(4 Suppl):S1–S8
16. Chalon S, Vancassel S, Zimmer L, Guilloteau D, Durand G. Polyunsaturated fatty acids and cerebral function: focus on monoaminergic neurotransmission. Lipids 2001;36(9):937–944
17. Calder PC. Dietary modification of inflammation with lipids. Proc Nutr Soc 2002;61(3):345–358
18. Price PT, Nelson CM, Clarke SD. Omega-3 polyunsaturated fatty acid regulation of gene expression. Curr Opin Lipidol 2000;11(1):3–7
19. Sampath H, Ntambi JM. Polyunsaturated fatty acid regulation of gene expression. Nutr Rev 2004;62(9): 333–339
20. Jeppesen PB, Hoy CE, Mortensen PB. Essential fatty acid deficiency in patients receiving home parenteral nutrition. Am J Clin Nutr 1998;68(1):126–133
21. Smit EN, Muskiet FA, Boersma ER. The possible role of essential fatty acids in the pathophysiology of malnutrition: a review. Prostaglandins Leukot Essent Fatty Acids 2004;71(4):241–250
22. Mascioli EA, Lopes SM, Champagne C, Driscoll DF. Essential fatty acid deficiency and home total parenteral nutrition patients. Nutrition 1996;12(4): 245–249
23. Steglink LD, Freeman JB, Wispe J, Connor WE. Absence of the biochemical symptoms of essential fatty acid deficiency in surgical patients undergoing protein sparing therapy. Am J Clin Nutr 1977;30(3):388–393
24. Jeppesen PB, Hoy CE, Mortensen PB. Deficiencies of essential fatty acids, vitamin A and E and changes in plasma lipoproteins in patients with reduced fat absorption or intestinal failure. Eur J Clin Nutr 2000; 54(8):632–642
25. Lepage G, Levy E, Ronco N, Smith L, Galeano N, Roy CC. Direct transesterification of plasma fatty acids for the diagnosis of essential fatty acid deficiency in cystic fibrosis. J Lipid Res 1989;30(10):1483–1490

26. Holman RT, Johnson SB, Hatch TF. A case of human linolenic acid deficiency involving neurological abnormalities. Am J Clin Nutr 1982;35(3):617–623

27. Uauy R, Hoffman DR, Peirano P, Birch DG, Birch EE. Essential fatty acids in visual and brain development. Lipids 2001;36(9):885–895

28. Larque E, Demmelmair H, Koletzko B. Perinatal supply and metabolism of long-chain polyunsaturated fatty acids: importance for the early development of the nervous system. Ann N Y Acad Sci 2002; 967:299–310

29. Simmer K. Longchain polyunsaturated fatty acid supplementation in infants born at term. Cochrane Database Syst Rev 2001;4:CD000376

30. Simmer K, Patole S. Longchain polyunsaturated fatty acid supplementation in preterm infants. Cochrane Database Syst Rev 2004;1:CD000375

31. Uauy R, Hoffman DR, Mena P, Llanos A, Birch EE. Term infant studies of DHA and ARA supplementation on neurodevelopment: results of randomized controlled trials. J Pediatr 2003;143(4 Suppl):S17–S25

32. SanGiovanni JP, Parra-Cabrera S, Colditz GA, Berkey CS, Dwyer JT. Meta-analysis of dietary essential fatty acids and long-chain polyunsaturated fatty acids as they relate to visual resolution acuity in healthy preterm infants. Pediatrics 2000;105(6):1292–1298

33. Fewtrell MS, Morley R, Abbott RA, et al. Double-blind, randomized trial of long-chain polyunsaturated fatty acid supplementation in formula fed to preterm infants. Pediatrics 2002;110(1 Pt 1):73–82

34. O'Connor DL, Hall R, Adamkin D, et al. Growth and development in preterm infants fed long-chain polyunsaturated fatty acids: a prospective, randomized controlled trial. Pediatrics 2001;108(2):359–371

35. Gibson RA, Chen W, Makrides M. Randomized trials with polyunsaturated fatty acid interventions in preterm and term infants: functional and clinical outcomes. Lipids 2001;36(9):873–883

36. Auestad N, Scott DT, Janowsky JS, et al. Visual, cognitive, and language assessments at 39 months: a follow-up study of children fed formulas containing long-chain polyunsaturated fatty acids to 1 year of age. Pediatrics 2003;112(3 Pt 1):e177–e183

37. Birch EE, Castaneda YS, Wheaton DH, Birch DG, Uauy RD, Hoffman DR. Visual maturation of term infants fed long-chain polyunsaturated fatty acid-supplemented or control formula for 12 mo. Am J Clin Nutr 2005;81(4):871–879

38. Koo WW. Efficacy and safety of docosahexaenoic acid and arachidonic acid addition to infant formulas: can one buy better vision and intelligence? J Am Coll Nutr 2003;22(2):101–107

39. Makrides M, Gibson RA. Long-chain polyunsaturated fatty acid requirements during pregnancy and lactation. Am J Clin Nutr 2000;71(1 Suppl):307S–311S

40. Smuts CM, Huang M, Mundy D, Plasse T, Major S, Carlson SE. A randomized trial of docosahexaenoic acid supplementation during the third trimester of pregnancy. Obstet Gynecol 2003;101(3):469–479

41. Olsen SF, Sorensen JD, Secher NJ, et al. Randomised controlled trial of effect of fish-oil supplementation on pregnancy duration. Lancet 1992;339(8800): 1003–1007

42. Onwude JL, Lilford RJ, Hjartardottir H, Staines A, Tuffnell D. A randomised double blind placebo con-trolled trial of fish oil in high risk pregnancy. Br J Obstet Gynaecol 1995;102(2):95–100

43. Olsen SF, Secher NJ, Tabor A, Weber T, Walker JJ, Gluud C. Randomised clinical trials of fish oil supplementation in high risk pregnancies. Fish Oil Trials In Pregnancy (FOTIP) Team. BJOG 2000;107(3):382–395

44. Helland IB, Smith L, Saarem K, Saugstad OD, Drevon CA. Maternal supplementation with very-long-chain n-3 fatty acids during pregnancy and lactation augments children's IQ at 4 years of age. Pediatrics 2003;111(1):e39–e44

45. Kris-Etherton PM, Hecker KD, Binkoski AE. Polyunsaturated fatty acids and cardiovascular health. Nutr Rev 2004;62(11):414–426

46. Ascherio A, Rimm EB, Giovannucci EL, Spiegelman D, Stampfer M, Willett WC. Dietary fat and risk of coronary heart disease in men: cohort follow up study in the United States. BMJ 1996;313(7049):84–90

47. Oh K, Hu FB, Manson JE, Stampfer MJ, Willett WC. Dietary fat intake and risk of coronary heart disease in women: 20 years of follow-up of the nurses' health study. Am J Epidemiol 2005;161(7):672–679

48. Shekelle RB, Shryock AM, Paul O, et al. Diet, serum cholesterol, and death from coronary heart disease. The Western Electric study. N Engl J Med 1981; 304(2):65–70

49. Sacks FM, Katan M. Randomized clinical trials on the effects of dietary fat and carbohydrate on plasma lipoproteins and cardiovascular disease. Am J Med 2002;113(Suppl 9B):13S–24S

50. Mensink RP, Katan MB. Effect of dietary fatty acids on serum lipids and lipoproteins. A meta-analysis of 27 trials. Arterioscler Thromb 1992;12(8):911–919

51. Controlled trial of soya-bean oil in myocardial infarction. Lancet 1968;2(7570):693–699

52. Dayton S, Pearce ML, Goldman H, et al. Controlled trial of a diet high in unsaturated fat for prevention of atherosclerotic complications. Lancet 1968; 2(7577):1060–1062

53. Leren P. The Oslo diet-heart study. Eleven-year report. Circulation 1970;42(5):935–942

54. Turpeinen O, Karvonen MJ, Pekkarinen M, Miettinen M, Elosuo R, Paavilainen E. Dietary prevention of coronary heart disease: the Finnish Mental Hospital Study. Int J Epidemiol 1979;8(2):99–118

55. Frantz ID Jr, Dawson EA, Ashman PL, et al. Test of effect of lipid lowering by diet on cardiovascular risk. The Minnesota Coronary Survey. Arteriosclerosis 1989;9(1):129–135

56. Miettinen M, Turpeinen O, Karvonen MJ, Pekkarinen M, Paavilainen E, Elosuo R. Dietary prevention of coronary heart disease in women: the Finnish mental hospital study. Int J Epidemiol 1983;12(1):17–25

57. Mozaffarian D, Ascherio A, Hu FB, et al. Interplay between different polyunsaturated fatty acids and risk of coronary heart disease in men. Circulation 2005; 111(2):157–164

58. Hu FB, Stampfer MJ, Manson JE, et al. Dietary intake of alpha-linolenic acid and risk of fatal ischemic heart disease among women. Am J Clin Nutr 1999; 69(5):890–897

59. Dolecek TA. Epidemiological evidence of relationships between dietary polyunsaturated fatty acids and mortality in the multiple risk factor intervention trial. Proc Soc Exp Biol Med 1992;200(2):177–182

60. Oomen CM, Ocke MC, Feskens EJ, Kok FJ, Kromhout D. Alpha-linolenic acid intake is not beneficially associated with 10-y risk of coronary artery disease incidence: the Zutphen Elderly Study. Am J Clin Nutr 2001;74(4):457–463

61. Pietinen P, Ascherio A, Korhonen P, et al. Intake of fatty acids and risk of coronary heart disease in a cohort of Finnish men. The Alpha-Tocopherol, Beta-Carotene Cancer Prevention Study. Am J Epidemiol 1997;145(10):876–887

62. Mozaffarian D. Does alpha-linolenic acid intake reduce the risk of coronary heart disease? A review of the evidence. Altern Ther Health Med 2005;11(3): 24–30; quiz 31, 79

63. Bemelmans WJ, Lefrandt JD, Feskens EJ, et al. Increased alpha-linolenic acid intake lowers C-reactive protein, but has no effect on markers of atherosclerosis. Eur J Clin Nutr 2004;58(7):1083–1089

64. Rallidis LS, Paschos G, Liakos GK, Velissaridou AH, Anastasiadis G, Zampelas A. Dietary alpha-linolenic acid decreases C-reactive protein, serum amyloid A and interleukin-6 in dyslipidaemic patients. Atherosclerosis 2003;167(2):237–242

65. Zhao G, Etherton TD, Martin KR, West SG, Gillies PJ, Kris-Etherton PM. Dietary alpha-linolenic acid reduces inflammatory and lipid cardiovascular risk factors in hypercholesterolemic men and women. J Nutr 2004;134(11):2991–2997

66. Kris-Etherton PM, Harris WS, Appel LJ. Omega-3 fatty acids and cardiovascular disease: new recommendations from the American Heart Association. Arterioscler Thromb Vasc Biol 2003;23(2):151–152

67. Kromhout D, Bosschieter EB, de Lezenne Coulander C. The inverse relation between fish consumption and 20-year mortality from coronary heart disease. N Engl J Med 1985;312(19):1205–1209

68. Kromhout D, Feskens EJ, Bowles CH. The protective effect of a small amount of fish on coronary heart disease mortality in an elderly population. Int J Epidemiol 1995;24(2):340–345

69. Dolecek TA, Granditis G. Dietary polyunsaturated fatty acids and mortality in the Multiple Risk Factor Intervention Trial (MRFIT). World Rev Nutr Diet 1991;66:205–216

70. Daviglus ML, Stamler J, Orencia AJ, et al. Fish consumption and the 30-year risk of fatal myocardial infarction. N Engl J Med 1997;336(15):1046–1053

71. Yuan JM, Ross RK, Gao YT, Yu MC. Fish and shellfish consumption in relation to death from myocardial infarction among men in Shanghai, China. Am J Epidemiol 2001;154(9):809–816

72. Hu FB, Bronner L, Willett WC, et al. Fish and omega-3 fatty acid intake and risk of coronary heart disease in women. JAMA 2002;287(14):1815–1821

73. Leaf A, Xiao YF, Kang JX, Billman GE. Prevention of sudden cardiac death by n-3 polyunsaturated fatty acids. Pharmacol Ther 2003;98(3):355–377

74. Albert CM, Hennekens CH, O'Donnell CJ, et al. Fish consumption and risk of sudden cardiac death. JAMA 1998;279(1):23–28

75. Albert CM, Campos H, Stampfer MJ, et al. Blood levels of long-chain n-3 fatty acids and the risk of sudden death. N Engl J Med 2002;346(15):1113–1118

76. American Stroke Association. What is a stroke? 2002. Available at: http://www.strokeassociation.org/presenter.jhtml?identifier=2528

77. Keli SO, Feskens EJ, Kromhout D. Fish consumption and risk of stroke. The Zutphen Study. Stroke 1994;25(2):328–332

78. Gillum RF, Mussolino ME, Madans JH. The relationship between fish consumption and stroke incidence. The NHANES I Epidemiologic Follow-up Study (National Health and Nutrition Examination Survey). Arch Intern Med 1996;156(5):537–542

79. Morris MC, Manson JE, Rosner B, Buring JE, Willett WC, Hennekens CH. Fish consumption and cardiovascular disease in the physicians' health study: a prospective study. Am J Epidemiol 1995;142(2):166–175

80. Orencia AJ, Daviglus ML, Dyer AR, Shekelle RB, Stamler J. Fish consumption and stroke in men. 30-year findings of the Chicago Western Electric Study. Stroke 1996;27(2):204–209

81. Iso H, Rexrode KM, Stampfer MJ, et al. Intake of fish and omega-3 fatty acids and risk of stroke in women. JAMA 2001;285(3):304–312

82. He K, Rimm EB, Merchant A, et al. Fish consumption and risk of stroke in men. JAMA 2002;288(24):3130–3136

83. Austin MA, Hokanson JE, Edwards KL. Hypertriglyceridemia as a cardiovascular risk factor. Am J Cardiol 1998;81(4A):7B–12B

84. Harris WS. n-3 fatty acids and serum lipoproteins: human studies. Am J Clin Nutr 1997;65(5 Suppl):1645S–1654S

85. Burr ML, Fehily AM, Gilbert JF, et al. Effects of changes in fat, fish, and fibre intakes on death and myocardial reinfarction: diet and reinfarction trial (DART). Lancet 1989;2(8666):757–761

86. de Lorgeril M, Salen P, Martin JL, Monjaud I, Delaye J, Mamelle N. Mediterranean diet, traditional risk factors, and the rate of cardiovascular complications after myocardial infarction: final report of the Lyon Diet Heart Study. Circulation 1999;99(6):779–785

87. Dietary supplementation with n-3 polyunsaturated fatty acids and vitamin E after myocardial infarction: results of the GISSI-Prevenzione trial. Gruppo Italiano per lo Studio della Sopravvivenza nell'Infarto miocardico. Lancet 1999;354(9177):447–455

88. Marchioli R, Barzi F, Bomba E, et al. Early protection against sudden death by n-3 polyunsaturated fatty acids after myocardial infarction: time-course analysis of the results of the Gruppo Italiano per lo Studio della Sopravvivenza nell'Infarto Miocardico (GISSI)-Prevenzione. Circulation 2002;105(16): 1897–1903

89. Singh RB, Niaz MA, Sharma JP, Kumar R, Rastogi V, Moshiri M. Randomized, double-blind, placebo-controlled trial of fish oil and mustard oil in patients with suspected acute myocardial infarction: the Indian experiment of infarct survival-4. Cardiovasc Drugs Ther 1997;11(3):485–491

90. Nilsen DW, Albrektsen G, Landmark K, Moen S, Aarsland T, Woie L. Effects of a high-dose concentrate of n-3 fatty acids or corn oil introduced early after an acute myocardial infarction on serum triacylglycerol and HDL cholesterol. Am J Clin Nutr 2001;74(1):50–56

91. Bucher HC, Hengstler P, Schindler C, Meier G. N-3 polyunsaturated fatty acids in coronary heart disease: a meta-analysis of randomized controlled trials. Am J Med 2002;112(4):298–304

92. Sacks FM, Stone PH, Gibson CM, Silverman DI, Rosner B, Pasternak RC. Controlled trial of fish oil for regression of human coronary atherosclerosis. HARP Research Group. J Am Coll Cardiol 1995;25(7):1492–1498

93. von Schacky C, Angerer P, Kothny W, Theisen K, Mudra H. The effect of dietary omega-3 fatty acids on coronary atherosclerosis. A randomized, double-blind, placebo-controlled trial. Ann Intern Med 1999;130(7):554–562

94. Balk E, Chung M, Lichtenstein A, et al. Effects of omega-3 fatty acids on cardiovascular risk factors and intermediate markers of cardiovascular disease. Evid Rep Technol Assess (Summ) 2004;93:1–6

95. Montori VM, Farmer A, Wollan PC, Dinneen SF. Fish oil supplementation in type 2 diabetes: a quantitative systematic review. Diabetes Care 2000;23(9): 1407–1415

96. Glauber H, Wallace P, Griver K, Brechtel G. Adverse metabolic effect of omega-3 fatty acids in non-insulin-dependent diabetes mellitus. Ann Intern Med 1988;108(5):663–668

97. Friday KE, Childs MT, Tsunehara CH, Fujimoto WY, Bierman EL, Ensinck JW. Elevated plasma glucose and lowered triglyceride levels from omega-3 fatty acid supplementation in type II diabetes. Diabetes Care 1989;12(4):276–281

98. MacLean CH, Mojica WA, Morton SC, et al. Effects of omega-3 fatty acids on lipids and glycemic control in type II diabetes and the metabolic syndrome and on inflammatory bowel disease, rheumatoid arthritis, renal disease, systemic lupus erythematosus, and osteoporosis. Evid Rep Technol Assess (Summ) 2004;89:1–4

99. Hu FB, Cho E, Rexrode KM, Albert CM, Manson JE. Fish and long-chain omega-3 fatty acid intake and risk of coronary heart disease and total mortality in diabetic women. Circulation 2003;107(14):1852–1857

100. Nettleton JA, Katz R. n-3 long-chain polyunsaturated fatty acids in type 2 diabetes: a review. J Am Diet Assoc 2005;105(3):428–440

101. Friedberg CE, Janssen MJ, Heine RJ, Grobbee DE. Fish oil and glycemic control in diabetes. A meta-analysis. Diabetes Care 1998;21(4):494–500

102. Franz MJ, Bantle JP, Beebe CA, et al. Evidence-based nutrition principles and recommendations for the treatment and prevention of diabetes and related complications. Diabetes Care 2003;26(Suppl 1):S51–S61

103. Fortin PR, Lew RA, Liang MH, et al. Validation of a meta-analysis: the effects of fish oil in rheumatoid arthritis. J Clin Epidemiol 1995;48(11):1379–1390

104. Kremer JM. n-3 fatty acid supplements in rheumatoid arthritis. Am J Clin Nutr 2000;71(1 Suppl):349S–351S

105. Lorenz R, Weber PC, Szimnau P, Heldwein W, Strasser T, Loeschke K. Supplementation with n-3 fatty acids from fish oil in chronic inflammatory bowel disease–a randomized, placebo-controlled, double-blind cross-over trial. J Intern Med Suppl 1989;731:225–232

106. Lorenz-Meyer H, Bauer P, Nicolay C, et al. Omega-3 fatty acids and low carbohydrate diet for maintenance of remission in Crohn's disease. A randomized controlled multicenter trial. Study Group

Members (German Crohn's Disease Study Group). Scand J Gastroenterol 1996;31(8):778–785

107. Belluzzi A, Brignola C, Campieri M, Pera A, Boschi S, Miglioli M. Effect of an enteric-coated fish-oil preparation on relapses in Crohn's disease. N Engl J Med 1996;334(24):1557–1560

108. Aslan A, Triadafilopoulos G. Fish oil fatty acid supplementation in active ulcerative colitis: a double-blind, placebo-controlled, crossover study. Am J Gastroenterol 1992;87(4):432–437

109. Hawthorne AB, Daneshmend TK, Hawkey CJ, et al. Treatment of ulcerative colitis with fish oil supplementation: a prospective 12 month randomised controlled trial. Gut 1992;33(7):922–928

110. Stenson WF, Cort D, Rodgers J, et al. Dietary supplementation with fish oil in ulcerative colitis. Ann Intern Med 1992;116(8):609–614

111. Loeschke K, Ueberschaer B, Pietsch A, et al. n-3 fatty acids only delay early relapse of ulcerative colitis in remission. Dig Dis Sci 1996;41(10):2087–2094

112. Hodge L, Salome CM, Hughes JM, et al. Effect of dietary intake of omega-3 and omega-6 fatty acids on severity of asthma in children. Eur Respir J 1998;11(2):361–365

113. Okamoto M, Mitsunobu F, Ashida K, et al. Effects of dietary supplementation with n-3 fatty acids compared with n-6 fatty acids on bronchial asthma. Intern Med 2000;39(2):107–111

114. Wong KW. Clinical efficacy of n-3 fatty acid supplementation in patients with asthma. J Am Diet Assoc 2005;105(1):98–105

115. Schachter HM, Reisman J, Tran K, et al. Health effects of omega-3 fatty acids on asthma. Evid Rep Technol Assess (Summ) 2004;91:1–7

116. Woods RK, Thien FC, Abramson MJ. Dietary marine fatty acids (fish oil) for asthma in adults and children. Cochrane Database Syst Rev 2002;3:CD001283

117. Donadio JV, Grande JP. IgA nephropathy. N Engl J Med 2002;347(10):738–748

118. Donadio JV Jr, Bergstralh EJ, Offord KP, Spencer DC, Holley KE. A controlled trial of fish oil in IgA nephropathy. Mayo Nephrology Collaborative Group. N Engl J Med 1994;331(18):1194–1199

119. Donadio JV Jr, Grande JP, Bergstralh EJ, Dart RA, Larson TS, Spencer DC. The long-term outcome of patients with IgA nephropathy treated with fish oil in a controlled trial. Mayo Nephrology Collaborative Group. J Am Soc Nephrol 1999;10(8):1772–1777

120. Donadio JV Jr, Larson TS, Bergstralh EJ, Grande JP. A randomized trial of high-dose compared with low-dose omega-3 fatty acids in severe IgA nephropathy. J Am Soc Nephrol 2001;12(4):791–799

121. Bennett WM, Walker RG, Kincaid-Smith P. Treatment of IgA nephropathy with eicosapentanoic acid (EPA): a two-year prospective trial. Clin Nephrol 1989;31(3):128–131

122. Cheng IK, Chan PC, Chan MK. The effect of fish-oil dietary supplement on the progression of mesangial IgA glomerulonephritis. Nephrol Dial Transplant 1990;5(4):241–246

123. Pettersson EE, Rekola S, Berglund L, et al. Treatment of IgA nephropathy with omega-3-polyunsaturated fatty acids: a prospective, double-blind, randomized study. Clin Nephrol 1994;41(4):183–190

124. Branten AJ, Klasen IS, Wetzels JF. Short-term effects of fish oil treatment on urinary excretion of high-

and low-molecular weight proteins in patients with IgA nephropathy. Clin Nephrol 2002;58(4):267–274

125. Dillon JJ. Fish oil therapy for IgA nephropathy: efficacy and interstudy variability. J Am Soc Nephrol 1997;8(11):1739–1744

126. Strippoli GF, Manno C, Schena FP. An "evidence-based" survey of therapeutic options for IgA nephropathy: assessment and criticism. Am J Kidney Dis 2003;41(6):1129–1139

127. Hibbeln JR. Fish consumption and major depression. Lancet 1998;351(9110):1213

128. Noaghiul S, Hibbeln JR. Cross-national comparisons of seafood consumption and rates of bipolar disorders. Am J Psychiatry 2003;160(12):2222–2227

129. Maes M, Christophe A, Delanghe J, Altamura C, Neels H, Meltzer HY. Lowered omega3 polyunsaturated fatty acids in serum phospholipids and cholesteryl esters of depressed patients. Psychiatry Res 1999; 85(3):275–291

130. Peet M, Murphy B, Shay J, Horrobin D. Depletion of omega-3 fatty acid levels in red blood cell membranes of depressive patients. Biol Psychiatry 1998;43(5):315–319

131. Mamalakis G, Tornaritis M, Kafatos A. Depression and adipose essential polyunsaturated fatty acids. Prostaglandins Leukot Essent Fatty Acids 2002; 67(5):311–318

132. Locke CA, Stoll AL. Omega-3 fatty acids in major depression. World Rev Nutr Diet 2001;89:173–185

133. Silvers KM, Woolley CC, Hamilton FC, Watts PM, Watson RA. Randomised double-blind placebo-controlled trial of fish oil in the treatment of depression. Prostaglandins Leukot Essent Fatty Acids 2005; 72(3):211–218

134. Marangell LB, Martinez JM, Zboyan HA, Kertz B, Kim HF, Puryear LJ. A double-blind, placebo-controlled study of the omega-3 fatty acid docosahexaenoic acid in the treatment of major depression. Am J Psychiatry 2003;160(5):996–998

135. Su KP, Huang SY, Chiu CC, Shen WW. Omega-3 fatty acids in major depressive disorder. A preliminary double-blind, placebo-controlled trial. Eur Neuropsychopharmacol 2003;13(4):267–271

136. Zanarini MC, Frankenburg FR. Omega-3 fatty acid treatment of women with borderline personality disorder: a double-blind, placebo-controlled pilot study. Am J Psychiatry 2003;160(1):167–169

137. Stoll AL, Severus WE, Freeman MP, et al. Omega 3 fatty acids in bipolar disorder: a preliminary double-blind, placebo-controlled trial. Arch Gen Psychiatry 1999;56(5):407–412

138. Assies J, Lieverse R, Vreken P, Wanders RJ, Dingemans PM, Linszen DH. Significantly reduced docosahexaenoic and docosapentaenoic acid concentrations in erythrocyte membranes from schizophrenic patients compared with a carefully matched control group. Biol Psychiatry 2001;49(6):510–522

139. Horrobin DF, Manku MS, Hillman H, Iain A, Glen M. Fatty acid levels in the brains of schizophrenics and normal controls. Biol Psychiatry 1991;30(8):795–805

140. Laugharne JD, Mellor JE, Peet M. Fatty acids and schizophrenia. Lipids 1996;31(Suppl):S163–S165

141. Peet M, Brind J, Ramchand CN, Shah S, Vankar GK. Two double-blind placebo-controlled pilot studies of eicosapentaenoic acid in the treatment of schizophrenia. Schizophr Res 2001;49(3):243–251

142. Emsley R, Myburgh C, Oosthuizen P, van Rensburg SJ. Randomized, placebo-controlled study of ethyl-eicosapentaenoic acid as supplemental treatment in schizophrenia. Am J Psychiatry 2002;159(9):1596–1598

143. Fenton WS, Dickerson F, Boronow J, Hibbeln JR, Knable M. A placebo-controlled trial of omega-3 fatty acid (ethyl eicosapentaenoic acid) supplementation for residual symptoms and cognitive impairment in schizophrenia. Am J Psychiatry 2001; 158(12):2071–2074

144. Peet M, Horrobin DF. A dose-ranging exploratory study of the effects of ethyl-eicosapentaenoate in patients with persistent schizophrenic symptoms. J Psychiatr Res 2002;36(1):7–18

145. Joy CB, Mumby-Croft R, Joy LA. Polyunsaturated fatty acid supplementation for schizophrenia. Cochrane Database Syst Rev 2003;2:CD001257

146. U. S. Department of Agriculture, Agricultural Research Service. USDA Nutrient Database for Standard Reference, Release 18. 2005. Available at: http://www.nal.usda.gov/fnic/foodcomp. Accessed 7/26/06

147. Hendler SS, Rorvik DR, eds. PDR for Nutritional Supplements. Montvale: Medical Economics Company, Inc; 2001

148. U.S. Food and Drug Administration, Center for Food Safety and Applied Nutrition. Agency response letter: GRAS Notice No. GRN 000080. 2001. Available at: http://www.cfsan.fda.gov/~rdb/opa-g080.html

149. Zurier RB, Rossetti RG, Jacobson EW, et al. Gamma-linolenic acid treatment of rheumatoid arthritis. A randomized, placebo-controlled trial. Arthritis Rheum 1996;39(11):1808–1817

150. Vaddadi KS. The use of gamma-linolenic acid and linoleic acid to differentiate between temporal lobe epilepsy and schizophrenia. Prostaglandins Med 1981;6(4):375–379

151. Nordstrom DC, Honkanen VE, Nasu Y, Antila E, Friman C, Konttinen YT. Alpha-linolenic acid in the treatment of rheumatoid arthritis. A double-blind, placebo-controlled and randomized study: flaxseed vs. safflower seed. Rheumatol Int 1995;14(6):231–234

152. Alonso L, Marcos ML, Blanco JG, et al. Anaphylaxis caused by linseed (flaxseed) intake. J Allergy Clin Immunol 1996;98(2):469–470

153. Harbige LS. Fatty acids, the immune response, and autoimmunity: a question of n-6 essentiality and the balance between n-6 and n-3. Lipids 2003;38(4): 323–341

154. Carlson SE, Cooke RJ, Werkman SH, Tolley EA. First year growth of preterm infants fed standard compared to marine oil n-3 supplemented formula. Lipids 1992;27(11):901–907

155. Environmental Protection Agency. Fish advisories. 2003. Available at: http://www.epa.gov/waterscience/fish/. Accessed 7/26/06

156. U.S. Department of Health and Human Services, U.S. Environmental Protection Agency. What you need to know about mercury in fish and shellfish. 2004. Available at: http://www.cfsan.fda.gov/~dms/admehg3.html. Accessed 7/26/06

157. Omega-3 oil: fish or pills? Consum Rep 2003;68(7): 30–32

158. ConsumerLab. Product review: Omega-3 fatty acids (EPA and DHA) from fish/marine oils. 2005. Available at: http://www.consumerlab.com/results/omega3.asp. Accessed 7/26/06

159. Melanson SF, Lewandrowski EL, Flood JG, Lewandrowski KB. Measurement of organochlorines in commercial over-the-counter fish oil preparations: implications for dietary and therapeutic recommendations for omega-3 fatty acids and a review of the literature. Arch Pathol Lab Med 2005;129(1):74–77

160. Hilbert G, Lillemark L, Balchen S, Hojskov CS. Reduction of organochlorine contaminants from fish oil during refining. Chemosphere 1998;37(7):1241–1252

161. Bender NK, Kraynak MA, Chiquette E, Linn WD, Clark GM, Bussey HI. Effects of marine fish oils on the anticoagulation status of patients receiving chronic warfarin therapy. J Thromb Thrombolysis 1998;5(3):257–261

162. Buckley MS, Goff AD, Knapp WE. Fish oil interaction with warfarin. Ann Pharmacother 2004;38(1):50–52

163. Valk EE, Hornstra G. Relationship between vitamin E requirement and polyunsaturated fatty acid intake in man: a review. Int J Vitam Nutr Res 2000;70(2):31–42

164. Higdon JV, Liu J, Du SH, Morrow JD, Ames BN, Wander RC. Supplementation of postmenopausal women with fish oil rich in eicosapentaenoic acid and docosahexaenoic acid is not associated with greater in vivo lipid peroxidation compared with oils rich in oleate and linoleate as assessed by plasma malondialdehyde and F(2)-isoprostanes. Am J Clin Nutr 2000;72(3):714–722

165. Wander RC, Du SH, Ketchum SO, Rowe KE. Alpha-tocopherol influences in vivo indices of lipid peroxidation in postmenopausal women given fish oil. J Nutr 1996;126(3):643–652

166. Wander RC, Du SH. Oxidation of plasma proteins is not increased after supplementation with eicosapentaenoic and docosahexaenoic acids. Am J Clin Nutr 2000;72(3):731–737

167. European Commission Directorate General for Health and Consumer Protection. Eurodiet: nutrition and diet for healthy lifestyles in Europe. 2001. Available at: http://europa.eu.int/comm/health/ph/programmes/health/reports/report01_en.pdf

168. World Health Organization, Food And Agriculture Organization. Joint WHO/FAO Expert Consultation on Diet, Nutrition and the Prevention of Chronic Diseases. 2002. Available at: http://www.who.int/hpr/NPH/docs/who_fao_expert_report.pdf

169. Hamazaki T, Okuyama H. The Japan Society for Lipid Nutrition recommends to reduce the intake of linoleic acid. A review and critique of the scientific evidence. World Rev Nutr Diet 2003;92:109–132

12 Fiber

All fibers are resistant to digestion in the small intestine, meaning they arrive at the colon intact.[1] Although most fibers are carbohydrates, one important factor that determines their susceptibility to digestion by human enzymes is the conformation of the chemical bonds between sugar molecules (glycosidic bonds). Humans lack digestive enzymes capable of hydrolyzing most β-glycosidic bonds, which explains why amylose, a glucose polymer with α-1,4 glycosidic bonds, is digestible by human enzymes, whereas cellulose, a glucose polymer with β-1,4 glycosidic bonds, is indigestible (**Fig. 12–1**).

Definitions of Fiber

Although nutrition scientists and clinicians generally agree that a healthy diet should include plenty of fiber-rich foods, agreement on the actual definition of fiber has been more difficult to achieve.[2-4] In the 1970s, dietary fiber was defined as remnants of plant cells that are resistant to digestion by human enzymes.[5] This definition includes a component of some plant cell walls called lignin, as well as indigestible carbohydrates found in plants. However, this definition omits indigestible carbohydrates derived from animal sources (e. g., chitin) or synthetic (e. g., fructooligosaccharides) and digestible carbohy-

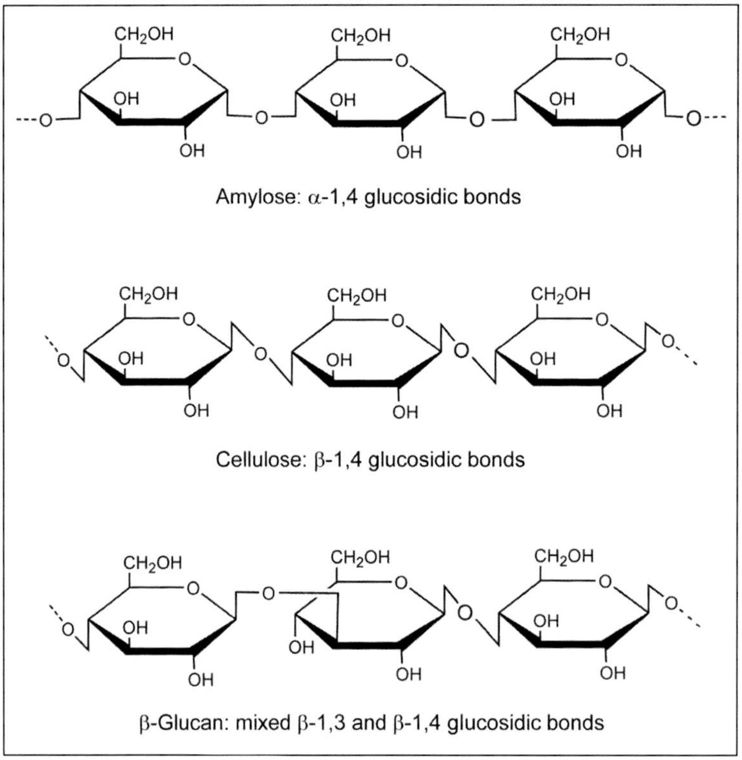

Figure 12–1 Chemical structures of amylose (a digestible carbohydrate), cellulose (a fiber that is not digestible by human enzymes), and β-glucan (a fiber).[7]

Amylose: α-1,4 glucosidic bonds

Cellulose: β-1,4 glucosidic bonds

β-Glucan: mixed β-1,3 and β-1,4 glucosidic bonds

drates that are inaccessible to human digestive enzymes (e. g., resistant starch).[6] These compounds share many of the characteristics of fiber present in plant foods.

Observational studies that have identified associations between high-fiber intakes and reductions in chronic disease risk have generally assessed only fiber-rich foods, rather than fiber per se, making it difficult to determine whether observed benefits are related to fiber or other nutrients and phytochemicals commonly found in fiber-rich foods. In contrast, intervention trials often use isolated fibers to determine whether a specific fiber component has beneficial health effects.

U.S. Institute of Medicine Classification System

Before establishing intake recommendations for fiber in 2001, a panel of experts convened by the U.S. Institute of Medicine developed definitions of fiber that made a distinction between fiber that occurs naturally in plant foods (dietary fiber) and isolated or synthetic fibers that may be added to foods or used as dietary supplements (functional fiber).[4]

Dietary Fiber

Lignin—Lignin is not a carbohydrate, but a polyphenolic compound with a complex three-dimensional structure that is found in the cell walls of woody plants and seeds.[7]

Cellulose—Cellulose is a glucose polymer with β-1,4 glycosidic bonds found in all plant cell walls (**Fig. 12–1**).[6]

β-glucans—β-Glucans are glucose polymers with a mixture of β-1,4 glycosidic bonds and β-1,3 glycosidic bonds (**Fig. 12–1**). Oats and barley are particularly rich in β-glucans.[7]

Hemicelluloses—Hemicelluloses are a diverse group of polysaccharides (sugar polymers) found in plant cell walls.[6]

Pectins—Pectins are viscous polysaccharides that are particularly abundant in fruits and berries.[4]

Gums—Gums are viscous polysaccharides often found in seeds.[4]

Inulin and oligofructose—Inulin is a mixture of fructose chains that vary in length and

often terminate with a glucose molecule.[8] Oligofructose is a mixture of shorter fructose chains that may terminate in glucose or fructose. Inulin and oligofructose occur naturally in plants, such as onions and Jerusalem artichokes.

Resistant starch—Naturally occurring resistant starch is starch that is sequestered in plant cell walls and, therefore, inaccessible to human digestive enzymes.[4] Bananas and legumes are sources of naturally occurring resistant starch. Resistant starch may also be formed by food processing or by cooling and reheating.

Functional Fiber

According to the U.S. Institute of Medicine's definition, functional fiber "consists of isolated, nondigestible carbohydrates that have beneficial physiological effects in humans."[4] Functional fibers may be nondigestible carbohydrates that have been isolated or extracted from a natural plant or animal source, or they may be manufactured or synthesized. However, designation as a functional fiber by the U.S. Institute of Medicine will require the presentation of sufficient evidence of physiological benefits in humans. Fibers identified as potential functional fibers by the Institute include:

Isolated fibers—Isolated fibers include isolated or extracted forms of the dietary fibers listed above.

Psyllium—Psyllium refers to viscous mucilage, isolated from the husks of psyllium seeds. The husks are usually isolated from the seeds of *Plantago ovata* or blond psyllium. Psyllium is also known as ispaghula husk.[4]

Chitin and chitosan—Chitin is a nondigestible carbohydrate extracted from the exoskeletons of crustaceans like crabs and lobsters. It is a long polymer of acetylated glucosamine units linked by β-1,4 glycosidic bonds. Deacetylation of chitin is used to produce chitosan, a nondigestible glucosamine polymer.[9]

Fructooligosaccharides—Fructooligosaccharides are short synthetic fructose chains terminating with a glucose unit. They are used as food additives.[8]

Polydextrose and polyols—Polydextrose and polyols are synthetic polysaccharides used as bulking agents and sugar substitutes in foods.[4]

Resistant dextrins—Resistant dextrins, also called resistant maltodextrins, are indigestible polysaccharides formed when starch is heated and treated with enzymes. They are used as food additives.[4]

Total Fiber

Total fiber is defined by the U.S. Institute of Medicine as "the sum of dietary fiber and functional fiber."[4]

Other Classification Systems

Viscous and Nonviscous Fiber

Some fibers form very viscous solutions or gels in water. This property is linked to the ability of some fibers to slow the emptying of the stomach, delay the absorption of some nutrients in the small intestine and lower serum cholesterol. Viscous fibers include pectins, β-glucans, some gums (e. g., guar gum), and mucilages (e. g., psyllium). Cellulose, lignin, and some hemicelluloses are nonviscous fibers.[6,7]

Fermentable and Nonfermentable Fiber

Bacteria that normally colonize the colon readily ferment some fibers. In addition to increasing the amount of bacteria in the colon, fermentation results in the formation of short-chain fatty acids (acetate, propionate, and butyrate) and gases.[1] Short-chain fatty acids can be absorbed and metabolized to produce energy. Interestingly, the preferred energy source for colonocytes (epithelial cells that line the colon) is butyrate. β-Glucans, pectins, guar gum, inulin, and oligofructose are readily fermented, whereas cellulose and lignin are resistant to fermentation in the colon.[6,7] Foods that are rich in fermentable fibers include oats, barley and fruits and vegetables. Cereal fibers that are rich in cellulose, such as wheat bran, are relatively resistant to bacterial fermentation.[1]

Soluble and Insoluble Fiber

Soluble fiber originated as an analytical term.[10] Soluble fibers are dispersible in water; insoluble fibers are not. Originally, the solubility of fiber was thought to predict its physiological effects. For example, soluble fibers were thought more likely to form viscous gels and were more easily fermented by colonic bacteria. Further research has revealed that solubility does not reliably predict the physiological effects of fiber. However, the terms "soluble" and "insoluble" fiber are still used by many nutrition and health care professionals, as well as the U.S. Food and Drug Administration (FDA) for nutrition labeling. β-Glucans, gums, mucilages (e. g., psyllium), pectins, and some hemicelluloses are soluble fibers, whereas cellulose, lignin, some pectins, and some hemicelluloses are insoluble fibers.[10] Oat products and legumes (dry beans, peas, and lentils) are rich sources of soluble fiber.

Biological Activities

Lowering Serum Cholesterol

Numerous controlled clinical trials have found that increasing intakes of viscous dietary fibers, particularly from legumes[11] and oat products,[12,13] decreases serum total and low-density lipoprotein (LDL) cholesterol. These findings led the FDA to approve health claims like the following: "Soluble fiber from foods such as oat bran, as part of a diet low in saturated fat and cholesterol, may reduce the risk of heart disease."[14] Supplementation with viscous fibers, such as pectin, guar gum, and psyllium, has also been found to decrease total and LDL cholesterol levels when compared with low-fiber placebos.[13,15] Although many of these studies examined relatively high-fiber intakes, a meta-analysis that combined the results of 67 controlled trials found that even a modest 10 g/d increase in viscous fiber intake resulted in reductions in LDL-cholesterol averaging 22 mg/dL (0.57 mmol/L) and reductions in total cholesterol averaging 17 mg/dL (0.45 mmol/L).[13]

Decreasing Postprandial Glycemia

The addition of viscous dietary fiber[16,17] and isolated viscous fibers[18,19] to a carbohydrate-containing meal has been found to result in significant improvements in blood glucose and insulin responses in numerous controlled clinical trials.[20] Large, rapid increases in blood glucose levels are potent signals to the β-cells of the pancreas to increase insulin secretion. When the carbohydrate content of two meals is equal, the presence of fiber, particularly viscous fiber, generally results in smaller but more sustained increases in blood glucose and significantly lower insulin levels.[20]

Softening Stool

Increasing intakes of dietary fibers and fiber supplements can prevent or ameliorate constipation by softening and adding bulk to stool and speeding its passage through the colon.[21] Wheat bran and fruits and vegetables are the fiber sources that have been most consistently found to increase stool bulk and shorten transit time.[22] Fiber supplements that have been found to be effective in treating constipation include cellulose and psyllium.[4] Sufficient fluid intake is also required to maximize the stool-softening effect of increased fiber intake.[23] In addition to increasing fiber intake, drinking at least 64 oz ($\sim$ 2 L) of fluid daily is usually recommended to help prevent and treat constipation.[24]

Prevention

Cardiovascular Disease

Prospective cohort studies have consistently found that high intakes of fiber-rich foods are associated with significant reductions in coronary heart disease (CHD) risk.[25-34] Recently, a pooled analysis of 10 prospective cohort studies of dietary fiber intake in the United States and Europe found that each 10 g/d increase in total dietary fiber intake was associated with a 14% decrease in the risk of coronary events, such as myocardial infarction (MI), and a 24% decrease in deaths from CHD.[35] This inverse association between fiber intake and CHD death

was particularly high for cereal fiber and fruit fiber. Findings from the three largest prospective cohort studies[29,30,32] that dietary fiber intakes of $\sim$ 14 g per 1000 kcal of energy were associated with substantial (16 to 33%) decreases in the risk of CHD are the basis for the Institute of Medicine's Adequate Intake (AI) recommendation for fiber (see the Intake Recommendations section below).[4]

Although the cholesterol-lowering effect of viscous dietary fibers and fiber supplements probably contributes to the cardioprotective effects of dietary fiber, other mechanisms are likely to play a role. Beneficial effects of fiber consumption on blood glucose and insulin responses may also contribute to observed reductions in CHD risk.[36] Low-fiber, high-glycemic load diets are associated with higher serum triglyceride levels and lower high-density lipoprotein (HDL) cholesterol levels, also risk factors for cardiovascular disease.[37,38] Diets that are rich in fiber may also help lower blood pressure, another important risk factor for cardiovascular disease. Some observational studies have found inverse associations between dietary fiber intake and blood pressure[39] or hypertension.[40] Two intervention trials found that increasing fiber intake from oat cereals[41] or oat bran[42] resulted in modest but significant reductions in blood pressure compared with low-fiber placebos. Although viscous dietary fibers and fiber supplements appear to be most effective in lowering LDL-cholesterol levels, large epidemiological studies provide strong and consistent evidence that diets rich in all fiber from whole grains, legumes, fruits, and nonstarchy vegetables can significantly reduce CHD risk.[43]

Type 2 Diabetes Mellitus

Increasing intakes of refined carbohydrates and decreasing intakes of fiber in the United States have paralleled the increasing prevalence of type 2 DM to near epidemic proportions.[44] Numerous prospective cohort studies have found that that diets rich in fiber, particularly cereal fiber from whole grains, are associated with significant reductions in the risk of developing type 2 DM.[45-50] Although no intervention trials have evaluated the effect of increasing dietary fiber intake alone on type 2

DM prevention, two important intervention trials found that a combination of lifestyle modifications that included increasing fiber intake decreased the risk of developing type 2 DM in adults with impaired glucose tolerance.[51,52] Although multiple factors, including obesity, inactivity, and genetic factors, increase the risk of developing type 2 DM, the results of observational studies and intervention trials indicate that fiber-rich diets improve glucose tolerance and decrease the risk of type 2 DM, particularly in high-risk individuals.

Cancer

Colorectal Cancer

The majority of case-control studies conducted prior to 1990 found the incidence of colorectal cancer was lower in people with higher fiber intakes.[53,54] In contrast, most prospective cohort studies conducted more recently have not found significant associations between measures of dietary fiber intake and colorectal cancer risk.[55-61] Three controlled clinical trials also failed to demonstrate a protective effect of fiber consumption on the recurrence of colorectal adenomas (precancerous polyps). The rate of recurrence of colorectal adenomas over a 4-year period was not significantly different between those who consumed ~ 33 g/d of fiber from a fruit and vegetable-rich, low-fat diet and those in a control group who consumed ~ 19 g/d.[62] In another trial, there was no significant difference in the rate of colorectal adenoma recurrence over a 3-year period between those supplemented with 13.5 g/d of wheat bran fiber and those supplemented with 2 g/d.[63] Surprisingly, supplementation with 3.5 g/d of psyllium for 3 years resulted in a significant increase in adenoma recurrence compared with placebo.[64]

The reasons for the discrepancies between the findings of early case-control studies with those of most prospective cohort studies and recent intervention trials have generated considerable debate among scientists. Potential reasons for the lack of a protective effect by dietary fiber observed in these studies include the possibility that the type or the amount of fiber consumed by most people in these studies was inadequate to prevent colorectal cancer,[4] or that other dietary factors like fat may interact with fiber, influencing its effects on colorectal cancer.[1,65] Clearly, more research is needed to sort out the complex effects of dietary fiber and fiber supplements on colorectal cancer risk and progression.

Breast Cancer

Although several early case-control studies found significant inverse associations between dietary fiber intake and breast cancer incidence,[66-69] the majority of prospective cohort studies have not found dietary fiber intake to be associated with significant reductions in breast cancer risk.[70-73] The only exception was a prospective cohort study in Sweden, which found that women with the highest fiber intakes (averaging ~ 26 g/d) had a risk of breast cancer that was 40% lower than women with the lowest fiber intakes (averaging ~ 13 g/d).[74] Those women with the highest fiber and lowest fat intakes had the very lowest risk of breast cancer. The results of small short-term intervention trials in premenopausal and postmenopausal women suggest that low-fat (10 to 25% of energy), high-fiber (25 to 40 g/d) diets could decrease circulating estrogen levels by increasing the excretion of estrogens and promoting the metabolism of estrogens to less estrogenic forms.[75,76] However, it is not known whether fiber-associated effects on endogenous estrogen levels have a clinically significant impact on breast cancer risk.[4] At present, the available evidence does not support the idea that high-fiber intakes significantly decrease the risk of breast cancer in women.

Diverticular Disease

High-fiber intakes are associated with decreased risk of diverticulosis, a relatively common condition that is characterized by the formation of small pouches (diverticula) in the colon. Although most people with diverticulosis experience no symptoms, ~ 15 to 20% may develop pain or inflammation, known as diverticulitis.[77] In a large prospective cohort study, men with the highest dietary fiber intakes had a risk of developing symptomatic diverticular disease that was 42% lower than men with the lowest dietary fiber intakes. The protective effect of dietary fiber against diverticular disease was strongest for nonviscous dietary fiber, particularly cellulose.[78]

Weight Control

In addition to providing less energy, there is some evidence that higher fiber intakes can help to prevent weight gain or promote weight loss by extending the feeling of fullness after a meal (satiety).[79] Observational studies have found that adults with higher dietary fiber intakes are leaner[80] and are less likely to be obese than adults with low-fiber intakes.[81] One large prospective cohort study found that women whose intake of high-fiber foods increased by an average of 9 g/d over a 12-year period were half as likely to experience a major weight gain of at least 55 lb (25 kg) than those whose intake of high-fiber foods decreased by an average of 3 g/d.[82] The results of short-term clinical trials examining the effect of increased fiber intake on weight loss have been mixed. Overall, a systematic review of clinical trials conducted prior to 2001 found that increasing fiber intake from foods or supplements by 14 g/d resulted in a 10% decrease in energy intake and weight losses averaging ~4 lb (1.9 kg) over 4 months.[79] However, more recent clinical trials did not find fiber-rich cereal[83] or fiber supplements[84] to enhance weight loss. Although people with higher intakes of fiber-rich foods, particularly whole grains, appear more likely to maintain a healthy bodyweight, the role of fiber alone in weight control is not yet clear.

Treatment

Diabetes Mellitus

Numerous controlled clinical trials in people who have type 1 or type 2 DM have found that increasing fiber intake from foods[85,86] and viscous fiber supplements[87-89] improves markers of glycemic control, particularly postprandial glucose levels, and serum lipid profiles. A recent meta-analysis that combined the results of 23 clinical trials comparing the effects of high-fiber diets ($\geq$20 g/1000 kcal) with those of low-fiber diets ($<$10 g/1000 kcal)

found that high-fiber diets lowered postprandial blood glucose concentrations by 13 to 21%, serum LDL cholesterol concentrations by 8 to 16%, and serum triglyceride concentrations by 8 to 13%.[90] Based on the evidence from this meta-analysis, the authors recommended a dietary fiber intake of 25 to 50 g/d (15 to 25 g/1000 kcal) for individuals with diabetes, which is consistent with the recommendations of many international diabetes organizations of at least 25 to 35 g/d.[91-93] In general, the results of controlled clinical trials support recommendations that people with diabetes aim for high-fiber intakes by increasing consumption of whole grains, legumes, nuts, fruits, and nonstarchy vegetables. Because there is little evidence from clinical trials that increasing nonviscous fiber alone is beneficial,[94] individuals with diabetes should avoid increasing fiber intake exclusively from nonviscous sources, such as wheat bran.[90]

Irritable Bowel Syndrome

Irritable bowel syndrome (IBS) is a functional disorder of the intestines, characterized by episodes of abdominal pain or discomfort associated with a change in bowel movements, such as constipation or diarrhea.[95] Although people diagnosed with IBS are often encouraged by health care providers to increase dietary fiber intake, the results of controlled clinical trials of psyllium, methylcellulose, and wheat bran have been mixed.[96] A systematic review of 17 randomized controlled trials of fiber supplements in IBS patients found that supplementation with soluble fiber, mainly from psyllium, significantly improved a global measure of IBS symptoms; supplementation with insoluble fiber, such as corn bran or wheat bran, did not improve IBS symptoms.[97] In general, fiber supplements improved constipation in IBS patients, but did not improve IBS-associated abdominal pain. Thus, the results of randomized controlled trials suggest that increasing soluble or viscous fiber intake gradually to 12 to 30 g/d may be beneficial for patients in whom constipation is the predominant symptom of IBS.[98] However, fiber supplements could actually exacerbate symptoms in those in whom diarrhea predominates.[99] IBS patients should be advised to increase fiber intake gradually because increasing intake of viscous, readily fermented fibers could increase gas production and bloating.

Sources

Food Sources

Dietary fiber intakes in the United States average from 16 to 18 g/d for men and 12 to 14 g/d for women—well below recommended intake levels[4] (see the Intake Recommendations section below). Good sources of dietary fiber include legumes, nuts, whole grains, bran products, fruits, and nonstarchy vegetables. Legumes, whole grains, and nuts are generally more concentrated sources of fiber than fruits and vegetables. All plant-based foods contain mixtures of soluble and insoluble fiber.[10] Oat products and legumes are rich sources of soluble and viscous fiber. Wheat bran and whole grains are rich sources of insoluble and nonviscous fiber. The total fiber content of some fiber-rich foods is presented in **Table 12–1**. Some strategies for increasing dietary fiber intake include increasing fruit and non-starchy vegetable intake, particularly legumes, eating whole grain cereal or oatmeal for breakfast, substituting whole grains for refined grains, and substituting nuts or popcorn for less healthful snacks.

Isolated Fibers and Fiber Supplements

β-Glucans

β-Glucans are viscous, easily fermented, soluble fibers found naturally in oats, barley, mushrooms, yeast, bacteria, and algae.[9] β-Glucans extracted from oats, mushrooms, and yeast are available in a variety of nutritional supplements without a prescription.

Pectin

Pectins are viscous fibers, most often extracted from citrus peels and apple pulp. Pectins are widely used as gelling agents in foods, but are also available as dietary supplements without a prescription.[9]

Table 12–1   Total Fiber Content of Selected Fiber-Rich Foods[129]

Food	Serving	Total Dietary Fiber (g)
Navy beans, cooked from dried Navy beans	¹/₂ cup	9.5
100% (wheat) bran cereal	¹/₂ cup	8.8
Kidney beans, canned	¹/₂ cup	8.2
Split peas, cooked from dried split peas	¹/₂ cup	8.1
Lentils, cooked from dried lentils	¹/₂ cup	7.8
Bran cereals (various brands)	~1 oz	2.6–5.0
Sweet potato, baked with peel	1 medium	4.8
Asian pear	1 small	4.4
English muffin, whole wheat	1	4.4
Bulgur, cooked	¹/₂ cup	4.1
Raspberries, raw	¹/₂ cup	4.0
Spinach, frozen, cooked	¹/₂ cup	3.5
Shredded wheat cereals, various	~1 oz	2.8–3.4
Almonds	1 oz	3.3
Apple with skin	1 medium	3.3

Inulins and Oligofructose

Inulins and oligofructose, extracted from chicory root or synthesized from sucrose, are used as food additives.[8] Isolated inulin is added to replace fat in products, such as salad dressing; sweet-tasting oligofructose is added to products, such as fruit yogurts and desserts. Inulins and oligofructose are highly fermentable fibers that are also classified as prebiotics because of their ability to stimulate the growth of potentially beneficial *Bifidobacteria* species in the human colon.[100] Encouraging the growth of *Bifidobacteria* could promote intestinal health by suppressing the growth of pathogenic bacteria known to cause diarrhea or enhancing the immune response.[101] Although several dietary supplements containing inulins and oligofructose are marketed as prebiotics, the health benefits of prebiotics have not yet been convincingly demonstrated in humans.[102,103]

Guar Gum

Guar gum is a viscous, fermentable fiber derived from the Indian cluster bean. It is used as a thickener or emulsifier in many food products. Dietary supplements containing guar gum have been marketed as weight-loss aids, but a meta-analysis that combined the results of 11 randomized controlled trials found that guar gum supplements were not effective in reducing body weight.[104]

Psyllium

Psyllium, a viscous, soluble fiber isolated from psyllium seed husks, is available without a prescription in laxatives, ready-to-eat cereals, and dietary supplements.[9] The FDA has approved health claims like the following on the labels of foods containing at least 1.7 g/serving of soluble fiber from psyllium: "Diets low in saturated fat and cholesterol that include 7 g/d of soluble fiber from psyllium may reduce the risk of heart disease".[14]

Chitosan

Chitosan is an indigestible glucosamine polymer derived from chitin. When administered with food, chitosan decreased fat absorption in animal studies.[105] Consequently, chitosan has been marketed as a dietary supplement to promote weight loss and lower cholesterol. Controlled clinical trials in humans have not generally found chitosan supplementation to be more effective than placebo in promoting weight loss.[106] Some clinical trials in humans have found chitosan supplementation to result in modest reductions in total and LDL cholesterol levels compared with placebo[107,108]; however, others found no improvement.[109,110] Chitosan is available as a dietary supplement without a prescription in the United States.

Safety

Adverse Reactions

Dietary Fiber

Some people experience abdominal cramping, bloating, or gas when they abruptly increase their dietary fiber intakes.[111,112] These symptoms can be minimized or avoided by increasing intake of fiber-rich foods gradually and increasing fluid intake to at least 64 oz/d (~2 L/d). There have been rare reports of intestinal obstruction related to large intakes of oat bran or wheat bran, usually in people with impaired intestinal motility or difficulty chewing.[113-116] The U.S. Institute of Medicine has not established a tolerable upper intake level (UL) for dietary or functional fiber.[4]

Isolated Fibers and Fiber Supplements

Gastrointestinal Symptoms

The following fibers have been found to cause gastrointestinal distress, including abdominal cramping, bloating, gas and diarrhea: guar gum, inulin, oligofructose, fructooligosaccharides, polydextrose, resistant starch, and psyllium.[4] Several cases of intestinal obstruction by psyllium have been reported when taken with insufficient fluids or by people with impaired swallowing or gastrointestinal motility.[117,118]

Colorectal Adenomas

One randomized controlled trial in patients with a history of colorectal adenomas found that supplementation with 3.5 g/d of psyllium for 3 years resulted in a significant increase in colorectal adenoma recurrence compared with placebo (see the Colorectal Cancer section above).[64]

Allergy and Anaphylaxis

Because chitin and chitosan may be isolated from the exoskeletons of crustaceans, such as crabs and lobsters, people with shellfish allergies should avoid taking chitin or chitosan supplements.[9] Anaphylaxis has been reported after intravenous administration of inulin,[119] as well as ingestion of margarine containing inulin extracted from chicory.[120] Anaphylaxis has also been reported after the ingestion of cereals containing psyllium, and asthma has occasionally been reported in people with occupational exposure to psyllium powder.[121]

Drug Interactions

Psyllium may reduce the absorption of lithium, carbamazepine (Tegretol), digoxin (Lanoxin), and warfarin (Coumadin) when taken at the same time.[9] Guar gum may slow the absorption of digoxin, acetaminophen (Tylenol), and bumetanide (Bumex), and decrease the absorption of metformin (Glucophage), penicillin, and some formulations of glyburide (Glynase) when taken at the same time.[122] Pectin may decrease the absorption of lovastatin (Mevacor) when taken at the same time.[123] Concomitant administration of kaolin-pectin has been reported to decrease the absorption of clindamycin, tetracyclines, and digoxin, but it is not known whether kaolin or pectin is responsible for the interaction.[9] In general, medications should be taken at least 1 hour before or 2 hours after fiber supplements.

Nutrient Interactions

The addition of cereal fiber to meals has generally been found to decrease the absorption of iron, zinc, calcium, and magnesium in the same meal, but this effect appears to be related to the phytate present in the cereal fiber supplements rather than the fiber itself.[124] In general, dietary fiber as part of a balanced diet has not been found to adversely affect the calcium, magnesium, iron, or zinc status of healthy people at recommended intake levels.[4] Evidence from animal studies and limited research in humans suggests that inulin and oligofructose may enhance calcium absorption.[125,126] The addition of pectin and guar gum to a meal significantly reduced the absorption of β-carotene, lycopene, and lutein from that meal.[127,128]

Intake Recommendations

Adequate Intake

In light of consistent evidence from prospective cohort studies that fiber-rich diets are associated with significant reductions in cardiovascular disease risk, the Food and Nutrition Board of the Institute of Medicine established its first recommended intake levels for fiber in 2001.[4] The Adequate Intake (AI) recommendations for total fiber intake are based on the findings of several large prospective cohort studies that dietary fiber intakes of ∼ 14 g/4184 kJ (1000 kcal) of energy were associated with significant reductions in the risk of CHD,[29,30,32] as well as type 2 DM.[45,46] For adults who are 50 years of age or younger, the AI for total fiber intake is 38 g/d for men and 25 g/d for women. For adults over 50 years of age, the recommendation is 30 g/d for men and 21 g/d for women. The AI recommendations for males and females of all ages are presented in **Table 12–2**.

Table 12–2   U.S. Institute of Medicine Adequate Intake Recommendations for Total Fiber[4]

Life Stage	Age	Males (g/d)	Females (g/d)
Infants	0–6 mo	ND*	ND
Infants	7–12 mo	ND	ND
Children	1–3 y	19	19
Children	4–8 y	25	25
Children	9–13 y	31	26
Adolescents	14–18 y	38	26
Adults	19–50 y	38	25
Adults	51 y and older	30	21
Pregnancy	All ages	–	28
Breastfeeding	All ages	–	29

* Not determined.

Summary

- Fiber is a diverse group of compounds, including lignin and complex carbohydrates that cannot be digested by human enzymes in the small intestine.
- Although each class of fiber is chemically unique, scientists have tried to classify fibers based on their solubility, viscosity, and fermentation ability, to understand their physiological effects better.
- Viscous fibers, such as those found in oat products and legumes, can lower serum LDL cholesterol levels and normalize blood glucose and insulin responses.
- High-fiber intakes promote bowel health by preventing constipation and diverticular disease.
- Large prospective cohort studies provide strong and consistent evidence that diets rich in fiber from whole grains, legumes, fruits, and nonstarchy vegetables can reduce the risk of cardiovascular disease and type 2 DM.
- Although the results of case-control studies suggested that breast and colorectal cancer were more prevalent in people with low-fiber intakes, the findings from most prospective cohort studies do not support an association between fiber intake and the risk of breast or colorectal cancer.
- Numerous controlled clinical trials in people with type 1 and type 2 DM have found that increasing fiber intake improves glycemic control and serum lipid profiles.
- In 2001, the Food and Nutrition Board of the U.S. Institute of Medicine established an Adequate Intake (AI) level for total fiber. For adults who are 50 years of age or younger, the AI for total fiber is 38 g/d for men and 25 g/d for women. For adults over 50 years of age, the AI for total fiber is 30 g/d for men and 21 g/d for women.

References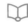

1. Lupton JR. Microbial degradation products influence colon cancer risk: the butyrate controversy. J Nutr 2004;134(2):479–482
2. Ha MA, Jarvis MC, Mann JI. A definition for dietary fibre. Eur J Clin Nutr 2000;54(12):861–864
3. DeVries JW. On defining dietary fibre. Proc Nutr Soc 2003;62(1):37–43
4. Institute of Medicine. Dietary, Functional, and Total Fiber. Dietary Reference Intakes for Energy, Carbohydrate, Fiber, Fat, Fatty Acids, Cholesterol, Protein, and Amino Acids. Washington, D.C.: National Academies Press; 2002:265–334
5. Trowell H. Dietary fibre, ischaemic heart disease and diabetes mellitus. Proc Nutr Soc 1973;32(3):151–157
6. Lupton JR, Turner ND. Dietary fiber. In: Stipanuk MH, ed. Biochemical and Physiological Aspects of Human Nutrition. Philadelphia: W.B. Saunders; 2000:143–154
7. Gallaher CM, Schneeman BO. Dietary fiber. In: Bowman BA, Russell RM, eds. Present Knowledge in Nutrition. 8th ed. Washington, D.C.: ILSI Press; 2001:83–91
8. Niness KR. Inulin and oligofructose: what are they? J Nutr 1999;129(7 Suppl):1402S–1406S
9. Hendler SS, Rorvik DR, eds. PDR for Nutritional Supplements. Montvale: Medical Economics Company, Inc; 2001
10. Marlett JA. Content and composition of dietary fiber in 117 frequently consumed foods. J Am Diet Assoc 1992;92(2):175–186
11. Anderson JW, Major AW. Pulses and lipaemia, short- and long-term effect: potential in the prevention of cardiovascular disease. Br J Nutr 2002;88(Suppl 3):S263–S271
12. Ripsin CM, Keenan JM, Jacobs DR Jr, et al. Oat products and lipid lowering. A meta-analysis. JAMA 1992;267(24):3317–3325
13. Brown L, Rosner B, Willett WW, Sacks FM. Cholesterol-lowering effects of dietary fiber: a meta-analysis. Am J Clin Nutr 1999;69(1):30–42
14. Food and Drug Administration. Food labeling: health claims; soluble dietary fiber from certain foods and coronary heart disease. Final rule. Fed Regist 2003;68(144):44207–44209

15. Anderson JW, Allgood LD, Lawrence A, et al. Cholesterol-lowering effects of psyllium intake adjunctive to diet therapy in men and women with hypercholesterolemia: meta-analysis of 8 controlled trials. Am J Clin Nutr 2000;71(2):472–479

16. Schafer G, Schenk U, Ritzel U, Ramadori G, Leonhardt U. Comparison of the effects of dried peas with those of potatoes in mixed meals on postprandial glucose and insulin concentrations in patients with type 2 diabetes. Am J Clin Nutr 2003;78(1):99–103

17. Kabir M, Oppert JM, Vidal H, et al. Four-week low-glycemic index breakfast with a modest amount of soluble fibers in type 2 diabetic men. Metabolism 2002;51(7):819–826

18. Williams JA, Lai CS, Corwin H, et al. Inclusion of guar gum and alginate into a crispy bar improves postprandial glycemia in humans. J Nutr 2004;134(4): 886–889

19. Sierra M, Garcia JJ, Fernandez N, Diez MJ, Calle AP, Sahagun AM. Effects of ispaghula husk and guar gum on postprandial glucose and insulin concentrations in healthy subjects. Eur J Clin Nutr 2001;55(4):235–243

20. Wolever TM, Jenkins DA. Effect of dietary fiber and foods on carbohydrate metabolism. In: Spiller GA, ed. CRC Handbook of Dietary Fiber in Human Nutrition. 3rd ed. Boca Raton: CRC Press; 2001:321–360

21. Marlett JA, McBurney MI, Slavin JL. Position of the American Dietetic Association: health implications of dietary fiber. J Am Diet Assoc 2002;102(7):993–1000

22. Cummings JH. The effect of dietary fiber on fecal weight and composition. In: Spiller GA, ed. Fiber in Human Nutrition. 3rd ed. Boca Raton: CRC Press; 2001:183–252

23. Anti M, Pignataro G, Armuzzi A, et al. Water supplementation enhances the effect of high-fiber diet on stool frequency and laxative consumption in adult patients with functional constipation. Hepatogastroenterology 1998;45(21):727–732

24. American Academy of Family Physicians. Constipation: Keeping Your Bowels Moving Smoothly. 2000. Available at: http://familydoctor.org/037.xml. Accessed 9/14/04

25. Fraser GE, Sabate J, Beeson WL, Strahan TM. A possible protective effect of nut consumption on risk of coronary heart disease. The Adventist Health Study. Arch Intern Med 1992;152(7):1416–1424

26. Humble CG, Malarcher AM, Tyroler HA. Dietary fiber and coronary heart disease in middle-aged hypercholesterolemic men. Am J Prev Med 1993;9(4):197–202

27. Jacobs DR Jr, Meyer KA, Kushi LH, Folsom AR. Whole-grain intake may reduce the risk of ischemic heart disease death in postmenopausal women: the Iowa Women's Health Study. Am J Clin Nutr 1998;68(2):248–257

28. Khaw KT, Barrett-Connor E. Dietary fiber and reduced ischemic heart disease mortality rates in men and women: a 12-year prospective study. Am J Epidemiol 1987;126(6):1093–1102

29. Pietinen P, Rimm EB, Korhonen P, et al. Intake of dietary fiber and risk of coronary heart disease in a cohort of Finnish men. The Alpha-Tocopherol, Beta-Carotene Cancer Prevention Study. Circulation 1996; 94(11):2720–2727

30. Rimm EB, Ascherio A, Giovannucci E, Spiegelman D, Stampfer MJ, Willett WC. Vegetable, fruit, and cereal fiber intake and risk of coronary heart disease among men. JAMA 1996;275(6):447–451

31. Todd S, Woodward M, Tunstall-Pedoe H, Bolton-Smith C. Dietary antioxidant vitamins and fiber in the etiology of cardiovascular disease and all-causes mortality: results from the Scottish Heart Health Study. Am J Epidemiol 1999;150(10):1073–1080

32. Wolk A, Manson JE, Stampfer MJ, et al. Long-term intake of dietary fiber and decreased risk of coronary heart disease among women. JAMA 1999;281(21): 1998–2004

33. Bazzano LA, He J, Ogden LG, Loria CM, Whelton PK. Dietary fiber intake and reduced risk of coronary heart disease in US men and women: the National Health and Nutrition Examination Survey I Epidemiologic Follow-up Study. Arch Intern Med 2003; 163(16):1897–1904

34. Mozaffarian D, Kumanyika SK, Lemaitre RN, Olson JL, Burke GL, Siscovick DS. Cereal, fruit, and vegetable fiber intake and the risk of cardiovascular disease in elderly individuals. JAMA 2003;289(13):1659–1666

35. Pereira MA, O'Reilly E, Augustsson K, et al. Dietary fiber and risk of coronary heart disease: a pooled analysis of cohort studies. Arch Intern Med 2004; 164(4):370–376

36. Liu S, Willett WC. Dietary glycemic load and atherothrombotic risk. Curr Atheroscler Rep 2002; 4(6):454–461

37. Ford ES, Liu S. Glycemic index and serum high-density lipoprotein cholesterol concentration among us adults. Arch Intern Med 2001;161(4):572–576

38. Liu S, Manson JE, Stampfer MJ, et al. Dietary glycemic load assessed by food-frequency questionnaire in relation to plasma high-density-lipoprotein cholesterol and fasting plasma triacylglycerols in postmenopausal women. Am J Clin Nutr 2001;73(3): 560–566

39. Ascherio A, Hennekens C, Willett WC, et al. Prospective study of nutritional factors, blood pressure, and hypertension among US women. Hypertension 1996;27(5):1065–1072

40. Ascherio A, Rimm EB, Giovannucci EL, et al. A prospective study of nutritional factors and hypertension among US men. Circulation 1992;86(5):1475–1484

41. Keenan JM, Pins JJ, Frazel C, Moran A, Turnquist L. Oat ingestion reduces systolic and diastolic blood pressure in patients with mild or borderline hypertension: a pilot trial. J Fam Pract 2002;51(4):369

42. He J, Streiffer RH, Muntner P, Krousel-Wood MA, Whelton PK. Effect of dietary fiber intake on blood pressure: a randomized, double-blind, placebo-controlled trial. J Hypertens 2004;22(1):73–80

43. Lupton JR, Turner ND. Dietary fiber and coronary disease: does the evidence support an association? Curr Atheroscler Rep 2003;5(6):500–505

44. Gross LS, Li L, Ford ES, Liu S. Increased consumption of refined carbohydrates and the epidemic of type 2 diabetes in the United States: an ecologic assessment. Am J Clin Nutr 2004;79(5):774–779

45. Salmeron J, Ascherio A, Rimm EB, et al. Dietary fiber, glycemic load, and risk of NIDDM in men. Diabetes Care 1997;20(4):545–550

46. Salmeron J, Manson JE, Stampfer MJ, Colditz GA, Wing AL, Willett WC. Dietary fiber, glycemic load, and risk of non-insulin-dependent diabetes mellitus in women. JAMA 1997;277(6):472–477

47. Meyer KA, Kushi LH, Jacobs DR Jr, Slavin J, Sellers TA, Folsom AR. Carbohydrates, dietary fiber, and incident type 2 diabetes in older women. Am J Clin Nutr 2000;71(4):921–930

48. Stevens J, Ahn K. Juhaeri, Houston D, Steffan L, Couper D. Dietary fiber intake and glycemic index and incidence of diabetes in African-American and white adults: the ARIC study. Diabetes Care 2002; 25(10):1715–1721

49. Montonen J, Knekt P, Jarvinen R, Aromaa A, Reunanen A. Whole-grain and fiber intake and the incidence of type 2 diabetes. Am J Clin Nutr 2003;77(3): 622–629

50. Schulze MB, Liu S, Rimm EB, Manson JE, Willett WC, Hu FB. Glycemic index, glycemic load, and dietary fiber intake and incidence of type 2 diabetes in younger and middle-aged women. Am J Clin Nutr 2004;80(2):348–356

51. Knowler WC, Barrett-Connor E, Fowler SE, et al. Reduction in the incidence of type 2 diabetes with lifestyle intervention or metformin. N Engl J Med 2002; 346(6):393–403

52. Tuomilehto J, Lindstrom J, Eriksson JG, et al. Prevention of type 2 diabetes mellitus by changes in lifestyle among subjects with impaired glucose tolerance. N Engl J Med 2001;344(18):1343–1350

53. Trock B, Lanza E, Greenwald P. Dietary fiber, vegetables, and colon cancer: critical review and meta-analyses of the epidemiologic evidence. J Natl Cancer Inst 1990;82(8):650–661

54. Howe GR, Benito E, Castelleto R, et al. Dietary intake of fiber and decreased risk of cancers of the colon and rectum: evidence from the combined analysis of 13 case-control studies. J Natl Cancer Inst 1992; 84(24):1887–1896

55. Steinmetz KA, Kushi LH, Bostick RM, Folsom AR, Potter JD. Vegetables, fruit, and colon cancer in the Iowa Women's Health Study. Am J Epidemiol 1994; 139(1):1–15

56. Kato I, Akhmedkhanov A, Koenig K, Toniolo PG, Shore RE, Riboli E. Prospective study of diet and female colorectal cancer: the New York University Women's Health Study. Nutr Cancer 1997;28(3): 276–281

57. Pietinen P, Malila N, Virtanen M, et al. Diet and risk of colorectal cancer in a cohort of Finnish men. Cancer Causes Control 1999;10(5):387–396

58. Terry P, Giovannucci E, Michels KB, et al. Fruit, vegetables, dietary fiber, and risk of colorectal cancer. J Natl Cancer Inst 2001;93(7):525–533

59. Mai V, Flood A, Peters U, Lacey JV Jr, Schairer C, Schatzkin A. Dietary fibre and risk of colorectal cancer in the Breast Cancer Detection Demonstration Project (BCDDP) follow-up cohort. Int J Epidemiol 2003;32(2):234–239

60. Lin J, Zhang SM, Cook NR, et al. Dietary intakes of fruit, vegetables, and fiber, and risk of colorectal cancer in a prospective cohort of women (United States). Cancer Causes Control 2005;16(3):225–233

61. Michels KB, Fuchs CS, Giovannucci E, et al. Fiber intake and incidence of colorectal cancer among 76,947 women and 47,279 men. Cancer Epidemiol Biomarkers Prev 2005;14(4):842–849

62. Schatzkin A, Lanza E, Corle D, et al. Lack of effect of a low-fat, high-fiber diet on the recurrence of colorectal adenomas. Polyp Prevention Trial Study Group. N Engl J Med 2000;342(16):1149–1155

63. Alberts DS, Martinez ME, Roe DJ, et al. Lack of effect of a high-fiber cereal supplement on the recurrence of colorectal adenomas. Phoenix Colon Cancer Prevention Physicians' Network. N Engl J Med 2000; 342(16):1156–1162

64. Bonithon-Kopp C, Kronborg O, Giacosa A, Rath U, Faivre J. Calcium and fibre supplementation in prevention of colorectal adenoma recurrence: a randomised intervention trial. European Cancer Prevention Organisation Study Group. Lancet 2000; 356(9238):1300–1306

65. Giovannucci E, Stampfer MJ, Colditz G, Rimm EB, Willett WC. Relationship of diet to risk of colorectal adenoma in men. J Natl Cancer Inst 1992;84(2):91–98

66. Van 't Veer P, Kolb CM, Verhoef P, et al. Dietary fiber, beta-carotene and breast cancer: results from a case-control study. Int J Cancer 1990;45(5):825–828

67. Baghurst PA, Rohan TE. High-fiber diets and reduced risk of breast cancer. Int J Cancer 1994;56(2):173–176

68. Yuan JM, Wang QS, Ross RK, Henderson BE, Yu MC. Diet and breast cancer in Shanghai and Tianjin, China. Br J Cancer 1995;71(6):1353–1358

69. Ronco A, De Stefani E, Boffetta P, Deneo-Pellegrini H, Mendilaharsu M, Leborgne F. Vegetables, fruits, and related nutrients and risk of breast cancer: a case-control study in Uruguay. Nutr Cancer 1999;35(2): 111–119

70. Graham S, Zielezny M, Marshall J, et al. Diet in the epidemiology of postmenopausal breast cancer in the New York State Cohort. Am J Epidemiol 1992; 136(11):1327–1337

71. Terry P, Jain M, Miller AB, Howe GR, Rohan TE. No association among total dietary fiber, fiber fractions, and risk of breast cancer. Cancer Epidemiol Biomarkers Prev 2002;11(11):1507–1508

72. Cho E, Spiegelman D, Hunter DJ, Chen WY, Colditz GA, Willett WC. Premenopausal dietary carbohydrate, glycemic index, glycemic load, and fiber in relation to risk of breast cancer. Cancer Epidemiol Biomarkers Prev 2003;12(11 Pt 1):1153–1158

73. Holmes MD, Liu S, Hankinson SE, Colditz GA, Hunter DJ, Willett WC. Dietary carbohydrates, fiber, and breast cancer risk. Am J Epidemiol 2004;159(8):732–739

74. Mattisson I, Wirfalt E, Johansson U, Gullberg B, Olsson H, Berglund G. Intakes of plant foods, fibre and fat and risk of breast cancer–a prospective study in the Malmo Diet and Cancer cohort. Br J Cancer 2004; 90(1):122–127

75. Rock CL, Flatt SW, Thomson CA, et al. Effects of a high-fiber, low-fat diet intervention on serum concentrations of reproductive steroid hormones in women with a history of breast cancer. J Clin Oncol 2004;22(12):2379–2387

76. Kasim-Karakas SE, Almario RU, Gregory L, Todd H, Wong R, Lasley BL. Effects of prune consumption on the ratio of 2-hydroxyestrone to 16alpha-hydroxyestrone. Am J Clin Nutr 2002;76(6):1422–1427

77. Farrell RJ, Farrell JJ, Morrin MM. Diverticular disease in the elderly. Gastroenterol Clin North Am 2001; 30(2):475–496

78. Aldoori WH, Giovannucci EL, Rockett HR, Sampson L, Rimm EB, Willett WC. A prospective study of dietary fiber types and symptomatic diverticular disease in men. J Nutr 1998;128(4):714–719

79. Howarth NC, Saltzman E, Roberts SB. Dietary fiber and weight regulation. Nutr Rev 2001;59(5):129–139

80. Appleby PN, Thorogood M, Mann JI, Key TJ. Low body mass index in non-meat eaters: the possible roles of animal fat, dietary fibre and alcohol. Int J Obes Relat Metab Disord 1998;22(5):454–460

81. Miller WC, Niederpruem MG, Wallace JP, Lindeman AK. Dietary fat, sugar, and fiber predict body fat content. J Am Diet Assoc 1994;94(6):612–615

82. Liu S, Willett WC, Manson JE, Hu FB, Rosner B, Colditz G. Relation between changes in intakes of dietary fiber and grain products and changes in weight and development of obesity among middle-aged women. Am J Clin Nutr 2003;78(5):920–927

83. Saltzman E, Moriguti JC, Das SK, et al. Effects of a cereal rich in soluble fiber on body composition and dietary compliance during consumption of a hypocaloric diet. J Am Coll Nutr 2001;20(1):50–57

84. Howarth NC, Saltzman E, McCrory MA, et al. Fermentable and nonfermentable fiber supplements did not alter hunger, satiety or body weight in a pilot study of men and women consuming self-selected diets. J Nutr 2003;133(10):3141–3144

85. Giacco R, Parillo M, Rivellese AA, et al. Long-term dietary treatment with increased amounts of fiber-rich low-glycemic index natural foods improves blood glucose control and reduces the number of hypoglycemic events in type 1 diabetic patients. Diabetes Care 2000;23(10):1461–1466

86. Chandalia M, Garg A, Lutjohann D, von Bergmann K, Grundy SM, Brinkley LJ. Beneficial effects of high dietary fiber intake in patients with type 2 diabetes mellitus. N Engl J Med 2000;342(19):1392–1398

87. Groop PH, Aro A, Stenman S, Groop L. Long-term effects of guar gum in subjects with non-insulin-dependent diabetes mellitus. Am J Clin Nutr 1993; 58(4):513–518

88. Sierra M, Garcia JJ, Fernandez N, Diez MJ, Calle AP. Therapeutic effects of psyllium in type 2 diabetic patients. Eur J Clin Nutr 2002;56(9):830–842

89. Anderson JW, Allgood LD, Turner J, Oeltgen PR, Daggy BP. Effects of psyllium on glucose and serum lipid responses in men with type 2 diabetes and hypercholesterolemia. Am J Clin Nutr 1999;70(4):466–473

90. Anderson JW, Randles KM, Kendall CW, Jenkins DJ. Carbohydrate and fiber recommendations for individuals with diabetes: a quantitative assessment and meta-analysis of the evidence. J Am Coll Nutr 2004;23(1):5–17

91. American Diabetes Association position statement: evidence-based nutrition principles and recommendations for the treatment and prevention of diabetes and related complications. J Am Diet Assoc 2002; 102(1):109–118

92. Dietary recommendations for people with diabetes: an update for the 1990s. Nutrition Subcommittee of the British Diabetic Association's Professional Advisory Committee. Diabet Med 1992;9(2):189–202

93. National Nutrition Committee. Association CD. Guidelines for the Nutritional Management of Diabetes Mellitus in the New Millennium: A Position Statement of the Canadian Diabetes Association. Can J Diabetes Care. 1999;23(3):56–69

94. Jenkins DJ, Kendall CW, Augustin LS, et al. Effect of wheat bran on glycemic control and risk factors for cardiovascular disease in type 2 diabetes. Diabetes Care 2002;25(9):1522–1528

95. Horwitz BJ, Fisher RS. The irritable bowel syndrome. N Engl J Med 2001;344(24):1846–1850

96. Jailwala J, Imperiale TF, Kroenke K. Pharmacologic treatment of the irritable bowel syndrome: a systematic review of randomized, controlled trials. Ann Intern Med 2000;133(2):136–147

97. Bijkerk CJ, Muris JW, Knottnerus JA, Hoes AW, de Wit NJ. Systematic review: the role of different types of fibre in the treatment of irritable bowel syndrome. Aliment Pharmacol Ther 2004;19(3):245–251

98. Viera AJ, Hoag S, Shaughnessy J. Management of irritable bowel syndrome. Am Fam Physician 2002; 66(10):1867–1874

99. Mertz HR. Irritable bowel syndrome. N Engl J Med 2003;349(22):2136–2146

100. Gibson GR, Beatty ER, Wang X, Cummings JH. Selective stimulation of bifidobacteria in the human colon by oligofructose and inulin. Gastroenterology 1995; 108(4):975–982

101. Kolida S, Tuohy K, Gibson GR. Prebiotic effects of inulin and oligofructose. Br J Nutr 2002;87(Suppl 2):S193–S197

102. Cummings JH, Macfarlane GT. Gastrointestinal effects of prebiotics. Br J Nutr 2002;87(Suppl 2):S145–S151

103. Duggan C, Penny ME, Hibberd P, et al. Oligofructose-supplemented infant cereal: 2 randomized, blinded, community-based trials in Peruvian infants. Am J Clin Nutr 2003;77(4):937–942

104. Pittler MH, Ernst E. Guar gum for body weight reduction: meta-analysis of randomized trials. Am J Med 2001;110(9):724–730

105. Gallaher CM, Munion J, Hesslink R Jr, Wise J, Gallaher DD. Cholesterol reduction by glucomannan and chitosan is mediated by changes in cholesterol absorption and bile acid and fat excretion in rats. J Nutr 2000;130(11):2753–2759

106. Pittler MH, Ernst E. Dietary supplements for body-weight reduction: a systematic review. Am J Clin Nutr 2004;79(4):529–536

107. Bokura H, Kobayashi S. Chitosan decreases total cholesterol in women: a randomized, double-blind, placebo-controlled trial. Eur J Clin Nutr 2003; 57(5):721–725

108. Wuolijoki E, Hirvela T, Ylitalo P. Decrease in serum LDL cholesterol with microcrystalline chitosan. Methods Find Exp Clin Pharmacol 1999;21(5):357–361

109. Metso S, Ylitalo R, Nikkila M, Wuolijoki E, Ylitalo P, Lehtimaki T. The effect of long-term microcrystalline chitosan therapy on plasma lipids and glucose concentrations in subjects with increased plasma total cholesterol: a randomised placebo-controlled double-blind crossover trial in healthy men and women. Eur J Clin Pharmacol 2003;59(10):741–746

110. Ho SC, Tai ES, Eng PH, Tan CE, Fok AC. In the absence of dietary surveillance, chitosan does not reduce plasma lipids or obesity in hypercholesterolaemic obese Asian subjects. Singapore Med J 2001;42(1): 006–010

111. American Academy of Family Physicians. Fiber: How to increase the amount in your diet. 2004. Available at: http://familydoctor.org/099.xml. Accessed 9/13/04

112. Papazian R. Bulking up fiber's healthful reputation. Food and Drug Administration. 1998. Available at: http://www.fda.gov/fdac/features/1997/597_fiber.html. Accessed 9/14/04

113. Rosario PG, Gerst PH, Prakash K, Albu E. Dentureless distention: oat bran bezoars cause obstruction. J Am Geriatr Soc 1990;38(5):608

114. Miller DL, Miller PF, Dekker JJ. Small-bowel obstruction from bran cereal. JAMA 1990;263(6):813–814

115. Cooper SG, Tracey EJ. Small-bowel obstruction caused by oat-bran bezoar. N Engl J Med 1989;320(17):1148–1149

116. McClurken JB, Carp NZ. Bran-induced small-intestinal obstruction in a patient with no history of abdominal operation. Arch Surg 1988;123(1):98–100

117. Agha FP, Nostrant TT, Fiddian-Green RG. "Giant colonic bezoar:" a medication bezoar due to psyllium seed husks. Am J Gastroenterol 1984;79(4):319–321

118. Schneider RP. Perdiem causes esophageal impaction and bezoars. South Med J 1989;82(11):1449–1450

119. Chandra R, Barron JL. Anaphylactic reaction to intravenous sinistrin (Inutest). Ann Clin Biochem 2002;39(Pt 1):76

120. Gay-Crosier F, Schreiber G, Hauser C. Anaphylaxis from inulin in vegetables and processed food. N Engl J Med 2000;342(18):1372

121. Khalili B, Bardana EJ Jr, Yunginger JW. Psyllium-associated anaphylaxis and death: a case report and review of the literature. Ann Allergy Asthma Immunol 2003;91(6):579–584

122. Fugh-Berman A. Herb-drug interactions. Lancet 2000;355(9198):134–138

123. Richter WO, Jacob BG, Schwandt P. Interaction between fibre and lovastatin. Lancet 1991;338(8768):706

124. Greger JL. Nondigestible carbohydrates and mineral bioavailability. J Nutr 1999;129(7 Suppl):1434S–1435S

125. Bosscher D, Van Caillie-Bertrand M, Van Cauwenbergh R, Deelstra H. Availabilities of calcium, iron, and zinc from dairy infant formulas is affected by soluble dietary fibers and modified starch fractions. Nutrition 2003;19(7–8):641–645

126. Scholz-Ahrens KE, Schrezenmeir J. Inulin, oligofructose and mineral metabolism – experimental data and mechanism. Br J Nutr 2002;87(Suppl 2):S179–S186

127. Rock CL, Swendseid ME. Plasma beta-carotene response in humans after meals supplemented with dietary pectin. Am J Clin Nutr 1992;55(1):96–99

128. Riedl J, Linseisen J, Hoffmann J, Wolfram G. Some dietary fibers reduce the absorption of carotenoids in women. J Nutr 1999;129(12):2170–2176

129. U.S. Department of Agriculture, Agricultural Research Service. USDA Nutrient Database for Standard Reference, Release 17. 2004. Available at: http://www.nal.usda.gov/fnic/foodcomp. Accessed 7/26/06

13 Flavonoids

Flavonoids are a large family of compounds synthesized by plants that have a common chemical structure.[1] Flavonoids may be further divided into subclasses based on their chemical structure (**Fig. 13–1**). Over the past decade, scientists have become increasingly interested in the potential for various dietary flavonoids to explain some of the health bene-

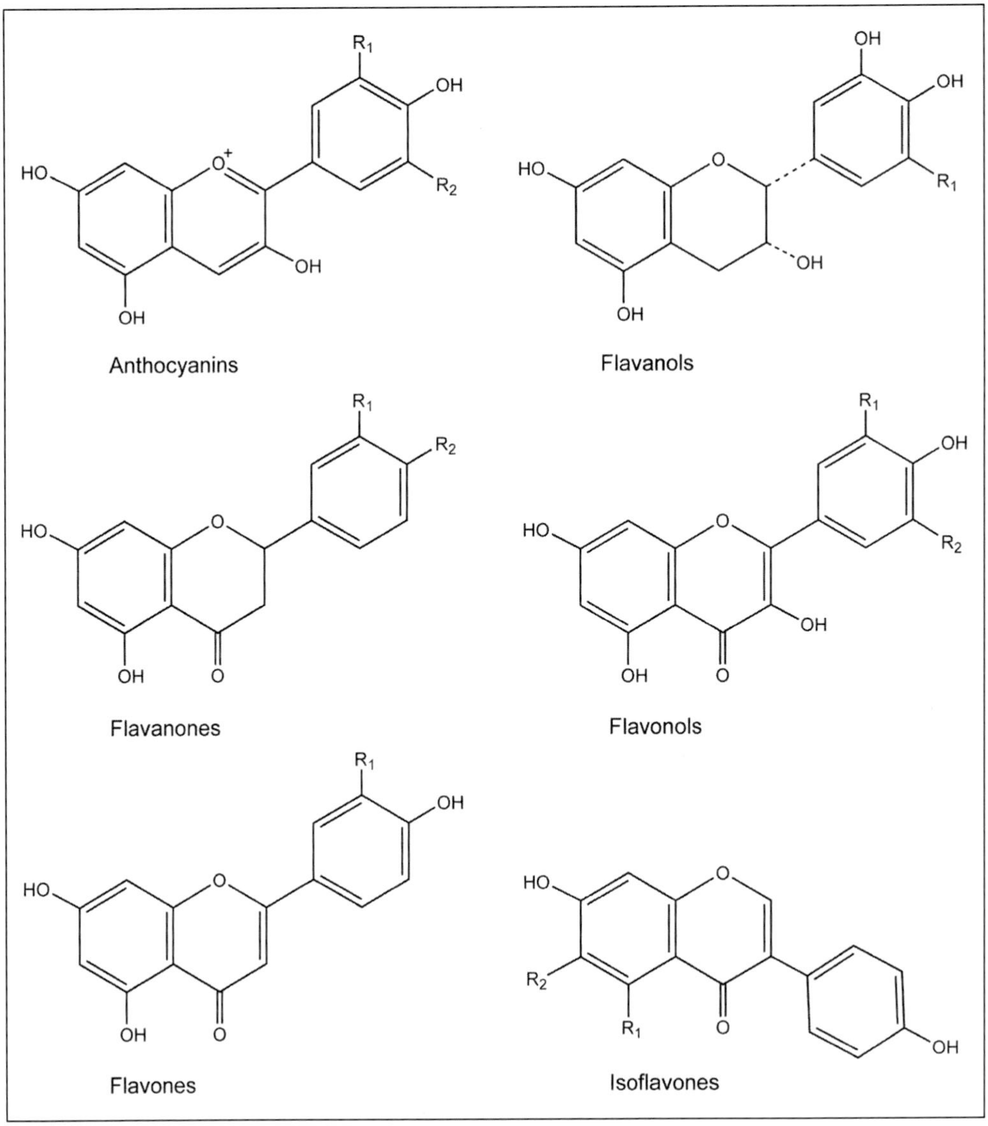

Figure 13–1 Basic chemical structures of the flavonoid subclasses.

fits associated with fruit and vegetable-rich diets. These potential health benefits are being used to promote the consumption of flavonoid-rich foods, beverages, and dietary supplements. The scientific evidence for the hypothesis that dietary flavonoids promote health and prevent disease in humans is reviewed in this chapter. See Chapter 14 on soy isoflavones for more detailed information on the health effects of isoflavones, a subclass of flavonoids with estrogenic activity.

Metabolism and Bioavailability

Absorption and Metabolism

Flavonoids bound to one or more sugar molecules are known as flavonoid glycosides; those that are not bound to a sugar molecule are called aglycones. With the exception of flavanols (catechins and proanthocyanidins), flavonoids occur in plants and most foods as glycosides.[2] Even after cooking, most flavonoid glycosides reach the small intestine intact. Only flavonoid aglycones and flavonoid glucosides (bound to glucose) are absorbed in the small intestine, where they are rapidly metabolized to form methylated, glucuronidated, or sulfated metabolites.[3] Bacteria that normally colonize the colon also play an important role in flavonoid metabolism and absorption. Flavonoids or flavonoid metabolites that reach the colon may be further metabolized by bacterial enzymes and absorbed. In general, the bioavailability of flavonoids is relatively low due to limited absorption and rapid elimination. Furthermore, flavonoids are rapidly and extensively metabolized, and the biological activities of flavonoid metabolites are not always the same as those of the parent compound.[4] When evaluating the results of flavonoid research in cultured cells, it is important to consider whether physiologically relevant flavonoid concentrations and flavonoid metabolites were used.[5] In humans, peak plasma concentrations of soy isoflavones and citrus flavanones have not been found to exceed 10 µmol/L after oral consumption. Peak plasma concentrations measured after the consumption of anthocyanins, flavonols, and flavanols (including those from tea) are generally less than 1 µmol/L.[3]

Biological Activities

Direct Antioxidant Activity

Flavonoids are effective scavengers of free radicals in the test tube (in vitro).[6,7] However, even with very high flavonoid intakes, plasma and intracellular flavonoid concentrations in humans are likely to be 100 to 1000 times lower than concentrations of other antioxidants, such as ascorbate (vitamin C) or glutathione. Moreover, most circulating flavonoids are actually flavonoid metabolites, some of which have lower antioxidant activity than the parent flavonoid. For these reasons, the relative contribution of dietary flavonoids to plasma and tissue antioxidant function in vivo is likely to be relatively minor.[8,9]

Metal Chelation

Metal ions, such as iron and copper, can catalyze the production of free radicals. The ability of flavonoids to chelate or bind metal ions appears to contribute to their antioxidant activity in vitro.[10,11] In living organisms, most iron and copper are bound to proteins, limiting their participation in reactions that produce free radicals. Although the metal-chelating activities of flavonoids may be beneficial in pathological conditions of iron or copper excess, it is not known whether flavonoids function as effective metal chelators in vivo.[8]

Effects on Cell Signaling Pathways

Cells are capable of responding to a variety of different stresses or signals by increasing or decreasing the availability of specific proteins. The complex cascades of events that lead to changes in the expression of specific genes are known as cell signaling pathways or signal transduction pathways. These pathways regulate numerous cell processes, including growth, proliferation, and death (apoptosis). Although it was initially hypothesized that the biological effects of flavonoids would be related to their antioxidant activity, available evidence from cell culture experiments suggests that many of the biological effects of flavonoids are related to their ability to modulate cell signaling pathways.[9] Intracellular concentrations of flavonoids required to affect cell signaling pathways are considerably lower than those required to impact cellular antioxidant capacity, and flavonoid metabolites may still retain their ability to interact with cell signaling proteins, even if their antioxidant activity is diminished.[12,13] Effective signal transduction requires proteins known as kinases that catalyze the phosphorylation of target proteins at specific sites. Cascades involving specific phosphorylations or dephosphorylations of signal transduction proteins ultimately affect the activity of transcription factors—proteins that bind to specific response elements on DNA and promote or inhibit the transcription of various genes. The results of numerous studies in cell culture suggest that flavonoids may affect chronic disease by selectively inhibiting kinases.[9,14] Cell growth and proliferation are also regulated by growth factors that initiate cell signaling cascades by binding to specific receptors in cell membranes. Flavonoids may alter growth factor signaling by inhibiting receptor phosphorylation or blocking receptor binding by growth factors.[15]

Biological Activities Related to Cancer Prevention

Stimulating Phase II Detoxification Enzyme Activity[16,17]

Phase II detoxification enzymes catalyze reactions that promote the excretion of potentially toxic or carcinogenic chemicals.

Preserving Normal Cell-Cycle Regulation[18,19]

Once a cell divides, it passes through a sequence of stages collectively known as the cell cycle before it divides again. Following DNA damage, the cell cycle can be transiently arrested at damage checkpoints, which allows for DNA repair or activation of pathways leading to cell death (apoptosis) if the damage is irreparable.[20] Defective cell-cycle regulation may result in the propagation of mutations that contribute to the development of cancer.

Inhibiting Proliferation and Inducing Apoptosis[21,22]

Unlike normal cells, cancer cells proliferate rapidly and lose the ability to respond to cell death signals by undergoing apoptosis.

Inhibiting Tumor Invasion and Angiogenesis[23,24]

Cancerous cells invade normal tissue aided by enzymes called matrix-metalloproteinases. Invasive tumors must also develop new blood vessels by a process known as angiogenesis to fuel their rapid growth.

Decreasing Inflammation[25–27]

Inflammation can result in locally increased production of free radicals by inflammatory enzymes, as well as the release of inflammatory mediators that promote cell proliferation and angiogenesis and inhibit apoptosis.[28]

Biological Activities Related to Cardiovascular Disease Prevention

Decreasing Inflammation[25–27]

Atherosclerosis is now recognized as an inflammatory disease, and several measures of inflammation are associated with increased risk of myocardial infarction (heart attack).[29]

Decreasing Vascular Cell Adhesion Molecule Expression[30,31]

One of the earliest events in the development of atherosclerosis is the recruitment of inflammatory white blood cells from the blood to the arterial wall. This event is dependent on the expression of adhesion molecules by the vascular endothelial cells that line the inner walls of blood vessels.[32]

Increasing Endothelial Nitric Oxide Synthase (eNOS) Activity[33]

eNOS is the enzyme that catalyzes the formation of nitric oxide by vascular endothelial cells. Nitric oxide is needed to maintain arterial relaxation (vasodilation). Impaired nitric oxide-dependent vasodilation is associated with increased risk of cardiovascular disease.[34]

Decreasing Platelet Aggregation[35,36]

Platelet aggregation is one of the first steps in the formation of a blood clot that can occlude a coronary or cerebral artery, resulting in myocardial infarction or stroke. Inhibiting platelet aggregation is considered an important strategy in the primary and secondary prevention of cardiovascular disease.[37]

Prevention

Cardiovascular Disease

Epidemiological Studies

At least eight prospective cohort studies conducted in the United States and Europe have examined the relationship between some measure of dietary flavonoid intake and coronary heart disease (CHD) risk.[38–45] Five of those studies found that higher flavonoid intakes were associated with significant reductions in CHD risk,[38–42] whereas three found no significant relationship.[43–45] In general, the foods that contributed most to total flavonoid intake in these cohorts were black tea, apples, and onions. One study in the Netherlands also found cocoa to be a significant source of dietary flavonoids. Of the six prospective cohort studies that examined relationships between dietary flavonoid intake and the risk of stroke, only two studies found that higher flavonoid intakes were associated with significant reductions in the risk of stroke,[41,46] whereas four found no relationship.[42,45,47,48] Although data from prospective cohort studies suggest that higher intakes of foods that are rich in flavonoids may help protect against CHD, it cannot be determined whether such protection is conferred by flavonoids, other nutrients, and phytochemicals in flavonoid-rich foods, or the whole foods themselves.[49]

Clinical Trials

Vascular Endothelial Function

Vascular endothelial cells play an important role in maintaining cardiovascular health by producing nitric oxide, a compound that promotes arterial relaxation (vasodilation).[50] Arterial vasodilation resulting from endothelial production of nitric oxide is termed endothelium-dependent vasodilation. Several clinical trials have examined the effect of flavonoid-rich foods and beverages on endothelium-dependent vasodilation. Two controlled clinical trials found that the daily consumption of 4 to 5 cups (900 to 1250 mL) of black tea for 4 weeks significantly improved endothelium-dependent vasodilation in patients with coronary artery disease[51] and patients with mildly elevated serum cholesterol levels[52] compared with the equivalent amount of caffeine alone or hot water. Other small clinical trials found similar improvements in endothelium-dependent vasodilation in response to daily consumption of ~3 cups (640 mL) of purple grape juice[53] or a high-flavonoid dark chocolate bar for 2 weeks.[54]

Platelet Aggregation

Endothelial nitric oxide production also inhibits the adhesion and aggregation of platelets, one of the first steps in blood clot formation.[50] Several clinical trials have examined the potential for high-flavonoid intakes to decrease various measures of platelet aggregation outside of the body (ex vivo) with mixed results. In general, increasing flavonoid intakes by increasing fruit and/or vegetable intake did not significantly affect ex vivo platelet aggregation,[37,55,56] nor did increasing black tea consumption.[57,58] However, several small clinical trials in healthy adults have reported significant decreases in ex vivo measures of platelet aggregation after consumption of grape juice (~500 mL/d) for 7 to 14 days[59–61] and dark chocolate.[62,63] The results of some controlled clinical trials suggest that relatively high intakes of some flavonoid-rich foods and beverages, including black tea, purple grape juice, and dark chocolate, may improve vascular endothelial function, but it is not known whether these short-term improvements will result in long-term reductions in cardiovascular disease risk.

Cancer

Although various flavonoids have been found to inhibit the development of chemically induced cancers in animal models of lung,[64] oral,[65] esophageal,[66] stomach,[67] colon,[68] skin,[69] prostate,[70] and breast cancer,[71] epidemiological studies do not provide convincing evidence that high intakes of dietary flavonoids are associated with substantial reductions in human cancer risk. Most prospective cohort studies that have assessed dietary flavonoid intake using food frequency questionnaires have not found flavonoid intake to be inversely associated with cancer risk.[72] Two prospective cohort studies in Europe found no relationship between the risk of various cancers and dietary intakes of flavones and flavonols,[73,74] catechins,[75] or tea.[76] In a cohort of postmenopausal women in the United States, catechin intake from tea but not fruits and vegetables was inversely associated with the risk of rectal cancer, but not other cancers.[77] Two prospective cohort studies in Finland, where average flavonoid intakes are relatively low, found that men with the highest dietary intakes of flavonols and flavones had a significantly lower risk of developing lung cancer than those with the lowest intakes.[40,41] When individual dietary flavonoids were analyzed, dietary quercetin intake, mainly from apples, was inversely associated with the risk of lung cancer, and myricetin intake was inversely associated with the risk of prostate cancer.[41] Tea is an important source of flavonoids (flavanols and flavonols) in some populations, but most prospective cohort studies have not found tea consumption to be inversely associated with cancer risk.[78] The results of case-control studies, which are more likely to be influenced by recall and selection bias, are mixed. Although some studies have observed lower flavonoid intakes in people diagnosed with lung,[79] gastric,[80,81] and breast cancer,[82] many others found no significant differences in flavonoid intake between cancer cases and controls.[83,84] There is limited evidence that low intakes of flavonoids from food are associated with in-

creased risk of certain cancers, but it is not clear whether these findings are related to insufficient intakes of flavonoids or other nutrients and phytochemicals in flavonoid-rich foods.

Neurodegenerative Disease

Inflammation, oxidative stress, and transition metal accumulation appear to play a role in the pathology of several neurodegenerative diseases, including Parkinson's disease and Alzheimer's disease. Because flavonoids have anti-inflammatory, antioxidant, and metal chelating properties, scientists are interested in the neuroprotective potential of flavonoid-rich diets or individual flavonoids. At present, the extent to which various dietary flavonoids and flavonoid metabolites cross the blood-brain barrier in humans is not known.[85] Although flavonoid-rich diets and flavonoid administration have been found to prevent cognitive impairment associated with aging and inflammation in some animal studies,[86-89] prospective cohort studies have not found consistent inverse associations between flavonoid intake and the risk of dementia or neurodegenerative disease in humans.[90-94] In a cohort of Japanese-American men followed for 25 to 30 years, flavonoid intake from tea during midlife was not associated with the risk of Alzheimer's or other types of dementia in late life.[90] Surprisingly, higher intakes of isoflavone-rich tofu during midlife were associated with cognitive impairment and brain atrophy in late life (see Chapter 14).[91] A prospective study of Dutch adults found that total dietary flavonoid intake was not associated with the risk of developing Parkinson's disease[92] or Alzheimer's disease,[93] except in current smokers whose risk of Alzheimer's disease decreased by 50% for every 12 mg increase in daily flavonoid intake. In contrast, a study of elderly French men and women found that those with the lowest flavonoid intakes had a risk of developing dementia over the next 5 years that was 50% higher than those with the highest intakes.[94] Although scientists are interested in the potential of flavonoids to protect the aging brain, it is not yet clear how flavonoid consumption affects neurodegenerative disease risk in humans.

Sources

Food Sources

Although some subclasses of dietary flavonoids like flavonols are found in many different fruits and vegetables, others are not as widely distributed (see **Table 13–1**).[3] Anthocyanins are most abundant in red, purple, and blue berries, and flavanones are limited to citrus fruits. Flavones are most commonly found in foods used as spices, such as parsley or chilies, while the principal dietary source of isoflavones is soybeans. Flavanols occur in foods as monomers, which are also called catechins, or as polymers. Tea is a rich source of flavanols. Unfermented teas, such as green and white teas, are rich in catechins. Black and oolong teas are fermented during processing, which results in the formation of catechin dimers and polymers known as theaflavins and thearubigins, respectively. See Chapter 7 for more information on tea and tea processing. Proanthocyanidins, also known as condensed tannins, are a family of flavanol polymers of varying lengths.[95] Recent research suggests that proanthocyanidins account for a substantial portion of the total flavonoids consumed in typical Western diets. Individual flavonoid intakes may vary considerably depending on whether tea, red wine, soy products, or fruits

and vegetables are commonly consumed.[3] Although individual flavonoid intakes may vary, total flavonoid intakes in Western populations appear to average ∼ 150 to 200 mg/d.[3,95] Information on the flavonoid content of some flavonoid-rich foods is presented in **Table 13–2**. These values should be considered approximate because several factors may affect the flavonoid content of foods, including agricultural practices, environmental factors, ripening, processing, storing, and cooking.

Supplements

Anthocyanins

Bilberry, elderberry, black currant, blueberry, red grape, and mixed berry extracts that are rich in anthocyanins are available as dietary supplements without a prescription in the United States. The anthocyanin content of these products may vary considerably. Standardized extracts that list the amount of anthocyanins per dose are available.

Flavanols

Numerous tea extracts are available in the United States as dietary supplements and may be labeled as tea catechins or tea polyphenols. Green tea extracts are the most commonly

Table 13–1   Subclasses of Common Dietary Flavonoids and Some Common Food Sources[3]

Flavonoid Subclass	Dietary Flavonoids	Some Common Food Sources
Anthocyanins	Cyanidin, delphinidin, malvidin, pelargonidin, peonidin, petunidin	Red, blue, and purple berries; red and purple grapes; red wine
Flavanols		
Monomers	Catechin, epicatechin, epigallo-catechin, epicatechin gallate, epigallocatechin gallate	Teas (green and white), chocolate, grapes, berries, apples
Polymers	Theaflavins, thearubigins, proanthocyanidins	Teas (black and oolong), chocolate, apples, berries, red grapes, red wine
Flavanones	Hesperetin, naringenin, eriodictyol	Citrus fruits and juices
Flavonols	Quercetin, kaempferol, myricetin, isorhamnetin	Yellow onions, scallions, kale, broccoli, apples, berries, teas
Flavones	Apigenin, luteolin	Parsley, thyme, celery, hot peppers
Isoflavones	Daidzein, genistein, glycitein	Soybeans, soy foods, legumes

Table 13–2   Flavonoid Content of 100 g or 100 mL of Selected Foods by Flavonoid Subclass[3,109–115]

100 g or 100 mL*	Anthocyanins (mg)	Flavanols (mg)	Proanthocya-nidins (mg)	Flavones (mg)	Flavonols (mg)	Flavanones (mg)
Blackberry	89–211	13–19	6–47	–	0–2	–
Blueberry	67–183	1	88–261	–	2–16	–
Grapes, red	25–92	2	44–76	–	3–4	–
Strawberry	15–75	–	97–183	–	1–4	–
Red wine	1–35	1–55	24–70	0	2–30	–
Plum	2–25	1–6	106–334	0	1–2	–
Onion, red	13–25	–	–	0	4–100	–
Onion, yellow	–	0	–	0	3–120	–
Green tea	–	24–216	–	0–1	3–9	–
Black tea	–	5–158	4	0	1–7	–
Chocolate, dark	–	43–63	90–322	–	–	–
Parsley, fresh	–	–	–	24–634	8–10	0
Grapefruit juice	–	–	–	0	0	10–104

* Per 100 g (fresh weight) or 100 mL (liquids); 100 g is equivalent to ~3.5 oz; 100 mL is equivalent to ~3.5 fl oz.

marketed, but black and oolong tea extracts are also available. Green tea extracts generally have higher levels of catechins; black tea extracts are richer in theaflavins and thearubigins. Oolong tea extracts fall somewhere in between green and black tea extracts with respect to their flavanol content. Some tea extracts contain caffeine; others are decaffeinated. Flavanol and caffeine content vary considerably among different products, so it is important to check the label or consult the manufacturer to determine the amounts of flavanols and caffeine that would be consumed daily with each supplement.

Flavanones

Citrus bioflavonoid supplements may contain glycosides of hesperetin (hesperidin), naringenin (naringin), and eriodictyol (eriocitrin). Hesperidin is also available in hesperidin-complex supplements.[96]

Flavones

The peels of citrus fruits are rich in the polymethoxylated flavones, tangeretin, nobiletin, and sinensetin.[3] Although dietary intakes of these naturally occurring flavones are generally low, they are often present in citrus bioflavonoid supplements.

Flavonols

The flavonol aglycone, quercetin, and its glycoside rutin are available as dietary supplements without a prescription in the United States. Other names for rutin include rutinoside, quercetin-3-rutinoside, and sophorin.[96] Citrus bioflavonoid supplements may also contain quercetin or rutin.

Safety

Adverse Effects

No adverse effects have been associated with high dietary intakes of flavonoids from plant-based foods. This lack of adverse effects may be explained by the relatively low bioavailability and rapid metabolism and elimination of most flavonoids.

Quercetin

Some men taking quercetin supplements (1000 mg/d for one month) reported nausea, headache, or tingling of the extremities.[97] Some cancer patients given intravenous quercetin in a phase I clinical trial reported nausea, vomiting, sweating, flushing, and dyspnea (difficulty breathing).[98] Intravenous administration of quercetin at doses of 945 mg/m^2 or more was associated with renal toxicity in that trial.

Tea Extracts

Cancer patients in clinical trials of caffeinated green tea extracts who took 6 g/d in 3 to 6 divided doses have reported mild-to-moderate gastrointestinal side effects, including nausea, vomiting, abdominal pain, and diarrhea.[99,100] Central nervous system symptoms including agitation, restlessness, insomnia, tremors, dizziness, and confusion have also been reported. In one case, confusion was severe enough to require hospitalization.[99] These side effects were likely related to the caffeine in the green tea extract.[100] In a 4-week clinical trial that assessed the safety of decaffeinated green tea extracts (800 mg/d of epigallocatechin gallate) to healthy individuals, a few of the participants reported mild nausea, stomach upset, dizziness, or muscle pain.[101]

Pregnancy and Lactation

The safety of flavonoid supplements in pregnancy and lactation has not been established.[96]

Drug Interactions

Inhibition of CYP 3A4 by Grapefruit Juice and Flavonoids

As little as 200 mL (7 fl oz) of grapefruit juice has been found to irreversibly inhibit the intestinal drug metabolizing enzyme, cytochrome P450 (CYP) 3A4.[102] Although the most potent inhibitors of CYP3A4 in grapefruit are thought to be furanocoumarins, particularly dihydroxybergamottin, the flavonoids naringenin and quercetin have also been found to inhibit CYP3A4 in vitro. Inhibition of intestinal CYP3A4 can increase the bioavailability and the risk of toxicity of several drugs, including but not limited to HMG-CoA reductase inhibitors (atorvastatin, lovastatin, and simvastatin), calcium channel antagonists (felodipine, nicardipine, nisoldipine, nitrendipine, and verapamil), antiarrhythmic agents (amiodarone), HIV protease inhibitors (saquinavir), immunosuppressants (cyclosporine), antihistamines (terfenadine), gastrointestinal stimulants (cisapride), benzodiazepines (diazepam, midazolam, and triazolam), anticonvulsants (carbamazepine), anxiolytics (buspirone), serotonin specific reuptake inhibitors (sertraline), and drugs used to treat erectile dysfunction (sildenafil).[103] Grapefruit juice may reduce the therapeutic effect of losartan, an angiotensin II receptor antagonist. Because of the potential for adverse drug interactions, some clinicians recommend that people taking medications that undergo extensive presystemic metabolism by CYP3A4 and have the potential for serious toxicity avoid consuming grapefruit juice altogether.[102]

Inhibition of P-glycoprotein by Grapefruit Juice and Flavonoids

P-glycoprotein is an efflux transporter that decreases the absorption of several drugs. There is some evidence that the consumption of grapefruit juice inhibits the activity of P-glycoprotein.[102] Quercetin, naringenin, and epigallocatechin gallate, have been found to inhibit the efflux activity of P-glycoprotein in cultured cells.[104] Thus, very high or supplemental intakes of these flavonoids could potentially increase the bioavailability and the risk of toxicity of drugs that are substrates of P-glycoprotein. Drugs known to be substrates of P-glycoprotein include digoxin, antihypertensive agents, antiarrhythmic agents, chemotherapeutic agents, antifungal agents, HIV protease inhibitors, immunosuppressive agents, H$_2$ receptor antagonists, and some antibiotics.[105]

Anticoagulant and Antiplatelet Drugs

High intakes of flavonoids from purple grape juice (500 mL/d) and dark chocolate (235 mg/d of flavanols) have been found to inhibit platelet aggregation in ex vivo assays.[59–61,63] Theoretically, high intakes of flavonoids (e.g., from supplements) could increase the risk of bleeding when taken with anticoagulant drugs, such as warfarin (Coumadin) and antiplatelet drugs, such as clopidogrel (Plavix), dipyridamole (Persantine), nonsteroidal antiinflammatory drugs (NSAIDs), and aspirin.

Nutrient Interactions

Iron

Flavonoids can bind nonheme iron, inhibiting its intestinal absorption. Nonheme iron is the principal form of iron in plant foods, dairy products, and iron supplements. The consumption of one cup of tea or cocoa with a meal has been found to decrease the absorption of nonheme iron in that meal by ∼ 70%.[106,107] To maximize iron absorption from a meal or iron supplements, flavonoid-rich beverages or flavonoid supplements should not be taken at the same time.

Vitamin C

Studies in cell culture indicate that several flavonoids inhibit the transport of vitamin C into cells, and supplementation of rats with quercetin and vitamin C decreased the intestinal absorption of the latter compound.[108] More research is needed to determine the significance of these findings in humans.

Summary

- Flavonoids are a large family of polyphenolic compounds synthesized by plants.
- Scientists are interested in the potential health benefits of flavonoids associated with fruit and vegetable-rich diets.
- Many of the biological effects of flavonoids appear to be related to their ability to modulate cell signaling pathways, rather than their antioxidant activity.
- Although higher intakes of flavonoid-rich foods are associated with reductions in cardiovascular disease risk, it is not yet known whether flavonoids themselves are cardioprotective.

- Despite promising results in animal studies, it is not clear whether high flavonoid intakes can help prevent cancer in humans.
- Although scientists are interested in the potential of flavonoids to protect the aging brain, it is not yet clear how flavonoid consumption affects neurodegenerative disease risk in humans.
- Higher intakes of flavonoid-rich foods have been associated with reduced risk of chronic disease in some studies, but it is not known whether isolated flavonoid supplements or extracts will confer the same benefits as flavonoid-rich foods.

References

1. Beecher GR. Overview of dietary flavonoids: nomenclature, occurrence and intake. J Nutr 2003;133(10):3248S–3254S
2. Williamson G. Common features in the pathways of absorption and metabolism of flavonoids. In: Meskin MS, R. BW, Davies AJ, Lewis DS, Randolph RK, eds. Phytochemicals: Mechanisms of Action. Boca Raton: CRC Press; 2004:21–33
3. Manach C, Scalbert A, Morand C, Remesy C, Jimenez L. Polyphenols: food sources and bioavailability. Am J Clin Nutr 2004;79(5):727–747
4. Spencer JP, Abd-el-Mohsen MM, Rice-Evans C. Cellular uptake and metabolism of flavonoids and their metabolites: implications for their bioactivity. Arch Biochem Biophys 2004;423(1):148–161
5. Kroon PA, Clifford MN, Crozier A, et al. How should we assess the effects of exposure to dietary polyphenols in vitro? Am J Clin Nutr 2004;80(1):15–21
6. Heijnen CG, Haenen GR, van Acker FA, van der Vijgh WJ, Bast A. Flavonoids as peroxynitrite scavengers: the role of the hydroxyl groups. Toxicol In Vitro 2001;15(1):3–6
7. Chun OK, Kim DO, Lee CY. Superoxide radical scavenging activity of the major polyphenols in fresh plums. J Agric Food Chem 2003;51(27):8067–8072
8. Frei B, Higdon JV. Antioxidant activity of tea polyphenols in vivo: evidence from animal studies. J Nutr 2003;133(10):3275S–3284S
9. Williams RJ, Spencer JP, Rice-Evans C. Flavonoids: antioxidants or signalling molecules? Free Radic Biol Med 2004;36(7):838–849
10. Mira L, Fernandez MT, Santos M, Rocha R, Florencio MH, Jennings KR. Interactions of flavonoids with iron and copper ions: a mechanism for their antioxidant activity. Free Radic Res 2002;36(11):1199–1208
11. Cheng IF, Breen K. On the ability of four flavonoids, baicilein, luteolin, naringenin, and quercetin, to suppress the Fenton reaction of the iron-ATP complex. Biometals 2000;13(1):77–83
12. Spencer JP, Rice-Evans C, Williams RJ. Modulation of pro-survival Akt/protein kinase B and ERK1/2 signaling cascades by quercetin and its in vivo metabolites

underlie their action on neuronal viability. J Biol Chem 2003;278(37):34783–34793

13. Spencer JP, Schroeter H, Crossthwaithe AJ, Kuhnle G, Williams RJ, Rice-Evans C. Contrasting influences of glucuronidation and O-methylation of epicatechin on hydrogen peroxide-induced cell death in neurons and fibroblasts. Free Radic Biol Med 2001;31(9): 1139–1146

14. Hou Z, Lambert JD, Chin KV, Yang CS. Effects of tea polyphenols on signal transduction pathways related to cancer chemoprevention. Mutat Res 2004; 555(1–2):3–19

15. Lambert JD, Yang CS. Mechanisms of cancer prevention by tea constituents. J Nutr 2003;133(10):3262S–3267S

16. Kong AN, Owuor E, Yu R, et al. Induction of xenobiotic enzymes by the MAP kinase pathway and the antioxidant or electrophile response element (ARE/EpRE). Drug Metab Rev 2001;33(3–4):255–271

17. Walle UK, Walle T. Induction of human UDP-glucuronosyltransferase UGT1A1 by flavonoids-structural requirements. Drug Metab Dispos 2002;30(5):564–569

18. Chen JJ, Ye ZQ, Koo MW. Growth inhibition and cell cycle arrest effects of epigallocatechin gallate in the NBT-II bladder tumour cell line. BJU Int 2004; 93(7):1082–1086

19. Wang W, VanAlstyne PC, Irons KA, Chen S, Stewart JW, Birt DF. Individual and interactive effects of apigenin analogs on G2/M cell-cycle arrest in human colon carcinoma cell lines. Nutr Cancer 2004;48(1): 106–114

20. Stewart ZA, Westfall MD, Pietenpol JA. Cell-cycle dysregulation and anticancer therapy. Trends Pharmacol Sci 2003;24(3):139–145

21. Sah JF, Balasubramanian S, Eckert RL, Rorke EA. Epigallocatechin-3-gallate inhibits epidermal growth factor receptor signaling pathway. Evidence for direct inhibition of ERK1/2 and AKT kinases. J Biol Chem 2004;279(31):12755–12762

22. Kavanagh KT, Hafer LJ, Kim DW, et al. Green tea extracts decrease carcinogen-induced mammary tumor burden in rats and rate of breast cancer cell proliferation in culture. J Cell Biochem 2001;82(3): 387–398

23. Bagli E, Stefaniotou M, Morbidelli L, et al. Luteolin inhibits vascular endothelial growth factor-induced angiogenesis; inhibition of endothelial cell survival and proliferation by targeting phosphatidylinositol 3′-kinase activity. Cancer Res 2004;64(21):7936–7946

24. Kim MH. Flavonoids inhibit VEGF/bFGF-induced angiogenesis in vitro by inhibiting the matrix-degrading proteases. J Cell Biochem 2003;89(3):529–538

25. O'Leary KA, de Pascual-Tereasa S, Needs PW, Bao YP, O'Brien NM, Williamson G. Effect of flavonoids and vitamin E on cyclooxygenase-2 (COX-2) transcription. Mutat Res 2004;551(1–2):245–254

26. Sakata K, Hirose Y, Qiao Z, Tanaka T, Mori H. Inhibition of inducible isoforms of cyclooxygenase and nitric oxide synthase by flavonoid hesperidin in mouse macrophage cell line. Cancer Lett 2003; 199(2):139–145

27. Cho SY, Park SJ, Kwon MJ, et al. Quercetin suppresses proinflammatory cytokines production through MAP kinases andNF-kappaB pathway in lipopolysac-

charide-stimulated macrophage. Mol Cell Biochem 2003;243(1–2):153–160

28. Steele VE, Hawk ET, Viner JL, Lubet RA. Mechanisms and applications of non-steroidal anti-inflammatory drugs in the chemoprevention of cancer. Mutat Res 2003;523–524:137–144

29. Blake GJ, Ridker PM. C-reactive protein and other inflammatory risk markers in acute coronary syndromes. J Am Coll Cardiol 2003; 41 (4, Suppl S)37S–42S

30. Choi JS, Choi YJ, Park SH, Kang JS, Kang YH. Flavones mitigate tumor necrosis factor-alpha-induced adhesion molecule upregulation in cultured human endothelial cells: role of nuclear factor-kappa B. J Nutr 2004;134(5):1013–1019

31. Ludwig A, Lorenz M, Grimbo N, et al. The tea flavonoid epigallocatechin-3-gallate reduces cytokine-induced VCAM-1 expression and monocyte adhesion to endothelial cells. Biochem Biophys Res Commun 2004;316(3):659–665

32. Stocker R, Keaney JF Jr. Role of oxidative modifications in atherosclerosis. Physiol Rev 2004;84(4): 1381–1478

33. Anter E, Thomas SR, Schulz E, Shapira OM, Vita JA, Keaney JF Jr. Activation of endothelial nitric-oxide synthase by the p38 MAP kinase in response to black tea polyphenols. J Biol Chem 2004;279(45):46637–46643

34. Duffy SJ, Vita JA. Effects of phenolics on vascular endothelial function. Curr Opin Lipidol 2003;14(1):21–27

35. Deana R, Turetta L, Donella-Deana A, et al. Green tea epigallocatechin-3-gallate inhibits platelet signalling pathways triggered by both proteolytic and non-proteolytic agonists. Thromb Haemost 2003; 89(5):866–874

36. Bucki R, Pastore JJ, Giraud F, Sulpice JC, Janmey PA. Flavonoid inhibition of platelet procoagulant activity and phosphoinositide synthesis. J Thromb Haemost 2003;1(8):1820–1828

37. Hubbard GP, Wolffram S, Lovegrove JA, Gibbins JM. The role of polyphenolic compounds in the diet as inhibitors of platelet function. Proc Nutr Soc 2003; 62(2):469–478

38. Geleijnse JM, Launer LJ, Van der Kuip DA, Hofman A, Witteman JC. Inverse association of tea and flavonoid intakes with incident myocardial infarction: the Rotterdam Study. Am J Clin Nutr 2002; 75(5):880–886

39. Hertog MG, Feskens EJ, Kromhout D. Antioxidant flavonols and coronary heart disease risk. Lancet 1997;349(9053):699

40. Hirvonen T, Pietinen P, Virtanen M, et al. Intake of flavonols and flavones and risk of coronary heart disease in male smokers. Epidemiology 2001;12(1):62–67

41. Knekt P, Kumpulainen J, Jarvinen R, et al. Flavonoid intake and risk of chronic diseases. Am J Clin Nutr 2002;76(3):560–568

42. Yochum L, Kushi LH, Meyer K, Folsom AR. Dietary flavonoid intake and risk of cardiovascular disease in postmenopausal women. Am J Epidemiol 1999; 149(10):943–949

43. Hertog MG, Sweetnam PM, Fehily AM, Elwood PC, Kromhout D. Antioxidant flavonols and ischemic heart disease in a Welsh population of men: the

Caerphilly Study. Am J Clin Nutr 1997;65(5):1489–1494

44. Rimm EB, Katan MB, Ascherio A, Stampfer MJ, Willett WC. Relation between intake of flavonoids and risk for coronary heart disease in male health professionals. Ann Intern Med 1996;125(5):384–389

45. Sesso HD, Gaziano JM, Liu S, Buring JE. Flavonoid intake and the risk of cardiovascular disease in women. Am J Clin Nutr 2003;77(6):1400–1408

46. Keli SO, Hertog MG, Feskens EJ, Kromhout D. Dietary flavonoids, antioxidant vitamins, and incidence of stroke: the Zutphen study. Arch Intern Med 1996; 156(6):637–642

47. Hirvonen T, Virtamo J, Korhonen P, Albanes D, Pietinen P. Intake of flavonoids, carotenoids, vitamins C and E, and risk of stroke in male smokers. Stroke 2000;31(10):2301–2306

48. Knekt P, Isotupa S, Rissanen H, et al. Quercetin intake and the incidence of cerebrovascular disease. Eur J Clin Nutr 2000;54(5):415–417

49. Liu RH. Health benefits of fruit and vegetables are from additive and synergistic combinations of phytochemicals. Am J Clin Nutr 2003;78(3 Suppl):517S–520S

50. Vita JA. Tea consumption and cardiovascular disease: effects on endothelial function. J Nutr 2003; 133(10):3293S–3297S

51. Duffy SJ, Keaney JF Jr, Holbrook M, et al. Short- and long-term black tea consumption reverses endothelial dysfunction in patients with coronary artery disease. Circulation 2001;104(2):151–156

52. Hodgson JM, Puddey IB, Burke V, Watts GF, Beilin LJ. Regular ingestion of black tea improves brachial artery vasodilator function. Clin Sci (Lond) 2002; 102(2):195–201

53. Stein JH, Keevil JG, Wiebe DA, Aeschlimann S, Folts JD. Purple grape juice improves endothelial function and reduces the susceptibility of LDL cholesterol to oxidation in patients with coronary artery disease. Circulation 1999;100(10):1050–1055

54. Engler MB, Engler MM, Chen CY, et al. Flavonoid-rich dark chocolate improves endothelial function and increases plasma epicatechin concentrations in healthy adults. J Am Coll Nutr 2004;23(3):197–204

55. Freese R, Vaarala O, Turpeinen AM, Mutanen M. No difference in platelet activation or inflammation markers after diets rich or poor in vegetables, berries and apple in healthy subjects. Eur J Nutr 2004; 43(3):175–182

56. Janssen K, Mensink RP, Cox FJ, et al. Effects of the flavonoids quercetin and apigenin on hemostasis in healthy volunteers: results from an in vitro and a dietary supplement study. Am J Clin Nutr 1998;67(2): 255–262

57. Duffy SJ, Vita JA, Holbrook M, Swerdloff PL, Keaney JF Jr. Effect of acute and chronic tea consumption on platelet aggregation in patients with coronary artery disease. Arterioscler Thromb Vasc Biol 2001;21(6): 1084–1089

58. Hodgson JM, Puddey IB, Burke V, Beilin LJ, Mori TA, Chan SY. Acute effects of ingestion of black tea on postprandial platelet aggregation in human subjects. Br J Nutr 2002;87(2):141–145

59. Freedman JE, Parker C III, Li L, et al. Select flavonoids and whole juice from purple grapes inhibit platelet function and enhance nitric oxide release. Circulation 2001;103(23):2792–2798

60. Keevil JG, Osman HE, Reed JD, Folts JD. Grape juice, but not orange juice or grapefruit juice, inhibits human platelet aggregation. J Nutr 2000;130(1):53–56

61. Polagruto JA, Schramm DD, Wang-Polagruto JF, Lee L, Keen CL. Effects of flavonoid-rich beverages on prostacyclin synthesis in humans and human aortic endothelial cells: association with ex vivo platelet function. J Med Food 2003;6(4):301–308

62. Innes AJ, Kennedy G, McLaren M, Bancroft AJ, Belch JJ. Dark chocolate inhibits platelet aggregation in healthy volunteers. Platelets 2003;14(5):325–327

63. Murphy KJ, Chronopoulos AK, Singh I, et al. Dietary flavanols and procyanidin oligomers from cocoa (Theobroma cacao) inhibit platelet function. Am J Clin Nutr 2003;77(6):1466–1473

64. Yang CS, Yang GY, Landau JM, Kim S, Liao J. Tea and tea polyphenols inhibit cell hyperproliferation, lung tumorigenesis, and tumor progression. Exp Lung Res 1998;24(4):629–639

65. Balasubramanian S, Govindasamy S. Inhibitory effect of dietary flavonol quercetin on 7,12-dimethylbenz[a]anthracene-induced hamster buccal pouch carcinogenesis. Carcinogenesis 1996;17(4):877–879

66. Li ZG, Shimada Y, Sato F, et al. Inhibitory effects of epigallocatechin-3-gallate on N-nitrosomethylbenzylamine-induced esophageal tumorigenesis in F344 rats. Int J Oncol 2002;21(6):1275–1283

67. Yamane T, Nakatani H, Kikuoka N, et al. Inhibitory effects and toxicity of green tea polyphenols for gastrointestinal carcinogenesis. Cancer 1996;77(8 Suppl):1662–1667

68. Guo JY, Li X, Browning JD Jr, et al. Dietary soy isoflavones and estrone protect ovariectomized ERalphaKO and wild-type mice from carcinogen-induced colon cancer. J Nutr 2004;134(1):179–182

69. Huang MT, Xie JG, Wang ZY, et al. Effects of tea, decaffeinated tea, and caffeine on UVB light-induced complete carcinogenesis in SKH-1 mice: demonstration of caffeine as a biologically important constituent of tea. Cancer Res 1997;57(13):2623–2629

70. Gupta S, Hastak K, Ahmad N, Lewin JS, Mukhtar H. Inhibition of prostate carcinogenesis in TRAMP mice by oral infusion of green tea polyphenols. Proc Natl Acad Sci U S A 2001;98(18):10350–10355

71. Yamagishi M, Natsume M, Osakabe N, et al. Effects of cacao liquor proanthocyanidins on PhIP-induced mutagenesis in vitro, and in vivo mammary and pancreatic tumorigenesis in female Sprague-Dawley rats. Cancer Lett 2002;185(2):123–130

72. Ross JA, Kasum CM. Dietary flavonoids: bioavailability, metabolic effects, and safety. Annu Rev Nutr 2002;22:19–34

73. Goldbohm RA, Van den Brandt PA, Hertog MG, Brants HA, Van Poppel G. Flavonoid intake and risk of cancer: a prospective cohort study. Am J Epidemiol 1995;41:S61

74. Hertog MG, Feskens EJ, Hollman PC, Katan MB, Kromhout D. Dietary flavonoids and cancer risk in the Zutphen Elderly Study. Nutr Cancer 1994;22(2): 175–184

75. Arts IC, Hollman PC, Bueno De Mesquita HB, Feskens EJ, Kromhout D. Dietary catechins and epithelial cancer incidence: the Zutphen elderly study. Int J Cancer 2001;92(2):298–302

76. Goldbohm RA, Hertog MG, Brants HA, van Poppel G, van den Brandt PA. Consumption of black tea and

cancer risk: a prospective cohort study. J Natl Cancer Inst 1996;88(2):93–100

77. Arts IC, Jacobs DR Jr, Gross M, Harnack LJ, Folsom AR. Dietary catechins and cancer incidence among postmenopausal women: the Iowa Women's Health Study (United States). Cancer Causes Control 2002; 13(4):373–382

78. Higdon JV, Frei B. Tea catechins and polyphenols: health effects, metabolism, and antioxidant functions. Crit Rev Food Sci Nutr 2003;43(1):89–143

79. De Stefani E, Ronco A, Mendilaharsu M, Deneo-Pellegrini H. Diet and risk of cancer of the upper aerodigestive tract–II. Nutrients. Oral Oncol 1999;35(1): 22–26

80. Garcia-Closas R, Gonzalez CA, Agudo A, Riboli E. Intake of specific carotenoids and flavonoids and the risk of gastric cancer in Spain. Cancer Causes Control 1999;10(1):71–75

81. Lagiou P, Samoli E, Lagiou A, et al. Flavonoids, vitamin C and adenocarcinoma of the stomach. Cancer Causes Control 2004;15(1):67–72

82. Peterson J, Lagiou P, Samoli E, et al. Flavonoid intake and breast cancer risk: a case–control study in Greece. Br J Cancer 2003;89(7):1255–1259

83. Garcia R, Gonzalez CA, Agudo A, Riboli E. High intake of specific carotenoids and flavonoids does not reduce the risk of bladder cancer. Nutr Cancer 1999; 35(2):212–214

84. Garcia-Closas R, Agudo A, Gonzalez CA, Riboli E. Intake of specific carotenoids and flavonoids and the risk of lung cancer in women in Barcelona, Spain. Nutr Cancer 1998;32(3):154–158

85. Youdim KA, Qaiser MZ, Begley DJ, Rice-Evans CA, Abbott NJ. Flavonoid permeability across an in situ model of the blood-brain barrier. Free Radic Biol Med 2004;36(5):592–604

86. Goyarzu P, Malin DH, Lau FC, et al. Blueberry supplemented diet: effects on object recognition memory and nuclear factor-kappa B levels in aged rats. Nutr Neurosci 2004;7(2):75–83

87. Joseph JA, Denisova NA, Arendash G, et al. Blueberry supplementation enhances signaling and prevents behavioral deficits in an Alzheimer disease model. Nutr Neurosci 2003;6(3):153–162

88. Joseph JA, Shukitt-Hale B, Denisova NA, et al. Reversals of age-related declines in neuronal signal transduction, cognitive, and motor behavioral deficits with blueberry, spinach, or strawberry dietary supplementation. J Neurosci 1999;19(18):8114–8121

89. Patil CS, Singh VP, Satyanarayan PS, Jain NK, Singh A, Kulkarni SK. Protective effect of flavonoids against aging- and lipopolysaccharide-induced cognitive impairment in mice. Pharmacology 2003;69(2):59–67

90. Laurin D, Masaki KH, Foley DJ, White LR, Launer LJ. Midlife dietary intake of antioxidants and risk of late-life incident dementia: the Honolulu-Asia Aging Study. Am J Epidemiol 2004;159(10):959–967

91. White LR, Petrovitch H, Ross GW, et al. Brain aging and midlife tofu consumption. J Am Coll Nutr 2000; 19(2):242–255

92. de Rijk MC, Breteler MM, den Breeijen JH, et al. Dietary antioxidants and Parkinson disease. The Rotterdam Study. Arch Neurol 1997;54(6):762–765

93. Engelhart MJ, Geerlings MI, Ruitenberg A, et al. Dietary intake of antioxidants and risk of Alzheimer disease. JAMA 2002;287(24):3223–3229

94. Commenges D, Scotet V, Renaud S, Jacqmin-Gadda H, Barberger-Gateau P, Dartigues JF. Intake of flavonoids and risk of dementia. Eur J Epidemiol 2000; 16(4):357–363

95. Gu L, Kelm MA, Hammerstone JF, et al. Concentrations of proanthocyanidins in common foods and estimations of normal consumption. J Nutr 2004; 134(3):613–617

96. Hendler SS, Rorvik DR, eds. PDR for Nutritional Supplements. Montvale: Medical Economics Company, Inc; 2001

97. Shoskes DA, Zeitlin SI, Shahed A, Rajfer J. Quercetin in men with category III chronic prostatitis: a preliminary prospective, double-blind, placebo-controlled trial. Urology 1999;54(6):960–963

98. Ferry DR, Smith A, Malkhandi J, et al. Phase I clinical trial of the flavonoid quercetin: pharmacokinetics and evidence for in vivo tyrosine kinase inhibition. Clin Cancer Res 1996;2(4):659–668

99. Jatoi A, Ellison N, Burch PA, et al. A phase II trial of green tea in the treatment of patients with androgen independent metastatic prostate carcinoma. Cancer 2003;97(6):1442–1446

100. Pisters KM, Newman RA, Coldman B, et al. Phase I trial of oral green tea extract in adult patients with solid tumors. J Clin Oncol 2001;19(6):1830–1838

101. Chow HH, Cai Y, Hakim IA, et al. Pharmacokinetics and safety of green tea polyphenols after multiple-dose administration of epigallocatechin gallate and polyphenon E in healthy individuals. Clin Cancer Res 2003;9(9):3312–3319

102. Bailey DG, Dresser GK. Interactions between grapefruit juice and cardiovascular drugs. Am J Cardiovasc Drugs 2004;4(5):281–297

103. Dahan A, Altman H. Food-drug interaction: grapefruit juice augments drug bioavailability–mechanism, extent and relevance. Eur J Clin Nutr 2004; 58(1):1–9

104. Zhou S, Lim LY, Chowbay B. Herbal modulation of P-glycoprotein. Drug Metab Rev 2004;36(1):57–104

105. Marzolini C, Paus E, Buclin T, Kim RB. Polymorphisms in human MDR1 (P-glycoprotein): recent advances and clinical relevance. Clin Pharmacol Ther 2004;75(1):13–33

106. Hurrell RF, Reddy M, Cook JD. Inhibition of non-haem iron absorption in man by polyphenolic-containing beverages. Br J Nutr 1999;81(4):289–295

107. Zijp IM, Korver O, Tijburg LB. Effect of tea and other dietary factors on iron absorption. Crit Rev Food Sci Nutr 2000;40(5):371–398

108. Song J, Kwon O, Chen S, et al. Flavonoid inhibition of sodium-dependent vitamin C transporter 1 (SVCT1) and glucose transporter isoform 2 (GLUT2), intestinal transporters for vitamin C and Glucose. J Biol Chem 2002;277(18):15252–15260

109. U.S. Department of Agriculture. USDA database for the flavonoid content of selected foods. 2003. Available at: http://www.nal.usda.gov/fnic/foodcomp/ Data/Flav/flav.html. Accessed 9/13/04

110. U.S. Department of Agriculture. USDA database for the proanthocyanidin content of selected foods. 2004. Available at: http://www.nal.usda.gov/fnic/ foodcomp/Data/PA/PA.html. Accessed 9/13/04

111. Vrhovsek U, Rigo A, Tonon D, Mattivi F. Quantitation of polyphenols in different apple varieties. J Agric Food Chem 2004;52(21):6532–6538

112. Moyer RA, Hummer KE, Finn CE, Frei B, Wrolstad RE. Anthocyanins, phenolics, and antioxidant capacity in diverse small fruits: vaccinium, rubus, and ribes. J Agric Food Chem 2002;50(3):519–525

113. Lee HS. Characterization of major anthocyanins and the color of red-fleshed Budd Blood orange (Citrus sinensis). J Agric Food Chem 2002;50(5):1243–1246

114. Ryan JM, Revilla E. Anthocyanin composition of Cabernet Sauvignon and Tempranillo grapes at different stages of ripening. J Agric Food Chem 2003;51(11): 3372–3378

115. Henning SM, Fajardo-Lira C, Lee HW, Youssefian AA, Go VL, Heber D. Catechin content of 18 teas and a green tea extract supplement correlates with the antioxidant capacity. Nutr Cancer 2003;45(2):226–235

14 Soy Isoflavones

Isoflavones are polyphenolic compounds that are capable of exerting estrogen-like effects. For this reason, they are classified as phytoestrogens—compounds with estrogenic activity derived from plants.[1] Legumes, particularly soybeans, are the richest sources of isoflavones in the human diet. In soybeans, isoflavones are present as glycosides (bound to a sugar molecule). Fermentation or digestion of soybeans or soy products results in the release of the sugar molecule from the isoflavone glycoside, leaving an isoflavone aglycone. Soy isoflavone glycosides are called genistin, daidzin, and glycitin; the aglycones are called genistein, daidzein, and glycitein, respectively (**Fig. 14–1**). Unless otherwise indicated, quantities of isoflavones specified in this chapter refer to aglycones.

Metabolism and Bioavailability

The biological effects of soy isoflavones are strongly influenced by their metabolism, which is dependent on the activity of bacteria that colonize the human intestine.[2] For example, the soy isoflavone daidzein may be metabolized by colonic bacteria to equol (**Fig. 14–2**), a metabolite that has greater estrogenic activity than daidzein, and to other metabolites that are less estrogenic. Studies that measure urinary equol excretion after soy consumption indicate that only ~ 33 % of individuals from Western populations metabolize daidzein to equol.[3] Thus, individual differences in the metabolism of isoflavones could have important implications for the biological activities of these phytoestrogens.

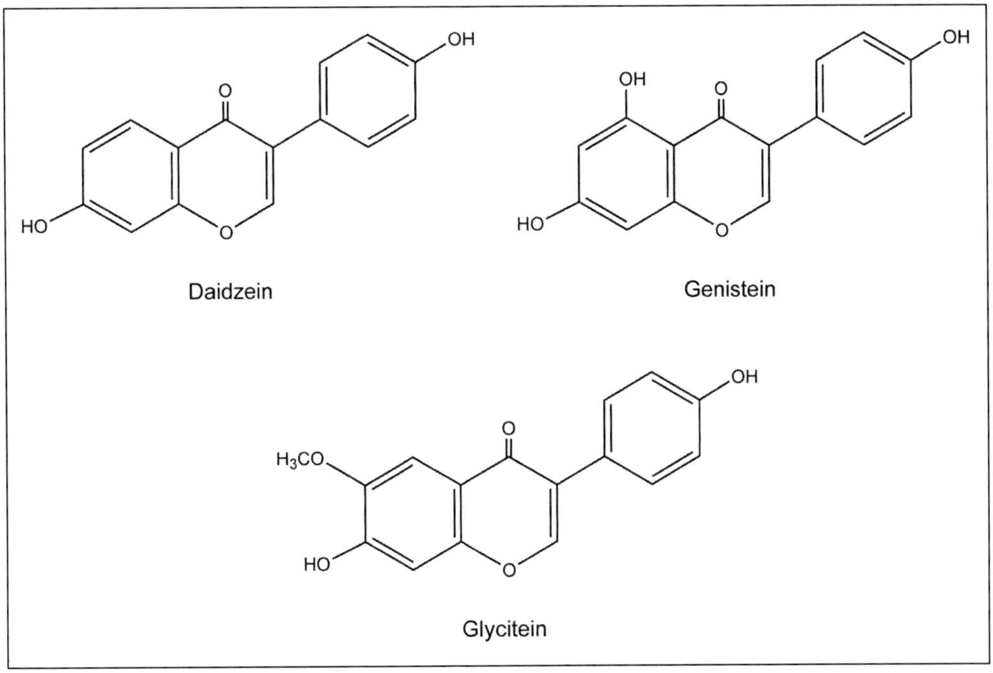

Figure 14–1 Chemical structures of the soy isoflavones, daidzein, genistein, and glycitein, in their aglycone forms.

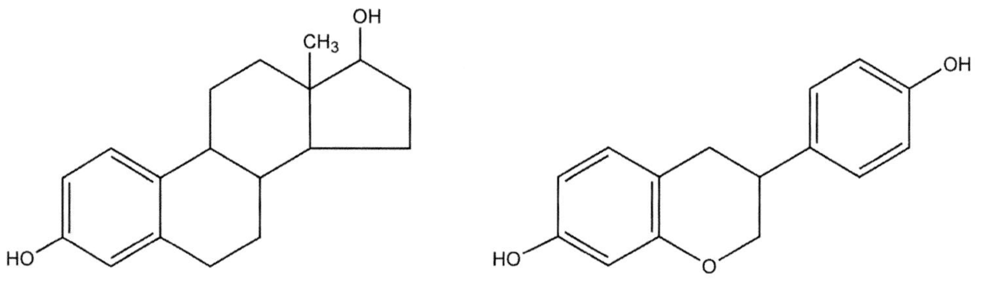

Figure 14–2   Chemical structures of 17β-estradiol, an endogenous estrogen, and equol, a bacterial metabolite of daidzein, that has estrogenic activity.

Biological Activity

Estrogenic and Antiestrogenic Activities

Soy isoflavones are known to have weak estrogenic activity. Estrogens are signaling molecules that exert their effects by binding to estrogen receptors within cells. The estrogen-receptor complex interacts with DNA to change the expression of estrogen-responsive genes. Estrogen receptors are present in numerous tissues other than those associated with reproduction, including bone, liver, heart, and brain.[4] Soy isoflavones and other phytoestrogens can bind to estrogen receptors, mimicking the effects of estrogen in some tissues and antagonizing the effects of estrogen in others.[5] Scientists are interested in the tissue-selective activities of phytoestrogens because anti-estrogenic effects in reproductive tissue could help reduce the risk of hormone-associated cancers (breast, uterine, and prostate), whereas estrogenic effects in other tissues could help maintain bone density and improve blood lipid profiles (cholesterol levels). The extent to which soy isoflavones exert estrogenic and anti-estrogenic effects in humans is currently the focus of considerable scientific research.

Estrogen Receptor-Independent Activities

Soy isoflavones and their metabolites also have biological activities that are unrelated to their interactions with estrogen receptors.[6] By inhibiting the synthesis and activity of enzymes involved in estrogen and testosterone metabolism, soy isoflavones may alter the biological activity of endogenous estrogens and testosterones.[7–9] Soy isoflavones have also been found to inhibit tyrosine kinases,[10] enzymes that play critical roles in the signaling pathways that stimulate cell proliferation. Additionally, isoflavones can act as antioxidants in vitro,[11] but the extent to which they contribute to the antioxidant status of humans is not yet clear. Plasma F_2-isoprostanes, biomarkers of lipid peroxidation in vivo, were lower after 2 weeks of daily consumption of soy protein containing 56 mg of isoflavones than after consumption of soy protein providing only 2 mg of isoflavones.[12] However, daily supplementation with 50 to 100 mg of isolated soy isoflavones did not significantly alter plasma or urinary F_2-isoprostane levels.[13,14]

Prevention

Cardiovascular Disease

Serum Cholesterol

Although controlled clinical trials conducted prior to 1995 suggested that substituting 25 to 50 g/d of soy protein for animal protein lowered serum low-density lipoprotein (LDL) cholesterol by ~ 13%,[15] more recent and better controlled trials indicate that the LDL cholesterol-lowering effect of soy protein is much more modest. A recent review of 22 randomized controlled trials concluded that substituting 50 g/d of soy protein for animal protein lowered LDL cholesterol by only ~ 3%.[16] There is limited evidence that soy protein containing isoflavones is more effective than soy protein without isoflavones in lowering LDL cholesterol,[17,18] but the consumption of soy isoflavones alone (as supplements or extracts) does not appear to have favorable effects on serum lipid profiles.[19,20] For more information on soy protein and cholesterol, see Chapter 3.

Arterial Function

The preservation of normal arterial function plays an important role in cardiovascular disease prevention. The ability of arteries to dilate in response to nitric oxide produced by the endothelial cells that line their inner surface (endothelium-mediated vasodilation) is compromised in people at high risk for cardiovascular disease.[21] However, most placebo-controlled trials found no significant improvement in endothelium-mediated vasodilation when postmenopausal women were supplemented with up to 80 mg/d of soy isoflavones[22-24] or up to 60 g/d of soy protein containing isoflavones.[25-28] Measures of arterial stiffness assess the distensibility of arteries, and a strong association between arterial stiffness and atherosclerosis has been observed.[29] In placebo-controlled clinical trials, supplementation of postmenopausal women with 80 mg/d of a soy isoflavone extract for 5 weeks significantly decreased arterial stiffness,[23] as did supplementation of men and postmenopausal women with 40 g/d of soy protein providing 118 mg/d of soy isoflavones for 3

months.[28] Although most studies have not found supplementation with soy protein or isoflavones to improve endothelium-mediated vasodilation, preliminary research suggests that soy isoflavone supplementation may decrease arterial stiffness.

Hormone-Associated Cancers

Breast Cancer

Breast cancer rates in Asia, where average isoflavone intakes from soy foods range from 11 to 47 mg/d,[30] are lower than breast cancer rates in the Western countries, where average isoflavone intakes in non-Asian women may be less than 2 mg/d.[31,32] However, many other hereditary and lifestyle factors could contribute to this difference in breast cancer rates. Most epidemiological studies have not found that women with higher soy intakes are at lower risk of breast cancer, with the possible exception of women who had higher soy intakes during adolescence.[33] See Chapter 3 for more information about soy consumption and breast cancer risk. At present, there is no evidence that taking soy isoflavone supplements decreases breast cancer risk.

Endometrial Cancer

Because the development of endometrial cancer is related to prolonged exposure to unopposed estrogens, it has been suggested that high intakes of phytoestrogens with anti-estrogenic activity in uterine tissue could be protective against endometrial cancer.[34] In support of this idea, two retrospective case-control studies found that women with endometrial cancer had lower intakes of soy isoflavones from foods compared with cancer-free control groups.[34,35] However, supplementation of postmenopausal women with soy protein providing 120 mg/d of isoflavones for 6 months did not prevent endometrial hyperplasia induced by the administration of exogenous estradiol.[36] Although limited evidence from case-control studies suggests that higher dietary intakes of soy foods may be associated with lower endometrial cancer risk, there is no evidence that taking soy isoflavone supplements decreases endometrial cancer risk.

Prostate Cancer

Mortality from prostate cancer is much higher in the United States than in Asian countries, such as Japan and China.[37] However, epidemiological studies do not provide consistent evidence that high intakes of soy foods are associated with reduced prostate cancer risk. See Chapter 3 for more information about soy foods and prostate cancer risk. The results of cell culture and animal studies suggest a potential role for soy isoflavones in limiting the progression of prostate cancer. Although soy isoflavone supplementation for up to one year did not significantly decrease serum prostate specific antigen (PSA) concentrations in men without confirmed prostate cancer,[38-40] soy isoflavone supplementation appeared to slow rising serum PSA concentrations, associated with prostate tumor growth, in two small studies of prostate cancer patients.[41,42] Although such preliminary findings are encouraging, the results of larger randomized controlled trials, which are currently ongoing, are needed to determine whether soy isoflavone supplementation can play a role in the prevention or treatment of prostate cancer.

Osteoporosis

Although hip fracture rates are generally lower among Asian populations consuming soy foods than among Western populations, it is not yet clear whether increasing soy isoflavone consumption in Western populations helps to prevent osteoporosis.[43] The results of short-term clinical trials (≤ 6 months) assessing the effects of increased soy intake on biochemical markers of bone formation and bone resorption are inconsistent. Although some controlled trials in postmenopausal women found that increasing intakes of soy foods, soy protein, or soy isoflavones improved markers of bone resorption and formation,[44-47] others found no improvement.[48-50] Randomized controlled trials of longer duration are required to determine whether increased soy intake can actually prevent losses in bone mineral density (BMD) or osteoporotic fracture. Two controlled clinical trials found that BMD losses over 6 months were lower in postmenopausal women supplemented with soy protein containing isoflavones than in those supplemented with equal amounts of milk protein,[49,51] but two longer trials found that BMD loss did not differ between postmenopausal women supplemented with soy protein containing isoflavones and those supplemented with milk protein.[52,53] A 2-year clinical trial found that daily consumption of soy milk containing isoflavones decreased BMD loss in the lumbar spine compared with daily consumption of soymilk without isoflavones,[54] but two other studies found that BMD loss did not differ between postmenopausal women taking soy protein supplements containing isoflavones and those taking soy protein supplements without isoflavones.[55,56] Loss of bone mineral content at the hip over one year was lower in Taiwanese women who took 80 mg/d of isolated soy isoflavones compared with placebo, but the difference was significant only in those women who were at least 4 years past menopause, had lower body weights or lower calcium intakes.[57] There is some evidence that isoflavone-rich diets have bone-sparing effects; however, it is not known whether increasing soy isoflavone intake appreciably decreases the risk of osteoporosis or osteoporotic fracture.

Cognitive Decline

Scientific research on the effect of soy isoflavones on cognitive function is limited. The only published observational study that examined the relationship between soy intake and cognitive function found that Hawaiian men who reported consuming tofu at least twice weekly during midlife were more likely to have poor cognitive test stores 20 to 25 years later than those who reported consuming tofu less than twice a week.[58] In contrast, the results of several small clinical trials in postmenopausal women suggest that increasing soy isoflavone intake may result in modest improvements in performance on some cognitive tests for up to 6 months. Postmenopausal women given soy extracts providing 60 mg/d of soy isoflavones for 6 to 12 weeks performed better than women given a placebo on cognitive tests of picture recall (short-term memory), learning rule reversals (mental flexibility), and a planning task.[59,60] In a longer trial, postmenopausal women given supplements that provided 110 mg/d of soy isoflavones for 6 months performed better than women given placebos on a test of verbal fluency.[61] However, in the largest placebo-controlled trial in post-menopausal women to date, daily intake of soy protein providing 99 mg of isoflavones for one year did not affect performance on a battery of cognitive function tests, including tests for memory, attention, verbal fluency, and dementia.[53]

Treatment

Menopausal Symptoms

Hot flushes (flashes) are the primary reason that women seek medical attention for menopausal symptoms.[62] Concern over potential adverse effects of hormone replacement therapy[63] has led to increased interest in the use of phytoestrogen supplements by women experiencing menopausal symptoms. The effects of increasing soy isoflavone intake on the frequency of hot flushes have been examined in several randomized controlled trials.[64] Out of eight randomized controlled trials of soy foods, only one found a significant reduction in the frequency of hot flushes, whereas three out of five controlled trials of soy isoflavone extracts reported a significant reduction in hot flush frequency.[65] In general, any reductions observed were modest (10 to 20%) compared with placebo. Breast cancer survivors in particular may experience more frequent and severe hot flushes related to therapies aimed at preventing breast cancer recurrence.[66] However, none of the randomized controlled trials in breast cancer survivors found that soy isoflavone supplementation was significantly more effective than a placebo in decreasing the frequency or severity of hot flushes.[67-70] Overall, there is little evidence that increasing soy isoflavone intake from food or supplements substantially improves menopausal hot flushes.[65]

Sources

Food Sources

Isoflavones are found in small amounts in several legumes, grains, and vegetables, but soybeans are by far the most concentrated source of isoflavones in the human diet.[30,71] Recent surveys suggest that average dietary isoflavone intakes in Japan, China, and other Asian countries range from 11 to 47 mg/d.[72,73] Dietary isoflavone intakes are considerably lower in Western countries, where studies have found average isoflavone intakes to be as low as 2 mg/d.[32,74] Traditional Asian foods made from soybeans include tofu, tempeh, miso, and natto. Edamame refers to varieties of soybeans that are harvested and eaten in their green phase. Soy products that are gaining popularity in Western countries include soy-based meat substitutes, soy milk, soy cheese, and soy yogurt. The isoflavone content of soy protein isolates depends on the method used to isolate it. Soy protein isolates prepared by an ethanol wash process generally lose most of their associated isoflavones, whereas those prepared by aqueous wash processes tend to retain them.[75] Some foods that are rich in soy isoflavones are listed in **Table 14–1** along with their isoflavone content.[76] Because the isoflavone content of soy foods can vary considerably between brands and between different lots of the same brand,[75] these values should be viewed only as a guide. Given the potential health implications of diets rich in soy isoflavones, accurate and consistent labeling of the soy isoflavone content of soy foods is needed.

Supplements

Soy isoflavone extracts and supplements are available as dietary supplements without a prescription in the United States. These products are not standardized, and the amounts of soy isoflavones they provide may vary considerably. Moreover, quality control may be an issue with some of these products. When isoflavone supplements available in the United States were tested for their isoflavone content by independent laboratories, the isoflavone content in the product differed by more than

Table 14–1   Total Isoflavone Aglycone, Daidzein, and Genistein Content of Selected Foods[76]

Food	Serving	Total Isoflavones (mg)	Daidzein (mg)	Genistein (mg)
Soy protein concentrate, aqueous washed	3.5 oz (100 g)	102	43	56
Miso	$1/2$ cup	59	22	34
Soybeans, boiled	$1/2$ cup	47	23	24
Tempeh	3 oz	37	15	21
Soybeans, dry roasted	1 oz	37	15	19
Soy milk	1 cup	30	12	17
Tofu yogurt	$1/2$ cup	21	7	12
Tofu	3 oz	20	8	12
Soy protein concentrate, alcohol washed	3.5 oz (100 g)	12	7	5
Meatless (soy) hot dog	1 hot dog	11	3	6
Meatless (soy) sausage	3 links	3	0.6	2
Soy cheese, mozzarella	1 oz	2	0.3	1

10% from the amount claimed on the label in 30 to 50% of the products tested.[77,78]

Infant Formulas

Soy-based infant formulas are made from soy protein isolate and contain significant amounts of soy isoflavones. In 1997, the total isoflavone content of soy-based infant formulas, commercially available in the United States, ranged from 32 to 47 mg/liter (~ 34 fl oz).[79]

Safety

Soy isoflavones have been consumed by humans as part of soy-based diets for many years without any evidence of adverse effects.[30] The 75th percentile of dietary isoflavone intake has been reported to be as high as 65 mg/d in some Asian populations.[80] Although diets rich in soy or soy-containing products appear safe and potentially beneficial, the long-term safety of very high supplemental doses of soy isoflavones is not yet known.

Adverse Effects

Safety for Breast Cancer Survivors

The safety of high intakes of soy isoflavones and other phytoestrogens for breast cancer survivors is an area of considerable debate among scientists and clinicians.[66,81] The effects of high intakes of soy isoflavones on breast cancer survival and breast cancer recurrence in humans have not been studied. The results of cell culture and animal studies are conflicting, but some have found that soy isoflavones can stimulate the growth of estrogen receptor positive (ER+) breast cancer cells.[82,83] The effects of high intakes of soy isoflavones in breast cancer survivors who are taking tamoxifen (an anti-estrogenic drug) have not been studied, but high intakes of the soy isoflavone, genistein, interfered with the ability of tamoxifen to inhibit the growth of ER+ breast cancer cells implanted in mice.[84] Very limited data from clinical trials suggests that increased consumption of soy isoflavones (38 to 45 mg/d) can have estrogenic effects in human breast tissue.[85,86] However, a recent study in women with biopsy-confirmed breast cancer found that supplementation with 200 mg/d of soy isoflavones did not increase tumor growth over the next 2 to 6 weeks before surgery when compared with a control group that did not take soy isoflavones.[87] Given the available data, some experts think that women with a history of breast cancer, particularly ER+ breast cancer, should not increase their consumption of phytoestrogens, including soy isoflavones.[66] However, other experts argue that there is not enough evidence to discourage breast cancer survivors from consuming soy foods in moderation.[81]

Soy-Based Infant Formulas

Infant formula made from soy protein isolate has been commercially available since the mid-1960s.[88] As much as 25% of the infant formula sold in the United States is soy-based formula. Because infants fed soy-based formulas are exposed to relatively high levels of isoflavones, which they can absorb and metabolize, concern has been raised regarding potential long-term effects on growth, development, reproductive, and immune function.[79,89] The results of at least six clinical trials comparing infants fed soy-based formula with infants fed cow's milk-based formula indicate that soy-based formula supports normal growth and development in the first year of life.[90] Limited data are available on the long-term effects of feeding infants soy-based formula. One retrospective study of 811 men and women at 20 to 34 years of age found no differences in height, weight, time of puberty, general health or pregnancy outcomes between those fed soy-based formula as infants and those fed cow's milk-based formula, although women fed soy-based formula reported significantly greater use of asthma or allergy drugs than women fed cow's milk formula.[91] At present, there is no convincing evidence that infants fed soy-based formula are at greater risk for adverse effects than infants fed cow's milk-based formula. However, long-term studies on the growth and development of infants fed soy-based formulas are currently ongoing.[92]

Thyroid Function

Soy isoflavones have been found to inhibit the activity of thyroid peroxidase, an enzyme required for thyroid hormone synthesis in cell culture and animal studies.[93,94] However, high intakes of soy isoflavones do not appear to increase the risk of hypothyroidism as long as dietary iodine consumption is adequate. Since the addition of iodine to soy-based formulas in the 1960s, there have been no further reports of hypothyroidism developing in soy formula-fed infants.[95] Several clinical trials in premenopausal and postmenopausal women with sufficient iodine intakes have not found high intakes of soy isoflavones to result in clinically significant changes in circulating thyroid hormone levels.[96–99]

Pregnancy

Although there is no evidence that diets rich in soy isoflavones have adverse effects on fetal development or pregnancy outcomes in humans, the safety of isoflavone supplements during pregnancy has not been established.

Drug Interactions

Because colonic bacteria play an important role in the metabolism of soy isoflavones, antibiotic therapy could decrease their biological activity.[100] Some evidence from animal studies suggests that high intakes of soy isoflavones, particularly genistein, can interfere with the antitumor effects of tamoxifen (Novaldex).[84] Until more is known about potential interactions in humans, those taking tamoxifen or other selective estrogen receptor modulators (SERMs) to treat or prevent breast cancer should avoid soy protein supplements or isoflavone extracts (see the Safety for Breast Cancer Survivors section). High intakes of soy protein may interfere with the efficacy of the anticoagulant medication warfarin. There is one case report of an individual on warfarin who developed subtherapeutic INR (international normalized ratio; prothrombin time) values upon consuming ~16 ounces of soy milk daily for 4 weeks.[101] INR values returned to therapeutic levels 2 weeks after discontinuing soy milk. The amount of levothyroxine required for adequate thyroid hormone replacement has been found to increase in infants with congenital hypothyroidism fed soy formula.[95,102] Taking levothyroxine at the same time as a soy protein supplement also increased the levothyroxine dose required for adequate thyroid hormone replacement in an adult with hypothyroidism.[103]

Summary

- Isoflavones are a class of phytoestrogens—plant-derived compounds with estrogenic activity.
- Soybeans and soy products are the richest sources of isoflavones in the human diet.
- The results of recent randomized controlled trials suggest that substituting 50 g/d of soy protein for animal protein results in only a modest 3% reduction of LDL cholesterol. Isolated soy isoflavone supplements do not appear to have favorable effects on serum lipid profiles.
- Overall, the results of numerous observational studies do not support the idea that high soy isoflavone intakes in adults are protective against breast cancer. Limited research suggests that higher intakes of soy foods early in life may decrease the risk of breast cancer in adulthood.
- Although scientists are interested in the potential for soy isoflavones to prevent or inhibit the progression of prostate cancer, evidence from observational studies that soy isoflavones are protective against prostate cancer is limited and inconsistent.
- Although hip fracture rates are generally lower among Asian populations consuming soy foods than among Western populations, it is not yet clear whether increasing soy isoflavone consumption in Western populations will help prevent osteoporosis.
- Overall, there is little evidence that increasing soy isoflavone intake from food or supplements substantially improves menopausal hot flushes.
- Although diets rich in soy foods appear safe and potentially beneficial, the long-term safety of high doses of soy isoflavone supplements is not yet known.
- At present, there is no convincing evidence that infants fed soy-based formula are at greater risk for adverse effects than infants fed cow's milk-based formula.

References

1. Lampe JW. Isoflavonoid and lignan phytoestrogens as dietary biomarkers. J Nutr 2003;133(Suppl 3): 956S–964S
2. Rowland I, Faughnan M, Hoey L, Wahala K, Williamson G, Cassidy A. Bioavailability of phyto-oestrogens. Br J Nutr 2003;89(Suppl 1):S45–S58
3. Setchell KD, Brown NM, Lydeking-Olsen E. The clinical importance of the metabolite equol-a clue to the effectiveness of soy and its isoflavones. J Nutr 2002; 132(12):3577–3584
4. Kleinsmith LJ, Kerrigan D, Kelly J. Science behind the news: understanding estrogen receptors, tamoxifen and raloxifene. National Cancer Institute; 2003. Available at: http://press2.nci.nih.gov/sciencebehind/estrogen/estrogen01.htm
5. Wang LQ. Mammalian phytoestrogens: enterodiol and enterolactone. J Chromatogr B Analyt Technol Biomed Life Sci 2002;777(1–2):289–309
6. Barnes S, Boersma B, Patel R, et al. Isoflavonoids and chronic disease: mechanisms of action. Biofactors 2000;12(1–4):209–215
7. Kao YC, Zhou C, Sherman M, Laughton CA, Chen S. Molecular basis of the inhibition of human aromatase (estrogen synthetase) by flavone and isoflavone phytoestrogens: a site-directed mutagenesis study. Environ Health Perspect 1998;106(2):85–92
8. Whitehead SA, Cross JE, Burden C, Lacey M. Acute and chronic effects of genistein, tyrphostin and lavendustin A on steroid synthesis in luteinized human granulosa cells. Hum Reprod 2002;17(3): 589–594
9. Holzbeierlein JM, McIntosh J, Thrasher JB. The role of soy phytoestrogens in prostate cancer. Curr Opin Urol 2005;15(1):17–22
10. Akiyama T, Ishida J, Nakagawa S, et al. Genistein, a specific inhibitor of tyrosine-specific protein kinases. J Biol Chem 1987;262(12):5592–5595
11. Ruiz-Larrea MB, Mohan AR, Paganga G, Miller NJ, Bolwell GP, Rice-Evans CA. Antioxidant activity of phytoestrogenic isoflavones. Free Radic Res 1997; 26(1):63–70
12. Wiseman H, O'Reilly JD, Adlercreutz H, et al. Isoflavone phytoestrogens consumed in soy decrease F(2)-isoprostane concentrations and increase resistance of low-density lipoprotein to oxidation in humans. Am J Clin Nutr 2000;72(2):395–400
13. Hodgson JM, Puddey IB, Croft KD, Mori TA, Rivera J, Beilin LJ. Isoflavonoids do not inhibit in vivo lipid peroxidation in subjects with high-normal blood pressure. Atherosclerosis 1999;145(1):167–172
14. Djuric Z, Chen G, Doerge DR, Heilbrun LK, Kucuk O. Effect of soy isoflavone supplementation on markers of oxidative stress in men and women. Cancer Lett 2001;172(1):1–6
15. Anderson JW, Johnstone BM, Cook-Newell ME. Meta-analysis of the effects of soy protein intake on serum lipids. N Engl J Med 1995;333(5):276–282
16. Sacks FM, Lichtenstein A, Van Horn L, Harris W, Kris-Etherton P, Winston M. Soy protein, isoflavones, and cardiovascular health. An American Heart Association Science Advisory for Professionals from the Nutrition Committee. Circulation 2006;113(7):1034–1044

17. Zhan S, Ho SC. Meta-analysis of the effects of soy protein containing isoflavones on the lipid profile. Am J Clin Nutr 2005;81(2):397–408

18. Zhuo XG, Melby MK, Watanabe S. Soy isoflavone intake lowers serum LDL cholesterol: a meta-analysis of 8 randomized controlled trials in humans. J Nutr 2004;134(9):2395–2400

19. Lichtenstein AH, Jalbert SM, Adlercreutz H, et al. Lipoprotein response to diets high in soy or animal protein with and without isoflavones in moderately hypercholesterolemic subjects. Arterioscler Thromb Vasc Biol 2002;22(11):1852–1858

20. Weggemans RM, Trautwein EA. Relation between soy-associated isoflavones and LDL and HDL cholesterol concentrations in humans: a meta-analysis. Eur J Clin Nutr 2003;57(8):940–946

21. Landmesser U, Hornig B, Drexler H. Endothelial function: a critical determinant in atherosclerosis? Circulation 2004; 109 (21, Suppl 1)II27–II33

22. Squadrito F, Altavilla D, Crisafulli A, et al. Effect of genistein on endothelial function in postmenopausal women: a randomized, double-blind, controlled study. Am J Med 2003;114(6):470–476

23. Nestel PJ, Yamashita T, Sasahara T, et al. Soy isoflavones improve systemic arterial compliance but not plasma lipids in menopausal and perimenopausal women. Arterioscler Thromb Vasc Biol 1997; 17(12):3392–3398

24. Simons LA, von Konigsmark M, Simons J, Celermajer DS. Phytoestrogens do not influence lipoprotein levels or endothelial function in healthy, postmenopausal women. Am J Cardiol 2000;85(11): 1297–1301

25. Kreijkamp-Kaspers S, Kok L, Bots ML, Grobbee DE, Lampe JW, van der Schouw YT. Randomized controlled trial of the effects of soy protein containing isoflavones on vascular function in postmenopausal women. Am J Clin Nutr 2005;81(1):189–195

26. Steinberg FM, Guthrie NL, Villablanca AC, Kumar K, Murray MJ. Soy protein with isoflavones has favorable effects on endothelial function that are independent of lipid and antioxidant effects in healthy postmenopausal women. Am J Clin Nutr 2003;78(1): 123–130

27. Blum A, Lang N, Vigder F, et al. Effects of soy protein on endothelium-dependent vasodilatation and lipid profile in postmenopausal women with mild hypercholesterolemia. Clin Invest Med 2003;26(1):20–26

28. Teede HJ, Dalais FS, Kotsopoulos D, Liang YL, Davis S, McGrath BP. Dietary soy has both beneficial and potentially adverse cardiovascular effects: a placebo-controlled study in men and postmenopausal women. J Clin Endocrinol Metab 2001;86(7): 3053–3060

29. van Popele NM, Grobbee DE, Bots ML, et al. Association between arterial stiffness and atherosclerosis: the Rotterdam Study. Stroke 2001;32(2):454–460

30. Munro IC, Harwood M, Hlywka JJ, et al. Soy isoflavones: a safety review. Nutr Rev 2003;61(1):1–33

31. van Erp-Baart MA, Brants HA, Kiely M, et al. Isoflavone intake in four different European countries: the VENUS approach. Br J Nutr 2003;89(Suppl 1): S25–S30

32. de Kleijn MJ, van der Schouw YT, Wilson PW, et al. Intake of dietary phytoestrogens is low in postmenopausal women in the United States: the Framingham study (1–4). J Nutr 2001;131(6):1826–1832

33. Peeters PH, Keinan-Boker L, van der Schouw YT, Grobbee DE. Phytoestrogens and breast cancer risk. Review of the epidemiological evidence. Breast Cancer Res Treat 2003;77(2):171–183

34. Horn-Ross PL, John EM, Canchola AJ, Stewart SL, Lee MM. Phytoestrogen intake and endometrial cancer risk. J Natl Cancer Inst 2003;95(15):1158–1164

35. Goodman MT, Wilkens LR, Hankin JH, Lyu LC, Wu AH, Kolonel LN. Association of soy and fiber consumption with the risk of endometrial cancer. Am J Epidemiol 1997;146(4):294–306

36. Murray MJ, Meyer WR, Lessey BA, Oi RH, DeWire RE, Fritz MA. Soy protein isolate with isoflavones does not prevent estradiol-induced endometrial hyperplasia in postmenopausal women: a pilot trial. Menopause 2003;10(5):456–464

37. Messina MJ. Emerging evidence on the role of soy in reducing prostate cancer risk. Nutr Rev 2003;61(4): 117–131

38. Adams KF, Chen C, Newton KM, Potter JD, Lampe JW. Soy isoflavones do not modulate prostate-specific antigen concentrations in older men in a randomized controlled trial. Cancer Epidemiol Biomarkers Prev 2004;13(4):644–648

39. Jenkins DJ, Kendall CW, D'Costa MA, et al. Soy consumption and phytoestrogens: effect on serum prostate specific antigen when blood lipids and oxidized low-density lipoprotein are reduced in hyperlipidemic men. J Urol 2003;169(2):507–511

40. Urban D, Irwin W, Kirk M, et al. The effect of isolated soy protein on plasma biomarkers in elderly men with elevated serum prostate specific antigen. J Urol 2001; 165(1):294–300

41. Fischer L, Mahoney C, Jeffcoat AR, et al. Clinical characteristics and pharmacokinetics of purified soy isoflavones: multiple-dose administration to men with prostate neoplasia. Nutr Cancer 2004;48(2): 160–170

42. Hussain M, Banerjee M, Sarkar FH, et al. Soy isoflavones in the treatment of prostate cancer. Nutr Cancer 2003;47(2):111–117

43. Setchell KD, Lydeking-Olsen E. Dietary phytoestrogens and their effect on bone: evidence from in vitro and in vivo, human observational, and dietary intervention studies. Am J Clin Nutr 2003;78(3 Suppl): 593S–609S

44. Scheiber MD, Liu JH, Subbiah MT, Rebar RW, Setchell KD. Dietary inclusion of whole soy foods results in significant reductions in clinical risk factors for osteoporosis and cardiovascular disease in normal postmenopausal women. Menopause 2001;8(5): 384–392

45. Chiechi LM, Secreto G, D'Amore M, et al. Efficacy of a soy rich diet in preventing postmenopausal osteoporosis: the Menfis randomized trial. Maturitas 2002;42(4):295–300

46. Arjmandi BH, Khalil DA, Smith BJ, et al. Soy protein has a greater effect on bone in postmenopausal women not on hormone replacement therapy, as evidenced by reducing bone resorption and urinary calcium excretion. J Clin Endocrinol Metab 2003; 88(3):1048–1054

47. Harkness LS, Fiedler K, Sehgal AR, Oravec D, Lerner E. Decreased bone resorption with soy isoflavone sup-

plementation in postmenopausal women. J Womens Health (Larchmt) 2004;13(9):1000–1007

48. Wangen KE, Duncan AM, Merz-Demlow BE, et al. Effects of soy isoflavones on markers of bone turnover in premenopausal and postmenopausal women. J Clin Endocrinol Metab 2000;85(9):3043–3048

49. Alekel DL, Germain AS, Peterson CT, Hanson KB, Stewart JW, Toda T. Isoflavone-rich soy protein isolate attenuates bone loss in the lumbar spine of perimenopausal women. Am J Clin Nutr 2000;72(3): 844–852

50. Dalais FS, Ebeling PR, Kotsopoulos D, McGrath BP, Teede HJ. The effects of soy protein containing isoflavones on lipids and indices of bone resorption in postmenopausal women. Clin Endocrinol (Oxf) 2003;58(6):704–709

51. Potter SM, Baum JA, Teng H, Stillman RJ, Shay NF, Erdman JW Jr. Soy protein and isoflavones: their effects on blood lipids and bone density in postmenopausal women. Am J Clin Nutr 1998;68(6 Suppl):1375S–1379S

52. Arjmandi BH, Lucas EA, Khalil DA, et al. One-year soy protein supplementation has positive effects on bone formation markers but not bone density in postmenopausal women. Nutr J 2005;4(1):8

53. Kreijkamp-Kaspers S, Kok L, Grobbee DE, et al. Effect of soy protein containing isoflavones on cognitive function, bone mineral density, and plasma lipids in postmenopausal women: a randomized controlled trial. JAMA 2004;292(1):65–74

54. Lydeking-Olsen E, Beck-Jensen JE, Setchell KD, Holm-Jensen T. Soymilk or progesterone for prevention of bone loss–a 2 year randomized, placebo-controlled trial. Eur J Nutr 2004;43(4):246–257

55. Gallagher JC, Satpathy R, Rafferty K, Haynatzka V. The effect of soy protein isolate on bone metabolism. Menopause 2004;11(3):290–298

56. Vitolins M, Anthony M, Lenschik L, Bland DR, Burke GL. Does soy protein and its isoflavones prevent bone loss in peri- and post-menopausal women? Results of a two year randomized clinical trial. J Nutr 2002;132:582S (abstract)

57. Chen YM, Ho SC, Lam SS, Ho SS, Woo JL. Beneficial effect of soy isoflavones on bone mineral content was modified by years since menopause, body weight, and calcium intake: a double-blind, randomized, controlled trial. Menopause 2004;11(3):246–254

58. White LR, Petrovitch H, Ross GW, et al. Brain aging and midlife tofu consumption. J Am Coll Nutr 2000; 19(2):242–255

59. File SE, Hartley DE, Elsabagh S, Duffy R, Wiseman H. Cognitive improvement after 6 weeks of soy supplements in postmenopausal women is limited to frontal lobe function. Menopause 2005;12(2):193–201

60. Duffy R, Wiseman H, File SE. Improved cognitive function in postmenopausal women after 12 weeks of consumption of a soya extract containing isoflavones. Pharmacol Biochem Behav 2003;75(3): 721–729

61. Kritz-Silverstein D, Von Muhlen D, Barrett-Connor E, Bressel MA. Isoflavones and cognitive function in older women: the Soy and Postmenopausal Health in Aging (SOPHIA) Study. Menopause 2003;10(3): 196–202

62. Tice JA, Ettinger B, Ensrud K, Wallace R, Blackwell T, Cummings SR. Phytoestrogen supplements for the treatment of hot flashes: the Isoflavone Clover Extract (ICE) Study: a randomized controlled trial. JAMA 2003;290(2):207–214

63. Nelson HD, Humphrey LL, Nygren P, Teutsch SM, Allan JD. Postmenopausal hormone replacement therapy: scientific review. JAMA 2002;288(7):872–881

64. Kronenberg F, Fugh-Berman A. Complementary and alternative medicine for menopausal symptoms: a review of randomized, controlled trials. Ann Intern Med 2002;137(10):805–813

65. Krebs EE, Ensrud KE, MacDonald R, Wilt TJ. Phytoestrogens for treatment of menopausal symptoms: a systematic review. Obstet Gynecol 2004; 104(4):824–836

66. Duffy C, Cyr M. Phytoestrogens: potential benefits and implications for breast cancer survivors. J Womens Health (Larchmt) 2003;12(7):617–631

67. MacGregor CA, Canney PA, Patterson G, McDonald R, Paul J. A randomised double-blind controlled trial of oral soy supplements versus placebo for treatment of menopausal symptoms in patients with early breast cancer. Eur J Cancer 2005;41(5):708–714

68. Nikander E, Kilkkinen A, Metsa-Heikkila M, et al. A randomized placebo-controlled crossover trial with phytoestrogens in treatment of menopause in breast cancer patients. Obstet Gynecol 2003;101(6):1213–1220

69. Van Patten CL, Olivotto IA, Chambers GK, et al. Effect of soy phytoestrogens on hot flashes in postmenopausal women with breast cancer: a randomized, controlled clinical trial. J Clin Oncol 2002;20(6): 1449–1455

70. Quella SK, Loprinzi CL, Barton DL, et al. Evaluation of soy phytoestrogens for the treatment of hot flashes in breast cancer survivors: A North Central Cancer Treatment Group Trial. J Clin Oncol 2000;18(5): 1068–1074

71. Fletcher RJ. Food sources of phyto-oestrogens and their precursors in Europe. Br J Nutr 2003;89(Suppl 1):S39–S43

72. Ho SC, Woo JL, Leung SS, Sham AL, Lam TH, Janus ED. Intake of soy products is associated with better plasma lipid profiles in the Hong Kong Chinese population. J Nutr 2000;130(10):2590–2593

73. Arai Y, Watanabe S, Kimira M, Shimoi K, Mochizuki R, Kinae N. Dietary intakes of flavonols, flavones and isoflavones by Japanese women and the inverse correlation between quercetin intake and plasma LDL cholesterol concentration. J Nutr 2000;130(9):2243–2250

74. Strom SS, Yamamura Y, Duphorne CM, et al. Phytoestrogen intake and prostate cancer: a case-control study using a new database. Nutr Cancer 1999; 33(1):20–25

75. Setchell KD, Cole SJ. Variations in isoflavone levels in soy foods and soy protein isolates and issues related to isoflavone databases and food labeling. J Agric Food Chem 2003;51(14):4146–4155

76. U.S. Department of Agriculture. USDA-Iowa State University Isoflavones Database. 2002. Available at: http://www.nal.usda.gov/fnic/foodcomp/Data/isoflav/isoflav.html. Accessed 4/14/04

77. Setchell KD, Brown NM, Desai P, et al. Bioavailability of pure isoflavones in healthy humans and analysis of commercial soy isoflavone supplements. J Nutr 2001;131(4 Suppl):1362S–1375S

78. Consumer Lab. Product review: phytoestrogens–soy and red clover isoflavones. 2001. Available at: http://www.consumerlab.com/results/phytoestrogens2.asp? Accessed 7/26/06

79. Setchell KD, Zimmer-Nechemias L, Cai J, Heubi JE. Exposure of infants to phyto-oestrogens from soy-based infant formula. Lancet 1997;350(9070):23–27

80. Chen Z, Zheng W, Custer LJ, et al. Usual dietary consumption of soy foods and its correlation with the excretion rate of isoflavonoids in overnight urine samples among Chinese women in Shanghai. Nutr Cancer 1999;33(1):82–87

81. Messina MJ, Loprinzi CL. Soy for breast cancer survivors: a critical review of the literature. J Nutr 2001;131(11 Suppl):3095S–3108S

82. Allred CD, Allred KF, Ju YH, Virant SM, Helferich WG. Soy diets containing varying amounts of genistein stimulate growth of estrogen-dependent (MCF-7) tumors in a dose-dependent manner. Cancer Res 2001;61(13):5045–5050

83. Ju YH, Allred CD, Allred KF, Karko KL, Doerge DR, Helferich WG. Physiological concentrations of dietary genistein dose-dependently stimulate growth of estrogen-dependent human breast cancer (MCF-7) tumors implanted in athymic nude mice. J Nutr 2001;131(11):2957–2962

84. Ju YH, Doerge DR, Allred KF, Allred CD, Helferich WG. Dietary genistein negates the inhibitory effect of tamoxifen on growth of estrogen-dependent human breast cancer (MCF-7) cells implanted in athymic mice. Cancer Res 2002;62(9):2474–2477

85. Petrakis NL, Barnes S, King EB, et al. Stimulatory influence of soy protein isolate on breast secretion in pre- and postmenopausal women. Cancer Epidemiol Biomarkers Prev 1996;5(10):785–794

86. Hargreaves DF, Potten CS, Harding C, et al. Two-week dietary soy supplementation has an estrogenic effect on normal premenopausal breast. J Clin Endocrinol Metab 1999;84(11):4017–4024

87. Sartippour MR, Rao JY, Apple S, et al. A pilot clinical study of short-term isoflavone supplements in breast cancer patients. Nutr Cancer 2004;49(1):59–65

88. American Academy of Pediatrics Committee on Nutrition. Soy protein-based formulas: recommendations for use in infant feeding. Pediatrics 1998;101(1 Pt 1):148–153

89. Setchell KD, Zimmer-Nechemias L, Cai J, Heubi JE. Isoflavone content of infant formulas and the metabolic fate of these phytoestrogens in early life. Am J Clin Nutr 1998;68(6 Suppl):1453S–1461S

90. Mendez MA, Anthony MS, Arab L. Soy-based formulae and infant growth and development: a review. J Nutr 2002;132(8):2127–2130

91. Strom BL, Schinnar R, Ziegler EE, et al. Exposure to soy-based formula in infancy and endocrinological and reproductive outcomes in young adulthood. JAMA 2001;286(7):807–814

92. U.S. Department of Agriculture, Agricultural Research Service. Study examines long-term health effects of soy infant formula. 2004. Available at: http://www.ars.usda.gov/is/AR/archive/jan04/soy0104.htm. Accessed 7/26/06

93. Divi RL, Chang HC, Doerge DR. Anti-thyroid isoflavones from soybean: isolation, characterization, and mechanisms of action. Biochem Pharmacol 1997;54(10):1087–1096

94. Doerge DR, Sheehan DM. Goitrogenic and estrogenic activity of soy isoflavones. Environ Health Perspect 2002;110(Suppl 3):349–353

95. Chorazy PA, Himelhoch S, Hopwood NJ, Greger NG, Postellon DC. Persistent hypothyroidism in an infant receiving a soy formula: case report and review of the literature. Pediatrics 1995;96(1 Pt 1):148–150

96. Bruce B, Messina M, Spiller GA. Isoflavone supplements do not affect thyroid function in iodine-replete postmenopausal women. J Med Food 2003;6(4):309–316

97. Persky VW, Turyk ME, Wang L, et al. Effect of soy protein on endogenous hormones in postmenopausal women. Am J Clin Nutr 2002;75(1):145–153

98. Duncan AM, Merz BE, Xu X, Nagel TC, Phipps WR, Kurzer MS. Soy isoflavones exert modest hormonal effects in premenopausal women. J Clin Endocrinol Metab 1999;84(1):192–197

99. Duncan AM, Underhill KE, Xu X, Lavalleur J, Phipps WR, Kurzer MS. Modest hormonal effects of soy isoflavones in postmenopausal women. J Clin Endocrinol Metab 1999;84(10):3479–3484

100. Natural Medicines Comprehensive Database. Soy. 2004. Available at: http://www.naturaldatabase.com/monograph.asp?mono_id=975&brand_id=. Accessed 7/26/06

101. Cambria-Kiely JA. Effect of soy milk on warfarin efficacy. Ann Pharmacother 2002;36(12):1893–1896

102. Jabbar MA, Larrea J, Shaw RA. Abnormal thyroid function tests in infants with congenital hypothyroidism: the influence of soy-based formula. J Am Coll Nutr 1997;16(3):280–282

103. Bell DS, Ovalle F. Use of soy protein supplement and resultant need for increased dose of levothyroxine. Endocr Pract 2001;7(3):193–194

15 Isothiocyanates

Cruciferous vegetables, such as broccoli, cabbage, and kale, are rich sources of sulfur-containing compounds called glucosinolates. Isothiocyanates are biologically active hydrolysis (breakdown) products of glucosinolates. Cruciferous vegetables contain a variety of different glucosinolates, each of which forms a different isothiocyanate when hydrolyzed (**Fig. 15–1**).[1] For example, broccoli is a good source of glucoraphanin, the glucosinolate precursor of sulforaphane (SFN), and sinigrin, the glucosinolate precursor of allyl isothiocyanate (AITC).[2] Watercress is a rich source of gluconasturtiin, the precursor of phenethyl isothiocyanate (PEITC), whereas garden cress is rich in glucotropaeolin, the precursor of benzyl isothiocyanate (BITC). At present, scientists are interested in the cancer-preventive activities of vegetables that are rich in glucosinolates (see Chapter 2), as well as individual isothiocyanates.[3]

Metabolism and Bioavailability

Myrosinase, a class of enzymes that catalyzes the hydrolysis (breakdown) of glucosinolates, is physically separated from glucosinolates when plant cells are intact.[4] When cruciferous vegetables are chopped or chewed, myrosinase can interact with glucosinolates and release isothiocyanates from their precursors (**Fig. 15–1**). Thorough chewing of raw cruciferous vegetables increases glucosinolate contact with plant myrosinase and increases the amount of isothiocyanates absorbed.[5] Even when plant myrosinase is completely inactivated by heat, the myrosinase activity of human intestinal bacteria allows for some formation and absorption of isothiocyanates.[6] However, the absorption and excretion of isothiocyanates is substantially lower from cooked than from raw cruciferous vegetables[5,7,8] (see the Food Sources section below).

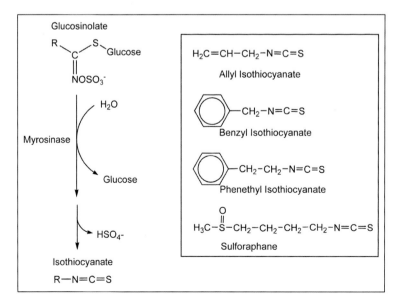

Figure 15–1 Myrosinase-catalyzed hydrolysis of glucosinolates and the chemical structures of allyl isothiocyanate, benzyl isothiocyanate, phenethyl isothiocyanate, and sulforaphane.

During metabolism, isothiocyanates are conjugated (bound) to glutathione, an activity that is promoted by a family of enzymes called glutathione-S-transferases (GSTs) and further metabolized to mercapturic acids. These isothiocyanate metabolites can be measured in the urine and are highly correlated with dietary intake of cruciferous vegetables.[9] There is also some evidence that isothiocyanate metabolites contribute to the biological activity of isothiocyanates.[3,10]

Biological Activities

Effects on Biotransformation Enzymes Involved in Carcinogen Metabolism

Biotransformation enzymes play important roles in the metabolism and elimination of a variety of chemicals, including drugs, toxins, and carcinogens. In general, phase I biotransformation enzymes catalyze reactions that increase the reactivity of hydrophobic (fat-soluble) compounds, preparing them for reactions catalyzed by phase II biotransformation enzymes. Reactions catalyzed by phase II enzymes generally increase water solubility and promote the elimination of the compound from the body.[11]

Inhibition of Phase I Biotransformation Enzymes

Some chemical carcinogens require biotransformation by phase I enzymes, such as those of the cytochrome P450 (CYP) family, to become active carcinogens that are capable of binding DNA and inducing mutations. Inhibition of specific CYP enzymes involved in carcinogen activation inhibits the development of cancer in animal models.[3] Isothiocyanates, including PEITC and BITC, have been found to inhibit carcinogen activation by CYP enzymes in animal studies.[12,13] A small clinical trial in smokers found evidence that consumption of 170 g/d (6 oz/d) of watercress, which is rich in the glucosinolate precursor of PEITC, decreased the activation of a procarcinogen found in tobacco.[14]

Induction of Phase II Biotransformation Enzymes

Many isothiocyanates, particularly SFN, are potent inducers of phase II enzymes in cultured human cells.[2] Phase II enzymes, including GSTs, UDP-glucuronosyl transferases (UGTs), quinone reductase, and glutamate cysteine ligase play important roles in protecting cells from DNA damage by carcinogens and reactive oxygen species.[15] The genes for these and other phase II enzymes contain a specific sequence of DNA called an antioxidant response element (ARE). Isothiocyanates have been shown to increase phase II enzyme activity by increasing the transcription of genes that contain an ARE.[16] Limited data from clinical trials suggest that glucosinolate-rich foods can increase phase II enzyme activity in humans. When smokers consumed 170 g/d (6 oz/d) of watercress, urinary excretion of glucuronidated nicotine metabolites increased significantly, suggesting UGT activity increased.[17] Brussels sprouts are rich in several glucosinolates, including precursors of AITC and SFN. Consumption of 300 g/d (11 oz/d) of Brussels sprouts for a week significantly increased plasma and intestinal GST levels in nonsmoking men.[18,19]

Preservation of Normal Cell-Cycle Regulation

After a cell divides, it passes through a sequence of stages known as the cell cycle before dividing again. Following DNA damage, the cell cycle can be transiently arrested to allow for DNA repair or activation of pathways leading to cell death (apoptosis) if the damage cannot be repaired.[20] Defective cell-cycle regulation may result in the propagation of mutations that contribute to the development of cancer. Several isothiocyanates, including AITC, BITC, PEITC, and SFN, have been found to induce cell-cycle arrest in cultured cells.[2]

Inhibition of Proliferation and Induction of Apoptosis

Unlike normal cells, cancer cells proliferate rapidly and lose the ability to respond to cell death signals by undergoing apoptosis.

Isothiocyanates has been found to inhibit proliferation and induce apoptosis in several cancer cell lines.[3]

Inhibition of Histone Deacetylation

In the nucleus of a cell, DNA is coiled around basic proteins called histones. In general, acetylation of histones by histone acetyl transferases makes DNA more accessible to transcription factors, which bind DNA and activate gene transcription. Deacetylation of histones by histone deacetylases restricts the access of transcription factors to DNA. Acetylation and deacetylation of nuclear histones is an important cellular mechanism for regulating gene transcription.[21] However, the balance between histone acetyl transferase and histone deacetylase activities that exists in normal cells may be disrupted in cancer cells. Compounds that inhibit histone deacetylases have the potential to suppress the development of cancer by inducing the transcription of tumor suppressor proteins that promote differentiation and apoptosis in transformed (precancerous) cells.[22] AITC and SFN metabolites have been found to inhibit histone deacetylase activity in cultured cancer cells.[10,23]

Anti-inflammatory Activity

Inflammation promotes cellular proliferation and inhibits apoptosis, increasing the risk of developing cancer.[24] SFN and PEITC have been found to decrease the secretion of inflammatory signaling molecules by white blood cells and to decrease DNA binding of NF-$\varkappa$B, a proinflammatory transcription factor.[25,26]

Antibacterial Activity:
Helicobacter pylori

Bacterial infection with Helicobacter pylori (H. pylori) is associated with a marked increase in the risk of gastric cancer.[27] Purified SFN inhibited the growth and killed multiple strains of H. pylori in the test tube and in tissue culture, including antibiotic resistant strains.[28] In an animal model of H. pylori infection, SFN administration for 5 days eradicated H. pylori from 8 out of 11 xenografts of human gastric tissue implanted in immune-compromised mice.[29] However, in a small clinical trial, consumption of up to 56 g/d (2 oz/d) of glucoraphanin-rich broccoli sprouts for a week was associated with H. pylori eradication in only 3 out of 9 gastritis patients.[30] Further research is needed to determine whether SFN or foods rich in its precursor glucobrassicin will be helpful in the treatment of H. pylori infection in humans.

Prevention

Cancer

Naturally occurring isothiocyanates and their metabolites have been found to inhibit the development of chemically induced cancers of the lung, liver, esophagus, stomach, small intestine, colon, and mammary gland (breast) in a variety of animal models.[3,12] Although epidemiological studies provide some evidence that higher intakes of cruciferous vegetables are associated with decreased cancer risk in humans,[31] it is difficult to determine whether such protective effects are related to isothiocyanates or other factors associated with cruciferous vegetable consumption (see Chapter 2). Investigators have attempted to calculate human isothiocyanate exposure based on assessments of cruciferous vegetable intake and measurements of the maximal amounts of isothiocyanates that can be liberated from various cruciferous vegetables in the laboratory.[32] Case-control studies using this technique found that dietary isothiocyanate intakes were significantly lower in Chinese women[33] and American men[34] diagnosed with lung cancer than in cancer-free control groups. Assessing dietary intake of cruciferous vegetables may not accurately measure an individual's exposure to isothiocyanates because other factors may alter the amount of isothiocyanates formed and absorbed (see the Metabolism and Bioavailability section above). Measuring urinary excretion of isothiocyanates and their metabolites may provide a better assessment of isothiocyanate exposure,[9,35] but few studies have examined relationships between urinary isothiocyanate excretion and cancer risk. In a prospective study,

Chinese men with detectable levels of urinary isothiocyanates at baseline were at significantly lower risk of developing lung cancer over the next 10 years than men with undetectable levels.[36] A case-control study found that urinary isothiocyanate excretion was significantly lower in Chinese women diagnosed with breast cancer than in a cancer-free control group.[37] In contrast, cruciferous vegetable intake estimated from a food frequency questionnaire was not associated with breast cancer risk in the same study.

Genetic Variation in Isothiocyanate Metabolism and Cancer Risk

GSTs are a family of phase II biotransformation enzymes that promote the metabolism and elimination of isothiocyanates and other compounds from the body. Genetic variations (polymorphisms) that affect the activity of GST enzymes have been identified in humans. Null variants of the GSTM1 gene and GSTT1 gene contain large deletions, and individuals who inherit two copies of the GSTM1-null or GSTT1-null gene cannot produce the corresponding GST enzyme.[38] Lower GST activity in such individuals could result in slower elimination and longer exposure to isothiocyanates after cruciferous vegetable consumption.[9] In support of this idea, several epidemiological studies found that inverse associations between isothiocyanate intake from cruciferous vegetables and the risk of lung cancer[33,34,36,39] or colon cancer[40–42] were more pronounced in GSTM1-null or GSTT1-null individuals. These findings suggest a protective role for isothiocyanates that may be enhanced in individuals who eliminate them from the body more slowly.

Sources

Food Sources

Cruciferous Vegetables

Cruciferous vegetables, such as bok choy, broccoli, brussel sprouts, cabbage, cauliflower, horseradish, kale, kohlrabi, mustard, radish, rutabaga, turnip, and watercress, are rich sources of glucosinolate precursors to isothio-

cyanates.[43] Unlike some other phytochemicals, glucosinolates are present in relatively high concentrations in commonly consumed portions of cruciferous vegetables. For example, 1/2 cup of raw broccoli might provide more than 25 mg of total glucosinolates. Total glucosinolate contents of selected cruciferous vegetables are presented in **Table 15–1**.[44] Some cruciferous vegetables are better sources of specific glucosinolates (and isothiocyanates) than others. Vegetables that are relatively good sources of some isothiocyanates currently under study for their cancer-preventive properties are listed in **Table 15–2**. Amounts of isothiocyanates formed from glucosinolates in foods are variable and depend partly on the processing and preparation of those foods (see the Effects of Cooking section below). Consumption of 5 or more weekly servings of cruciferous vegetables has been associated with significant reductions in cancer risk in some prospective cohort studies.[45–47]

Broccoli Sprouts

The amount of glucoraphanin, the precursor of SFN, in broccoli seeds remains more or less constant as those seeds germinate and grow into mature plants. Thus, 3-day-old broccoli sprouts are concentrated sources of glu-

Table 15–1   Total Glucosinolate Content of Selected Cruciferous Vegetables[44]

Vegetable (raw)	Serving	Total Glucosinolates (mg)
brussel sprouts	1/2 cup	104
Garden cress	1/2 cup	98
Mustard greens	1/2 cup	79
Turnip	1/2 cup	60
Kale	1/2 cup	34
Broccoli	1/2 cup	27
Cabbage, Savoy	1/2 cup	35
Cabbage, red	1/2 cup	29
Bok choy (pak choi)	1/2 cup	19
Watercress	1/2 cup	16

Table 15–2   Some Food Sources of Selected Isothiocyanates and Their Glucosinolate Precursors[12]

Isothiocyanate	Glucosinolate (Precursor)	Food Sources
Allyl-Isothiocyanate (AITC)	Sinigrin	Broccoli, brussel sprouts, cabbage, horseradish, mustard, radish
Benzyl-Isothiocyanate (BITC)	Glucotropaeolin	Cabbage, garden cress, Indian cress
Phenethyl-Isothiocyanate (PEITC)	Gluconasturtiin	Watercress
Sulforaphane (SFN)	Glucoraphanin	Broccoli, brussel sprouts, cabbage

coraphanin, which contain 10 to 100 times more glucoraphanin by weight than mature broccoli plants.[48] Broccoli sprouts that are certified to contain at least 73 mg of glucoraphanin (also called sulforaphane glucosinolate) per 1-oz serving are available in some health food and grocery stores.

Effects of Cooking

Glucosinolates are water-soluble compounds that may be leached into cooking water. Boiling cruciferous vegetables from 9 to 15 minutes resulted in 18 to 59% decreases in the total glucosinolate content of cruciferous vegetables.[44] Cooking methods that use less water, such as steaming or microwaving may reduce glucosinolate losses. However, some cooking practices, including boiling,[5] steaming,[7] and microwaving at high power (850 to 900 W)[8,49] may inactivate myrosinase, the enzyme that catalyzes glucosinolate hydrolysis. Even in the absence of plant myrosinase activity, the myrosinase activity of human intestinal bacteria results in some glucosinolate hydrolysis.[6] However, several studies in humans have found that inactivation of myrosinase in cruciferous vegetables substantially decreases the bioavailability of isothiocyanates.[5,7,8]

Supplements

Dietary supplements containing extracts of broccoli sprouts, broccoli, and other cruciferous vegetables are available without a prescription. Some products are standardized to contain a minimum amount of glucosinolates and/or sulforaphane. However, the bioavailability of isothiocyanates derived from these supplements is not known.

Safety

Adverse Effects

No serious adverse effects of isothiocyanates in humans have been reported. The majority of animal studies have found that isothiocyanates inhibited the development of cancer when given prior to the chemical carcinogen (pre-initiation) However, very high intakes of PEITC or BITC (25 to 250 times higher than average human dietary isothiocyanate intakes) have been found to promote bladder cancer in rats when given after a chemical carcinogen (post-initiation).[50] The relevance of these findings to human bladder cancer is not clear because at least one prospective cohort study found cruciferous vegetable consumption to be inversely associated with the risk of bladder cancer in men.[47]

Pregnancy and Lactation

Although high dietary intakes of glucosinolates from cruciferous vegetables are not known to have adverse effects during pregnancy or lactation, there is no information on the safety of purified isothiocyanates or supplements containing high doses of glucosinolates and/or isothiocyanates during pregnancy or lactation in humans.

Drug Interactions

Isothiocyanates are not known to interact with any drugs or medications. However, the potential for isothiocyanates to inhibit various isoforms of the CYP family of enzymes raises the potential for interactions with drugs that are CYP substrates.[51]

Summary

- Isothiocyanates are derived from the hydrolysis (breakdown) of glucosinolates—sulfur-containing compounds found in cruciferous vegetables.
- Cruciferous vegetables contain a variety of different glucosinolates, each of which forms a different isothiocyanate when hydrolyzed.
- Isothiocyanates, such as sulforaphane, may help prevent cancer by promoting the elimination of potential carcinogens from the body and enhancing the transcription of tumor suppressor proteins.
- Epidemiological studies provide some evidence that human exposure to isothiocyanates through cruciferous vegetable consumption may decrease cancer risk, but the protective effects may be influenced by individual genetic variation in the metabolism and elimination of isothiocyanates from the body.
- Glucosinolates are present in relatively high concentrations in cruciferous vegetables, but cooking, particularly boiling, and microwaving at high power, may decrease the bioavailability of isothiocyanates.

References

1. Fahey JW, Zalcmann AT, Talalay P. The chemical diversity and distribution of glucosinolates and isothiocyanates among plants. Phytochemistry 2001;56(1):5–51
2. Zhang Y. Cancer-preventive isothiocyanates: measurement of human exposure and mechanism of action. Mutat Res 2004;555(1–2):173–190
3. Hecht SS. Chemoprevention by isothiocyanates. In: Kelloff GJ, Hawk ET, Sigman CC, eds. Promising Cancer Chemopreventive Agents, Volume 1: Cancer Chemopreventive Agents. Totowa, NJ: Humana Press; 2004:21–35
4. Holst B, Williamson G. A critical review of the bioavailability of glucosinolates and related compounds. Nat Prod Rep 2004;21(3):425–447
5. Shapiro TA, Fahey JW, Wade KL, Stephenson KK, Talalay P. Chemoprotective glucosinolates and isothiocyanates of broccoli sprouts: metabolism and excretion in humans. Cancer Epidemiol Biomarkers Prev 2001;10(5):501–508
6. Shapiro TA, Fahey JW, Wade KL, Stephenson KK, Talalay P. Human metabolism and excretion of cancer chemoprotective glucosinolates and isothiocyanates of cruciferous vegetables. Cancer Epidemiol Biomarkers Prev 1998;7(12):1091–1100
7. Conaway CC, Getahun SM, Liebes LL, et al. Disposition of glucosinolates and sulforaphane in humans after ingestion of steamed and fresh broccoli. Nutr Cancer 2000;38(2):168–178
8. Rouzaud G, Young SA, Duncan AJ. Hydrolysis of glucosinolates to isothiocyanates after ingestion of raw or microwaved cabbage by human volunteers. Cancer Epidemiol Biomarkers Prev 2004;13(1):125–131
9. Seow A, Shi CY, Chung FL, et al. Urinary total isothiocyanate (ITC) in a population-based sample of middle-aged and older Chinese in Singapore: relationship with dietary total ITC and glutathione S-transferase M1/T1/P1 genotypes. Cancer Epidemiol Biomarkers Prev 1998;7(9):775–781
10. Myzak MC, Karplus PA, Chung FL, Dashwood RH. A novel mechanism of chemoprotection by sulforaphane: inhibition of histone deacetylase. Cancer Res 2004;64(16):5767–5774
11. Lampe JW, Peterson S. Brassica, biotransformation and cancer risk: genetic polymorphisms alter the preventive effects of cruciferous vegetables. J Nutr 2002;132(10):2991–2994
12. Conaway CC, Yang YM, Chung FL. Isothiocyanates as cancer chemopreventive agents: their biological activities and metabolism in rodents and humans. Curr Drug Metab 2002;3(3):233–255
13. Hecht SS. Inhibition of carcinogenesis by isothiocyanates. Drug Metab Rev 2000;32(3–4):395–411
14. Hecht SS, Chung FL, Richie JP Jr, et al. Effects of watercress consumption on metabolism of a tobacco-specific lung carcinogen in smokers. Cancer Epidemiol Biomarkers Prev 1995;4(8):877–884
15. Kensler TW, Talalay P. Inducers of enzymes that protect against carcinogens and oxidants: drug- and food-based approaches with dithiolethiones and sulforaphane. In: Kelloff GJ, Hawk ET, Sigman CC, eds. Promising Cancer Chemopreventive Agents, Volume 1: Cancer Chemopreventive Agents. Totowa, NJ: Humana Press; 2004:3–20
16. Dinkova-Kostova AT, Holtzclaw WD, Cole RN, et al. Direct evidence that sulfhydryl groups of Keap1 are the sensors regulating induction of phase 2 enzymes that protect against carcinogens and oxidants. Proc Natl Acad Sci U S A 2002;99(18):11908–11913
17. Hecht SS, Carmella SG, Murphy SE. Effects of watercress consumption on urinary metabolites of nicotine in smokers. Cancer Epidemiol Biomarkers Prev 1999;8(10):907–913
18. Nijhoff WA, Grubben MJ, Nagengast FM, et al. Effects of consumption of Brussels sprouts on intestinal and lymphocytic glutathione S-transferases in humans. Carcinogenesis 1995;16(9):2125–2128

19. Nijhoff WA, Mulder TP, Verhagen H, van Poppel G, Peters WH. Effects of consumption of Brussels sprouts on plasma and urinary glutathione S-transferase class-alpha and -pi in humans. Carcinogenesis 1995; 16(4):955–957

20. Stewart ZA, Westfall MD, Pietenpol JA. Cell-cycle dysregulation and anticancer therapy. Trends Pharmacol Sci 2003;24(3):139–145

21. Mei S, Ho AD, Mahlknecht U. Role of histone deacetylase inhibitors in the treatment of cancer (Review). Int J Oncol 2004;25(6):1509–1519

22. Marks PA, Richon VM, Miller T, Kelly WK. Histone deacetylase inhibitors. Adv Cancer Res 2004;91:137–168

23. Lea MA, Rasheed M, Randolph VM, Khan F, Shareef A. desBordes C. Induction of histone acetylation and inhibition of growth of mouse erythroleukemia cells by S-allylmercaptocysteine. Nutr Cancer 2002;43(1):90–102

24. Steele VE, Hawk ET, Viner JL, Lubet RA. Mechanisms and applications of non-steroidal anti-inflammatory drugs in the chemoprevention of cancer. Mutat Res 2003;523–524:137–144

25. Gerhauser C, Klimo K, Heiss E, et al. Mechanism-based in vitro screening of potential cancer chemopreventive agents. Mutat Res 2003;523–524:163–172

26. Heiss E, Herhaus C, Klimo K, Bartsch H, Gerhauser C. Nuclear factor kappa B is a molecular target for sulforaphane-mediated anti-inflammatory mechanisms. J Biol Chem 2001;276(34):32008–32015

27. Normark S, Nilsson C, Normark BH, Hornef MW. Persistent infection with Helicobacter pylori and the development of gastric cancer. Adv Cancer Res 2003; 90:63–89

28. Fahey JW, Haristoy X, Dolan PM, et al. Sulforaphane inhibits extracellular, intracellular, and antibiotic-resistant strains of Helicobacter pylori and prevents benzo[a]pyrene-induced stomach tumors. Proc Natl Acad Sci U S A 2002;99(11):7610–7615

29. Haristoy X, Angioi-Duprez K, Duprez A, Lozniewski A. Efficacy of sulforaphane in eradicating Helicobacter pylori in human gastric xenografts implanted in nude mice. Antimicrob Agents Chemother 2003;47(12): 3982–3984

30. Galan MV, Kishan AA, Silverman AL. Oral broccoli sprouts for the treatment of Helicobacter pylori infection: a preliminary report. Dig Dis Sci 2004;49(7–8): 1088–1090

31. Verhoeven DT, Goldbohm RA, van Poppel G, Verhagen H, van den Brandt PA. Epidemiological studies on brassica vegetables and cancer risk. Cancer Epidemiol Biomarkers Prev 1996;5(9):733–748

32. Jiao D, Yu MC, Hankin JH, Low SH, Chung FL. Total isothiocyanate contents in cooked vegetables frequently consumed in Singapore. J Agric Food Chem 1998;46(3):1055–1058

33. Zhao B, Seow A, Lee EJ, et al. Dietary isothiocyanates, glutathione S-transferase -M1, -T1 polymorphisms and lung cancer risk among Chinese women in Singapore. Cancer Epidemiol Biomarkers Prev 2001; 10(10):1063–1067

34. Spitz MR, Duphorne CM, Detry MA, et al. Dietary intake of isothiocyanates: evidence of a joint effect with glutathione S-transferase polymorphisms in lung cancer risk. Cancer Epidemiol Biomarkers Prev 2000; 9(10):1017–1020

35. Fowke JH, Hebert JR, Fahey JW. Urinary excretion of dithiocarbamates and self-reported cruciferous vegetable intake: application of the "method of triads" to a food-specific biomarker. Public Health Nutr 2002;5(6):791–799

36. London SJ, Yuan JM, Chung FL, et al. Isothiocyanates, glutathione S-transferase M1 and T1 polymorphisms, and lung-cancer risk: a prospective study of men in Shanghai, China. Lancet 2000;356(9231):724–729

37. Fowke JH, Shu XO, Dai Q, et al. Urinary isothiocyanate excretion, brassica consumption, and gene polymorphisms among women living in Shanghai, China. Cancer Epidemiol Biomarkers Prev 2003;12(12): 1536–1539

38. Coles BF, Kadlubar FF. Detoxification of electrophilic compounds by glutathione S-transferase catalysis: determinants of individual response to chemical carcinogens and chemotherapeutic drugs? Biofactors 2003;17(1–4):115–130

39. Lewis S, Brennan P, Nyberg F, et al. Re: Spitz, MR, Duphorne, CM, Detry, MA, Pillow, PC, Amos, CI, Lei, L, de Andrade, M, Gu, X, Hong, WK, and Wu, X. Dietary intake of isothiocyanates: evidence of a joint effect with glutathione S-transferase polymorphisms in lung cancer risk. Cancer Epidemiol Biomarkers Prev 2001; 10(10):1105–1106

40. Seow A, Yuan JM, Sun CL, Van Den Berg D, Lee HP, Yu MC. Dietary isothiocyanates, glutathione S-transferase polymorphisms and colorectal cancer risk in the Singapore Chinese Health Study. Carcinogenesis 2002;23(12):2055–2061

41. Slattery ML, Kampman E, Samowitz W, Caan BJ, Potter JD. Interplay between dietary inducers of GST and the GSTM-1 genotype in colon cancer. Int J Cancer 2000; 87(5):728–733

42. Turner F, Smith G, Sachse C, et al. Vegetable, fruit and meat consumption and potential risk modifying genes in relation to colorectal cancer. Int J Cancer 2004; 112(2):259–264

43. Fenwick GR, Heaney RK, Mullin WJ. Glucosinolates and their breakdown products in food and food plants. Crit Rev Food Sci Nutr 1983;18(2):123–201

44. McNaughton SA, Marks GC. Development of a food composition database for the estimation of dietary intakes of glucosinolates, the biologically active constituents of cruciferous vegetables. Br J Nutr 2003;90(3): 687–697

45. Feskanich D, Ziegler RG, Michaud DS, et al. Prospective study of fruit and vegetable consumption and risk of lung cancer among men and women. J Natl Cancer Inst 2000;92(22):1812–1823

46. Giovannucci E, Rimm EB, Liu Y, Stampfer MJ, Willett WC. A prospective study of cruciferous vegetables and prostate cancer. Cancer Epidemiol Biomarkers Prev 2003;12(12):1403–1409

47. Michaud DS, Spiegelman D, Clinton SK, Rimm EB, Willett WC, Giovannucci EL. Fruit and vegetable intake and incidence of bladder cancer in a male prospective cohort. J Natl Cancer Inst 1999;91(7):605–613

48. Fahey JW, Zhang Y, Talalay P. Broccoli sprouts: an exceptionally rich source of inducers of enzymes that protect against chemical carcinogens. Proc Natl Acad Sci U S A 1997;94(19):10367–10372

49. Verkerk R, Dekker M. Glucosinolates and myrosinase activity in red cabbage (Brassica oleracea L. var. Capitata f. rubra DC.) after various microwave treatments. J Agric Food Chem 2004;52(24):7318–7323

50. Okazaki K, Umemura T, Imazawa T, Nishikawa A, Masegi T, Hirose M. Enhancement of urinary bladder carcinogenesis by combined treatment with benzyl isothiocyanate and N-butyl-N-(4-hydroxybutyl)nitrosamine in rats after initiation. Cancer Sci 2003;94(11):948–952

51. Sulforaphane. Natural Medicines Online Database. 2005. Available at: http://naturaldatabase.com. Accessed 3/24/05

16 Indole-3-Carbinol

Cruciferous vegetables differ from other classes of vegetables in that they are rich sources of sulfur-containing compounds known as glucosinolates (see Chapter 2 and 15). Because epidemiological studies provide some evidence that diets rich in cruciferous vegetables are associated with lower risk of several types of cancer, scientists are interested in the potential cancer-preventive activities of compounds derived from glucosinolates.[1] Among these compounds is indole-3-carbinol (I3C), a compound derived from the enzymatic hydrolysis (breakdown) of an indole glucosinolate, commonly known as glucobrassicin.[2]

Metabolism and Bioavailability

Several commonly consumed cruciferous vegetables, including broccoli, brussels sprouts, and cabbage, are good sources of glucobrassicin, the glucosinolate precursor of I3C. Myrosinase, an enzyme that catalyzes the hydrolysis of glucosinolates, is physically separated from glucosinolates in intact plant cells.[3] When plant cells are damaged, as when cruciferous vegetables are chopped or chewed, the interaction of myrosinase and glucobrassicin results in the formation of I3C (**Fig. 16–1**). In the acidic environment of the stomach, I3C molecules can combine with each other to form a complex mixture of biologically active compounds, known collectively as acid con-

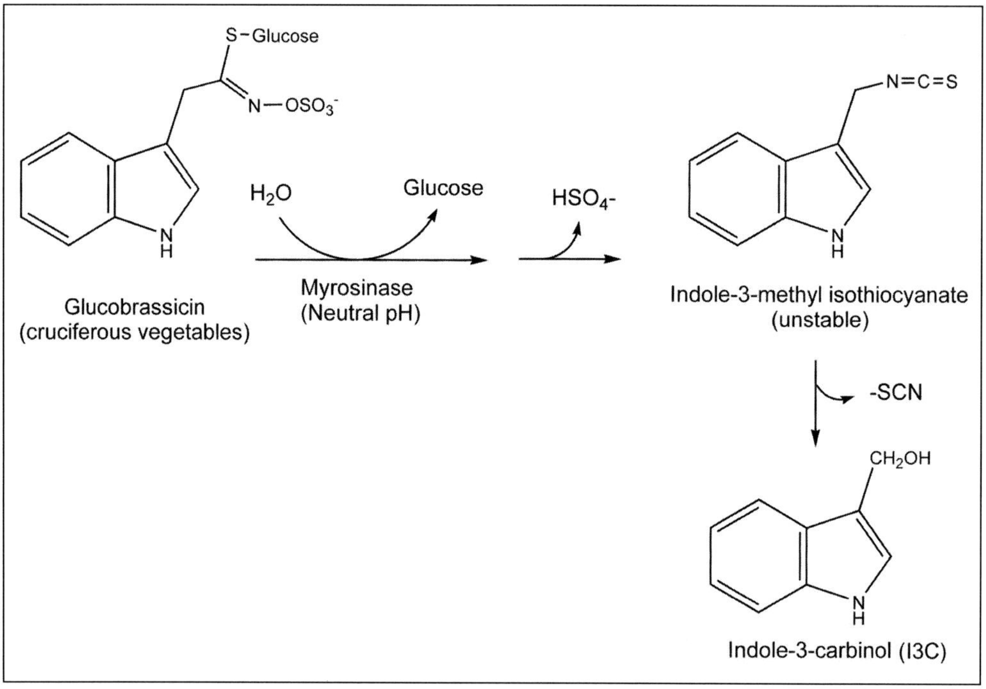

Figure 16–1 The hydrolysis of glucobrassicin by myrosinase at neutral pH results in an unstable indole isothiocyanate that degrades to form indole-3-carbinol and a thiocyanate ion.

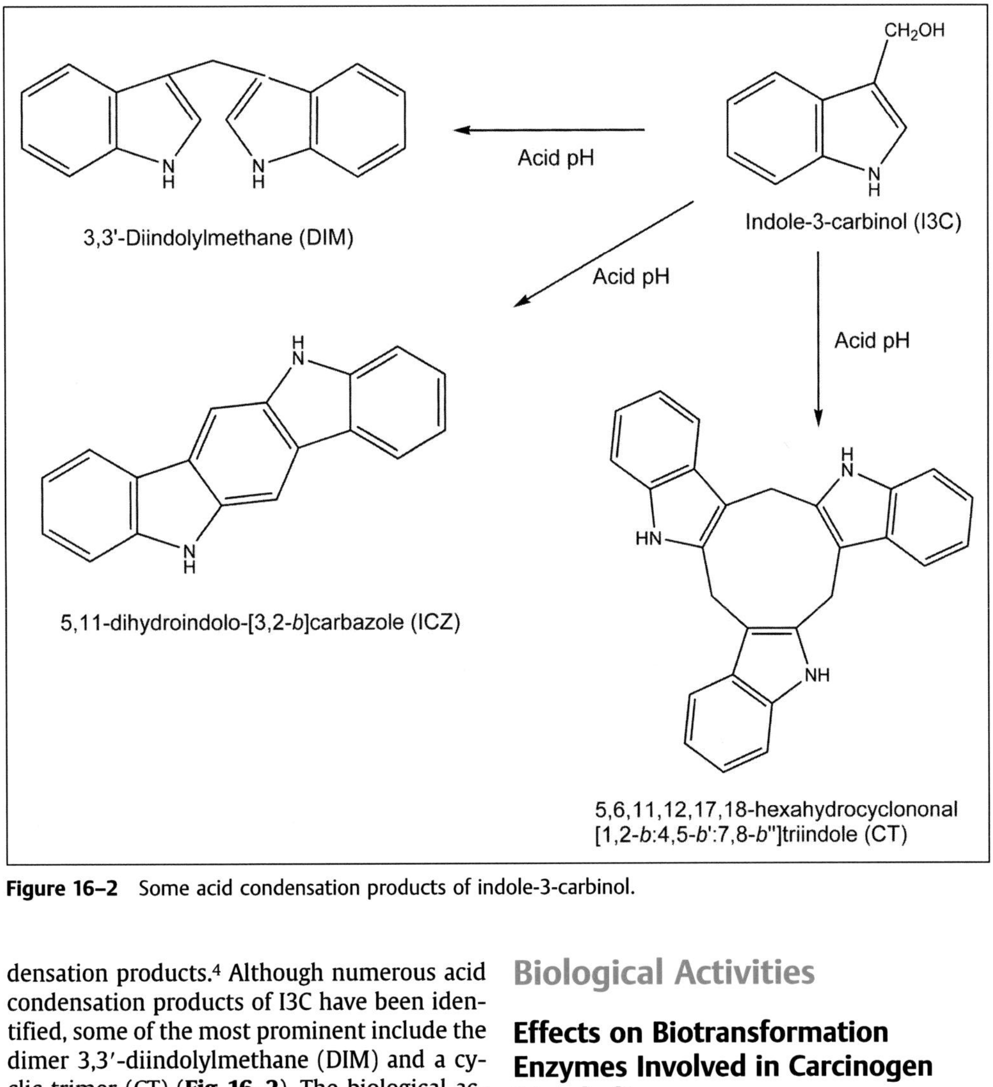

Figure 16–2 Some acid condensation products of indole-3-carbinol.

densation products.[4] Although numerous acid condensation products of I3C have been identified, some of the most prominent include the dimer 3,3'-diindolylmethane (DIM) and a cyclic trimer (CT) (**Fig. 16–2**). The biological activities of individual acid condensation products differ from those of I3C and are responsible for the biological effects attributed to I3C.[5] When plant myrosinase is inactivated (e.g., by boiling), glucosinolate hydrolysis still occurs to a lesser degree, due to the myrosinase activity of human intestinal bacteria.[6] Thus, when cruciferous vegetables are cooked in a manner that inactivates myrosinase, glucobrassicin hydrolysis by intestinal bacteria still results in some I3C formation (see the Food Sources section). However, acid condensation products would be less likely to form in the more alkaline environment of the intestine.

Biological Activities

Effects on Biotransformation Enzymes Involved in Carcinogen Metabolism

Biotransformation enzymes play major roles in the metabolism and elimination of many biologically active compounds, including steroid hormones, carcinogens, toxins, and drugs. In general, phase I biotransformation enzymes, including the cytochrome P450 (CYP) family, catalyze reactions that increase the reactivity of hydrophobic (fat-soluble) compounds, preparing them for reactions catalyzed by phase II biotransformation enzymes. Reactions catalyzed by phase II enzymes generally increase water solubility and promote the elimination of these compounds.[7]

Acid-condensation products of I3C, particularly DIM and indole[3,2-b]carbazole (ICZ), can bind to a protein in the cytoplasm of cells called the aryl hydrocarbon receptor (AhR).[5,8] Binding allows the AhR to enter the nucleus where it forms a complex with the Ahr nuclear translocator (Arnt) protein. This Ahr/Arnt complex binds to specific DNA sequences in genes known as xenobiotic response elements (XRE) and enhances their transcription.[9] Genes for several CYP enzymes and several phase II enzymes are known to contain XREs. Thus, oral consumption of I3C results in the formation of acid condensation products that can increase the activity of certain phase I and phase II enzymes.[8,10,11] Increasing the activity of biotransformation enzymes is generally considered a beneficial effect because the elimination of potential carcinogens or toxins is enhanced. However, there is a potential for adverse effects because some procarcinogens require biotransformation by phase I enzymes to become active carcinogens.[12]

Alterations in Estrogen Activity and Metabolism

Endogenous estrogens, including 17β-estradiol, exert their estrogenic effects by binding to estrogen receptors (ERs). Within the nucleus, the estrogen-ER complex can bind to DNA sequences in genes known as estrogen response elements (EREs), recruit coactivator molecules, and enhance the transcription of estrogen-responsive genes.[13] Some ER-mediated effects, such as those that promote cellular proliferation in the breast and uterus, can increase the risk of developing estrogen-sensitive cancers.[14]

Effects on Estrogen Receptor Activity

When added to breast cancer cells in culture, I3C has been found to inhibit the transcription of estrogen-responsive genes stimulated by 17β-estradiol.[15,16] Acid condensation products of I3C that bind and activate AhR may also inhibit the transcription of estrogen-responsive genes by competing for coactivators or increasing ER degradation.[9,17] In contrast, some studies in cell culture[18,19] and animal models[20] have found that acid-condensation products of

I3C enhance the transcription of estrogen-responsive genes. Further research is needed to determine the nature of the stimulatory and inhibitory effects of I3C and its acid-condensation products on estrogen-responsive gene transcription under conditions that are relevant to human cancer risk (see the Cancer section below).

Effects on Estrogen Metabolism

The endogenous estrogen 17β-estradiol can be irreversibly metabolized to 16α-hydroxyestrone ($16\alpha OHE_1$) or 2-hydroxyestrone ($2OHE_1$). In contrast to $2OHE_1$, $16\alpha OHE_1$ is highly estrogenic and has been found to stimulate the proliferation of several estrogen-sensitive cancer cell lines.[21,22] It has been hypothesized that shifting the metabolism of 17β-estradiol toward $2OHE_1$ and away from $16\alpha OHE_1$ could decrease the risk of estrogen-sensitive cancers, such as breast cancer.[23] In controlled clinical trials, oral supplementation with 300 to 400 mg/d of I3C has consistently increased urinary $2OHE_1$ levels or urinary $2OHE_1$:$16\alpha OHE_1$ ratios in women.[24–28] Supplementation with 108 mg/d of DIM also increased urinary $2OHE_1$ levels in postmenopausal women.[29] However, the relationship between urinary $2OHE_1$:$16\alpha OHE_1$ ratios and breast cancer risk is not clear. Although women with breast cancer had lower urinary ratios of $2OHE_1$:$16\alpha OHE_1$ in several small case-control studies,[30–32] larger case-control and prospective cohort studies have not found significant associations between urinary $2OHE_1$:$16\alpha OHE_1$ ratios and breast cancer risk.[33–35]

Induction of Cell-Cycle Arrest

Once a cell divides, it passes through a sequence of stages collectively known as the cell cycle before it divides again. Following DNA damage, the cell cycle can be transiently arrested at damage checkpoints that allow for DNA repair or activation of pathways leading to cell death (apoptosis) if the damage is irreparable.[36] Defective cell-cycle regulation may result in the propagation of mutations that contribute to the development of cancer. The addition of I3C to prostate and breast cancer cells in culture has been found to induce cell cycle arrest.[37,38] However, the physiological relevance of these cell culture studies is unclear because little or no I3C is available to the tissue after oral administration (see the Metabolism and Bioavailability section above).[39]

Induction of Apoptosis

Unlike normal cells, cancerous cells lose their ability to respond to death signals by undergoing apoptosis. I3C and DIM have been found to induce apoptosis when added to cultured prostate,[37] breast,[40,41] and cervical cancer cells.[42]

Inhibition of Tumor Invasion and Angiogenesis

Limited evidence in cell culture experiments suggests that I3C and DIM can inhibit the invasion of normal tissue by cancer cells[43] and inhibit the development of new blood vessels (angiogenesis) required by tumors to fuel their rapid growth.[44]

Prevention

Cancer

Epidemiological Studies

Epidemiological studies provide some support for the hypothesis that higher intakes of cruciferous vegetables are associated with lower risk for some types of cancer.[45] Cruciferous vegetables, however, are relatively good sources of other phytonutrients that may have protective effects against cancer, including vitamin C, folate, selenium, carotenoids, and fiber (see Chapter 2). Moreover, cruciferous vegetables provide a variety of glucosinolates that may be hydrolyzed to a variety of potentially protective isothiocyanates, in addition to indole-3-carbinol (see Chapter 15).[46,47] Consequently, evidence for an inverse association between cruciferous vegetable intake and cancer risk provides relatively little information about the specific effects of indole-3-carbinol on cancer risk.

Animal Studies

In most animal models, exposure to a chemical carcinogen is required to cause cancer. When administered before or at the same time as the carcinogen, oral I3C has been found to inhibit the development of cancer in a variety of animal models and tissues, including cancers of the mammary gland,[48,49] stomach,[50] colon,[51,52] lung,[53] and liver.[54] However, several studies have found that I3C actually promoted or enhanced the development of cancer when administered chronically after the carcinogen (postinitiation). The cancer promoting effects of I3C were first reported in a trout model of liver cancer.[55,56] However, I3C has also been found to promote cancer of the liver,[57,58] thyroid,[46] colon,[59] and uterus[60] in rats. Although the long-term effects of I3C supplementation on cancer risk in humans are not known, the contradictory results of animal studies have led several experts to caution against the widespread use of I3C and DIM supplements in humans until their potential risks and benefits are better understood.[58,61,62]

Treatment

Diseases Related to Human Papilloma Virus Infection

Cervical Intraepithelial Neoplasia

Infection with certain strains of human papilloma virus (HPV) is an important risk factor for cervical cancer.[63] Transgenic mice that express cancer-promoting HPV genes develop cervical cancer with chronic 17β-estradiol administration. In this model, feeding I3C markedly reduced the number of mice that developed cervical cancer.[64] A small placebo-controlled trial in women examined the effect of oral I3C supplementation on the progression of precancerous cervical lesions classified as cervical intraepithelial neoplasia (CIN) 2 or CIN 3.[65] After 12 weeks, 4 out of the 8 women who took 200 mg/d had complete regression of CIN, and 4 out of the 9 who took 400 mg/d had complete regression, while none of the 10 women who took a placebo had complete regression. Although these preliminary results are encouraging, larger controlled clinical trials are needed to determine the efficacy of I3C supplementation for preventing the progression of precancerous lesions of the cervix.[66]

Recurrent Respiratory Papillomatosis

Recurrent respiratory papillomatosis (RRP) is a rare disease of children and adults, characterized by generally benign growths (papillomas) in the respiratory tract caused by HPV infection.[67] These papillomas occur most commonly on or around the vocal cords in the larynx, but they may also affect the trachea, bronchi, and lungs. The most common treatment for RRP is surgical removal of the papillomas. Papillomas often recur; therefore, adjunct treatments may be used to help prevent or reduce recurrences.[68] In immune-compromised mice transplanted with HPV-infected laryngeal tissue, only 25% of the mice fed I3C developed laryngeal papillomas, compared with 100% of the control mice.[69] In a small observational study of RRP patients, increased ratios of urinary $2OHE_1:16\alpha OHE_1$ ratios resulting from increased cruciferous vegetable consumption were associated with less severe RRP.[70] An uncontrolled pilot study examined the effect of daily I3C supplementation (400 mg for adults and 10 mg/kg daily for children) on papilloma recurrence in RRP patients.[71] Over a 5-year follow-up period, 11 of the original 49 patients experienced no recurrence, 10 experienced a reduction in the rate of recurrence, 12 experienced no improvement, and 12 were lost to follow-up.[72] Although the low toxicity of I3C makes it an attractive adjunct therapy for RRP, controlled clinical trials are needed to determine whether I3C is effective in preventing or reducing the recurrence of respiratory papillomas.

Systemic Lupus Erythematosus

Systemic lupus erythematosus (SLE) is an autoimmune disorder characterized by chronic inflammation that may result in damage to the joints, skin, kidneys, heart, lungs, blood vessels, or brain.[73] Estrogen is thought to play a role in the pathology of SLE because the disorder is much more common in women than men, and its onset is most common during the reproductive years when endogenous estrogen levels are highest.[74] The potential for I3C supplementation to shift endogenous estrogen metabolism toward the less estrogenic metabolite $2OHE_1$ and away from the highly estrogenic metabolite $16\alpha OHE_1$ (see the Estrogen Metabolism section above) led to interest in its use in SLE.[25] In an animal model of SLE, I3C feeding decreased the severity of renal disease and prolonged survival.[75] A small uncontrolled trial of I3C supplementation (375 mg/d) in female SLE patients found that I3C supplementation increased urinary $2OHE_1:16\alpha OHE_1$ ratios, but found no significant change in SLE symptoms after 3 months.[25] Controlled clinical trials are needed to determine whether I3C supplementation will have beneficial effects in SLE patients.

Sources

Cruciferous Vegetables

Glucobrassicin, the glucosinolate precursor of I3C, is found in several cruciferous vegetables, including broccoli, Brussels sprouts, cabbage, cauliflower, collard greens, kale, kohlrabi, mustard greens, radish, rutabaga, and turnip.[76,77] Although glucosinolates are present in relatively high concentrations in cruciferous vegetables, glucobrassicin makes up only ~8 to 12% of the total glucosinolates.[78] The amount of indole-3-carbinol formed from glucobrassicin in foods is variable and depends, in part, on the processing and preparation of those foods. See Chapter 15 for the total glucosinolate contents of selected cruciferous vegetables.

Effects of Cooking

Glucosinolates are water-soluble compounds that may be leached into cooking water. Boiling cruciferous vegetables from 9 to 15 minutes resulted in 18 to 59% decreases in the total glucosinolate content of cruciferous vegetables.[79] Cooking methods that use less water, such as steaming or microwaving may reduce glucosinolate losses. Some cooking practices, including boiling,[80] steaming,[81] and microwaving at high power (850 to 900 W),[82,83] may inactivate myrosinase, the enzymes that catalyze glucosinolate hydrolysis. Even in the absence of plant myrosinase activity, the myrosinase activity of human intestinal bacteria results in some glucosinolate hydrolysis.[6] However, studies in humans have found that inactivation of myrosinase in cruciferous vegetables substantially decreases the bioavailability of glucosinolate hydrolysis products known as isothiocyanates.[80–82] The formation of I3C also depends on glucosinolate hydrolysis; hence, it is very likely that the bioavailability of I3C and its acid condensation products would also be decreased by myrosinase inactivation.

Supplements

Indole-3-Carbinol (I3C)

I3C is available without a prescription as a dietary supplement. I3C supplementation increased urinary 2OHE$_1$ levels in adults at doses of 300 to 400 mg/d.[28] I3C doses of 200 or 400 mg/d improved the regression of cervical intraepithelial neoplasia (CIN) in a preliminary clinical trial.[65] I3C in doses up to 400 mg/d has been used to treat recurrent respiratory papillomatosis.[71,72]

3,3'-Diindolylmethane (DIM)

DIM is available without a prescription as a dietary supplement. In a small clinical trial, DIM supplementation at a dose of 108 mg/d for 30 days increased urinary 2OHE$_1$ excretion in postmenopausal women with a history of breast cancer.[29]

Safety

Adverse Reactions

Slight increases in the serum concentrations of a liver enzyme (alanine aminotransferase; ALT) were observed in two women who took unspecified doses of I3C supplements for 4 weeks.[28] One person reported a skin rash while taking 375 mg/d of I3C.[25] High doses of I3C (800 mg/d) were associated with symptoms of disequilibrium and tremor, which resolved

when the dose was decreased.[71] I3C supplementation enhanced the development of cancer in some animal models when given after the carcinogen[46,58–60] (see the Cancer section above). The effects of I3C or DIM supplementation on cancer risk in humans are not known.

Pregnancy

The safety of I3C or DIM supplements during pregnancy or lactation has not been established.

Drug Interactions

No drug interactions in humans have been reported. However, preliminary evidence that I3C and DIM can increase the activity of CYP-1A2[84,85] suggests the potential for I3C or DIM supplementation to decrease serum concentrations of medications metabolized by CYP-1A2. Both I3C and DIM modestly increase the activity of CYP3A4 in rats when administered chronically.[86] This observation raises the potential for adverse drug interactions in humans because CYP3A4 is involved in the metabolism of ~60% of therapeutic drugs.

Summary

- Indole-3-carbinol (I3C) is derived from the hydrolysis (breakdown) of glucobrassicin, a compound found in cruciferous vegetables.
- In the acidic environment of the stomach, I3C molecules can combine with each other to form several biologically active acid condensation products, such as 3,3'-diindolylmethane (DIM).
- I3C has been found to inhibit the development of cancer in animals when given before or at the same time as a carcinogen. However, in some cases, I3C enhanced the development of cancer in animals when administered after a carcinogen.
- The contradictory results of animal studies have led some experts to caution against the widespread use of I3C and DIM supplements for cancer prevention in humans until their potential risks and benefits are better understood.

- Although I3C and DIM supplementation have been found to alter urinary estrogen metabolite profiles in women, the effects of I3C and DIM on breast cancer risk are not known.
- Small preliminary trials in humans suggest that I3C supplementation may be beneficial in treating conditions related to human papilloma virus (HPV) infection, such as cervical intraepithelial neoplasia (CIN) and recurrent respiratory papillomatosis (RRP), but larger randomized controlled trials are needed.

References

1. Verhoeven DT, Verhagen H, Goldbohm RA, van den Brandt PA, van Poppel G. A review of mechanisms underlying anticarcinogenicity by brassica vegetables. Chem Biol Interact 1997;103(2):79–129
2. Kim YS, Milner JA. Targets for indole-3-carbinol in cancer prevention. J Nutr Biochem 2005;16(2):65–73
3. Holst B, Williamson G. A critical review of the bioavailability of glucosinolates and related compounds. Nat Prod Rep 2004;21(3):425–447
4. Shertzer HG, Senft AP. The micronutrient indole-3-carbinol: implications for disease and chemoprevention. Drug Metabol Drug Interact 2000;17(1–4):159–188
5. Bjeldanes LF, Kim JY, Grose KR, Bartholomew JC, Bradfield CA. Aromatic hydrocarbon responsiveness-receptor agonists generated from indole-3-carbinol in vitro and in vivo: comparisons with 2,3,7,8-tetrachlorodibenzo-p-dioxin. Proc Natl Acad Sci U S A 1991;88(21):9543–9547
6. Shapiro TA, Fahey JW, Wade KL, Stephenson KK, Talalay P. Human metabolism and excretion of cancer chemoprotective glucosinolates and isothiocyanates of cruciferous vegetables. Cancer Epidemiol Biomarkers Prev 1998;7(12):1091–1100
7. Lampe JW, Peterson S. Brassica, biotransformation and cancer risk: genetic polymorphisms alter the preventive effects of cruciferous vegetables. J Nutr 2002; 132(10):2991–2994
8. Bonnesen C, Eggleston IM, Hayes JD. Dietary indoles and isothiocyanates that are generated from cruciferous vegetables can both stimulate apoptosis and confer protection against DNA damage in human colon cell lines. Cancer Res 2001;61(16):6120–6130
9. Safe S. Molecular biology of the Ah receptor and its role in carcinogenesis. Toxicol Lett 2001;120(1–3):1–7
10. Nho CW, Jeffery E. The synergistic upregulation of phase II detoxification enzymes by glucosinolate breakdown products in cruciferous vegetables. Toxicol Appl Pharmacol 2001;174(2):146–152
11. Wallig MA, Kingston S, Staack R, Jefferey EH. Induction of rat pancreatic glutathione S-transferase and quinone reductase activities by a mixture of glucosinolate breakdown derivatives found in Brussels sprouts. Food Chem Toxicol 1998;36(5):365–373
12. Baird WM, Hooven LA, Mahadevan B. Carcinogenic polycyclic aromatic hydrocarbon-DNA adducts and mechanism of action. Environ Mol Mutagen 2005; 45(2–3):106–114
13. Jordan VC, Gapstur S, Morrow M. Selective estrogen receptor modulation and reduction in risk of breast cancer, osteoporosis, and coronary heart disease. J Natl Cancer Inst 2001;93(19):1449–1457
14. Liehr JG. Is estradiol a genotoxic mutagenic carcinogen? Endocr Rev 2000;21(1):40–54
15. Ashok BT, Chen Y, Liu X, Bradlow HL, Mittelman A, Tiwari RK. Abrogation of estrogen-mediated cellular and biochemical effects by indole-3-carbinol. Nutr Cancer 2001;41(1–2):180–187
16. Meng Q, Yuan F, Goldberg ID, Rosen EM, Auborn K, Fan S. Indole-3-carbinol is a negative regulator of estrogen receptor-alpha signaling in human tumor cells. J Nutr 2000;130(12):2927–2931
17. Chen I, McDougal A, Wang F, Safe S. Aryl hydrocarbon receptor-mediated antiestrogenic and antitumorigenic activity of diindolylmethane. Carcinogenesis 1998;19(9):1631–1639
18. Leong H, Riby JE, Firestone GL, Bjeldanes LF. Potent ligand-independent estrogen receptor activation by 3,3′-diindolylmethane is mediated by cross talk between the protein kinase A and mitogen-activated protein kinase signaling pathways. Mol Endocrinol 2004;18(2):291–302
19. Riby JE, Feng C, Chang YC, Schaldach CM, Firestone GL, Bjeldanes LF. The major cyclic trimeric product of indole-3-carbinol is a strong agonist of the estrogen receptor signaling pathway. Biochemistry 2000;39(5):910–918
20. Shilling AD, Carlson DB, Katchamart S, Williams DE. 3,3′-Diindolylmethane, a major condensation product of indole-3-carbinol, is a potent estrogen in the rainbow trout. Toxicol Appl Pharmacol 2001;170(3):191–200
21. Telang NT, Suto A, Wong GY, Osborne MP, Bradlow HL. Induction by estrogen metabolite 16 alpha-hydroxyestrone of genotoxic damage and aberrant proliferation in mouse mammary epithelial cells. J Natl Cancer Inst 1992;84(8):634–638
22. Yuan F, Chen DZ, Liu K, Sepkovic DW, Bradlow HL, Auborn K. Anti-estrogenic activities of indole-3-carbinol in cervical cells: implication for prevention of cervical cancer. Anticancer Res 1999;19(3A):1673–1680
23. Bradlow HL, Telang NT, Sepkovic DW, Osborne MP. 2-Hydroxyestrone: the 'good' estrogen. J Endocrinol 1996;150(Suppl):S259–S265
24. Bradlow HL, Michnovicz JJ, Halper M, Miller DG, Wong GY, Osborne MP. Long-term responses of women to indole-3-carbinol or a high fiber diet. Cancer Epidemiol Biomarkers Prev 1994;3(7):591–595
25. McAlindon TE, Gulin J, Chen T, Klug T, Lahita R, Nuite M. Indole-3-carbinol in women with SLE: effect on estrogen metabolism and disease activity. Lupus 2001;10(11):779–783
26. Michnovicz JJ. Increased estrogen 2-hydroxylation in obese women using oral indole-3-carbinol. Int J Obes Relat Metab Disord 1998;22(3):227–229
27. Michnovicz JJ, Adlercreutz H, Bradlow HL. Changes in levels of urinary estrogen metabolites after oral indole-3-carbinol treatment in humans. J Natl Cancer Inst 1997;89(10):718–723

28. Wong GY, Bradlow L, Sepkovic D, Mehl S, Mailman J, Osborne MP. Dose-ranging study of indole-3-carbinol for breast cancer prevention. J Cell Biochem Suppl 1997;28–29:111–116

29. Dalessandri KM, Firestone GL, Fitch MD, Bradlow HL, Bjeldanes LF. Pilot study: effect of 3,3′-diindolyl-methane supplements on urinary hormone metabolites in postmenopausal women with a history of early-stage breast cancer. Nutr Cancer 2004;50(2): 161–167

30. Ho GH, Luo XW, Ji CY, Foo SC, Ng EH. Urinary 2/16 alpha-hydroxyestrone ratio: correlation with serum insulin-like growth factor binding protein-3 and a potential biomarker of breast cancer risk. Ann Acad Med Singapore 1998;27(2):294–299

31. Kabat GC, Chang CJ, Sparano JA, et al. Urinary estrogen metabolites and breast cancer: a case-control study. Cancer Epidemiol Biomarkers Prev 1997;6(7):505–509

32. Schneider J, Kinne D, Fracchia A, et al. Abnormal oxidative metabolism of estradiol in women with breast cancer. Proc Natl Acad Sci U S A 1982;79(9):3047–3051

33. Cauley JA, Zmuda JM, Danielson ME, et al. Estrogen metabolites and the risk of breast cancer in older women. Epidemiology 2003;14(6):740–744

34. Meilahn EN, De Stavola B, Allen DS, et al. Do urinary oestrogen metabolites predict breast cancer? Guernsey III cohort follow-up. Br J Cancer 1998;78(9):1250–1255

35. Ursin G, London S, Stanczyk FZ, et al. Urinary 2-hydroxyestrone/16alpha-hydroxyestrone ratio and risk of breast cancer in postmenopausal women. J Natl Cancer Inst 1999;91(12):1067–1072

36. Stewart ZA, Westfall MD, Pietenpol JA. Cell-cycle dysregulation and anticancer therapy. Trends Pharmacol Sci 2003;24(3):139–145

37. Chinni SR, Li Y, Upadhyay S, Koppolu PK, Sarkar FH. Indole-3-carbinol (I3C) induced cell growth inhibition, G1 cell cycle arrest and apoptosis in prostate cancer cells. Oncogene 2001;20(23):2927–2936

38. Cover CM, Hsieh SJ, Tran SH, et al. Indole-3-carbinol inhibits the expression of cyclin-dependent kinase-6 and induces a G1 cell cycle arrest of human breast cancer cells independent of estrogen receptor signaling. J Biol Chem 1998;273(7):3838–3847

39. Stresser DM, Williams DE, Griffin DA, Bailey GS. Mechanisms of tumor modulation by indole-3-carbinol. Disposition and excretion in male Fischer 344 rats. Drug Metab Dispos 1995;23(9):965–975

40. Hong C, Firestone GL, Bjeldanes LF. Bcl-2 family-mediated apoptotic effects of 3,3′-diindolylmethane (DIM) in human breast cancer cells. Biochem Pharmacol 2002;63(6):1085–1097

41. Howells LM, Gallacher-Horley B, Houghton CE, Manson MM, Hudson EA. Indole-3-carbinol inhibits protein kinase B/Akt and induces apoptosis in the human breast tumor cell line MDA MB468 but not in the nontumorigenic HBL100 line. Mol Cancer Ther 2002; 1(13):1161–1172

42. Chen D, Carter TH, Auborn KJ. Apoptosis in cervical cancer cells: implications for adjunct anti-estrogen therapy for cervical cancer. Anticancer Res 2004; 24(5A):2649–2656

43. Meng Q, Goldberg ID, Rosen EM, Fan S. Inhibitory effects of Indole-3-carbinol on invasion and migration in human breast cancer cells. Breast Cancer Res Treat 2000;63(2):147–152

44. Chang X, Tou JC, Hong C, et al. 3,3′-Diindolylmethane inhibits angiogenesis and the growth of transplantable human breast carcinoma in athymic mice. Carcinogenesis 2005;26(4):771–778

45. Verhoeven DT, Goldbohm RA, van Poppel G, Verhagen H, van den Brandt PA. Epidemiological studies on brassica vegetables and cancer risk. Cancer Epidemiol Biomarkers Prev 1996;5(9):733–748

46. Kim DJ, Han BS, Ahn B, et al. Enhancement by indole-3-carbinol of liver and thyroid gland neoplastic development in a rat medium-term multiorgan carcinogenesis model. Carcinogenesis 1997;18(2):377–381

47. Fahey JW, Zalcmann AT, Talalay P. The chemical diversity and distribution of glucosinolates and isothiocyanates among plants. Phytochemistry 2001;56(1): 5–51

48. Grubbs CJ, Steele VE, Casebolt T, et al. Chemoprevention of chemically-induced mammary carcinogenesis by indole-3-carbinol. Anticancer Res 1995;15(3):709–716

49. Bradlow HL, Michnovicz J, Telang NT, Osborne MP. Effects of dietary indole-3-carbinol on estradiol metabolism and spontaneous mammary tumors in mice. Carcinogenesis 1991;12(9):1571–1574

50. Wattenberg LW, Loub WD. Inhibition of polycyclic aromatic hydrocarbon-induced neoplasia by naturally occurring indoles. Cancer Res 1978;38(5):1410–1413

51. Wargovich MJ, Chen CD, Jimenez A, et al. Aberrant crypts as a biomarker for colon cancer: evaluation of potential chemopreventive agents in the rat. Cancer Epidemiol Biomarkers Prev 1996;5(5):355–360

52. Guo D, Schut HA, Davis CD, Snyderwine EG, Bailey GS, Dashwood RH. Protection by chlorophyllin and indole-3-carbinol against 2-amino-1-methyl-6-phenylimidazo[4,5-b]pyridine (PhIP)-induced DNA adducts and colonic aberrant crypts in the F344 rat. Carcinogenesis 1995;16(12):2931–2937

53. Morse MA, LaGreca SD, Amin SG, Chung FL. Effects of indole-3-carbinol on lung tumorigenesis and DNA methylation induced by 4-(methylnitrosamino)-1-(3-pyridyl)-1-butanone (NNK) and on the metabolism and disposition of NNK in A/J mice. Cancer Res 1990; 50(9):2613–2617

54. Dashwood RH, Arbogast DN, Fong AT, Hendricks JD, Bailey GS. Mechanisms of anti-carcinogenesis by indole-3-carbinol: detailed in vivo DNA binding dose-response studies after dietary administration with aflatoxin B1. Carcinogenesis 1988;9(3):427–432

55. Dashwood RH, Fong AT, Williams DE, Hendricks JD, Bailey GS. Promotion of aflatoxin B1 carcinogenesis by the natural tumor modulator indole-3-carbinol: influence of dose, duration, and intermittent exposure on indole-3-carbinol promotional potency. Cancer Res 1991;51(9):2362–2365

56. Oganesian A, Hendricks JD, Pereira CB, Orner GA, Bailey GS, Williams DE. Potency of dietary indole-3-carbinol as a promoter of aflatoxin B1-initiated hepatocarcinogenesis: results from a 9000 animal tumor study. Carcinogenesis 1999;20(3):453–458

57. Kim DJ, Lee KK, Han BS, Ahn B, Bae JH, Jang JJ. Biphasic modifying effect of indole-3-carbinol on diethylnitrosamine-induced preneoplastic glutathione S-

transferase placental form-positive liver cell foci in Sprague-Dawley rats. Jpn J Cancer Res 1994;85(6): 578–583

58. Stoner G, Casto B, Ralston S, Roebuck B, Pereira C, Bailey G. Development of a multi-organ rat model for evaluating chemopreventive agents: efficacy of indole-3-carbinol. Carcinogenesis 2002;23(2):265–272

59. Pence BC, Buddingh F, Yang SP. Multiple dietary factors in the enhancement of dimethylhydrazine carcinogenesis: main effect of indole-3-carbinol. J Natl Cancer Inst 1986;77(1):269–276

60. Yoshida M, Katashima S, Ando J, et al. Dietary indole-3-carbinol promotes endometrial adenocarcinoma development in rats initiated with N-ethyl-N'-nitro-N-nitrosoguanidine, with induction of cytochrome P450s in the liver and consequent modulation of estrogen metabolism. Carcinogenesis 2004;25(11): 2257–2264

61. Dashwood RH. Indole-3-carbinol: anticarcinogen or tumor promoter in brassica vegetables? Chem Biol Interact 1998;110(1–2):1–5

62. Lee BM, Park KK. Beneficial and adverse effects of chemopreventive agents. Mutat Res 2003;523–524:265–278

63. Bosch FX, de Sanjose S. Chapter 1: Human papillomavirus and cervical cancer–burden and assessment of causality. J Natl Cancer Inst Monogr 2003; 31:3–13

64. Jin L, Qi M, Chen DZ, et al. Indole-3-carbinol prevents cervical cancer in human papilloma virus type 16 (HPV16) transgenic mice. Cancer Res 1999;59(16): 3991–3997

65. Bell MC, Crowley-Nowick P, Bradlow HL, et al. Placebo-controlled trial of indole-3-carbinol in the treatment of CIN. Gynecol Oncol 2000;78(2):123–129

66. Stanley M. Chapter 17: Genital human papillomavirus infections–current and prospective therapies. J Natl Cancer Inst Monogr 2003;31:117–124

67. What is recurrent respiratory papillomatosis? Recurrent Respiratory Papillomatosis Foundation. 2004. Available at: http://rrpf.org/whatisRRP.html. Accessed 7/26/06

68. Auborn KJ. Therapy for recurrent respiratory papillomatosis. Antivir Ther 2002;7(1):1–9

69. Newfield L, Goldsmith A, Bradlow HL, Auborn K. Estrogen metabolism and human papillomavirus-induced tumors of the larynx: chemo-prophylaxis with indole-3-carbinol. Anticancer Res 1993;13(2):337–341

70. Auborn K, Abramson A, Bradlow HL, Sepkovic D, Mullooly V. Estrogen metabolism and laryngeal papillomatosis: a pilot study on dietary prevention. Anticancer Res 1998;18(6B):4569–4573

71. Rosen CA, Woodson GE, Thompson JW, Hengesteg AP, Bradlow HL. Preliminary results of the use of indole-3-carbinol for recurrent respiratory papillomatosis. Otolaryngol Head Neck Surg 1998;118(6):810–815

72. Rosen CA, Bryson PC. Indole-3-carbinol for recurrent respiratory papillomatosis: long-term results. J Voice 2004;18(2):248–253

73. Nass T. Lupus: a patient care guide for nurses and other health professionals. National Institute of Arthritis and Musculoskeletal and Skin Diseases. 2001. Available at: http://www.niams.nih.gov/hi/topics/lupus/lupusguide/outline.htm. Accessed 7/26/06

74. McMurray RW, May W. Sex hormones and systemic lupus erythematosus: review and meta-analysis. Arthritis Rheum 2003;48(8):2100–2110

75. Auborn KJ, Qi M, Yan XJ, et al. Lifespan is prolonged in autoimmune-prone (NZB/NZW) F1 mice fed a diet supplemented with indole-3-carbinol. J Nutr 2003; 133(11):3610–3613

76. Carlson DG, Kwolek WF, Williams PH. Glucosinolates in crucifer vegetables: broccoli, Brussels sprouts, cauliflower, collards, kale, mustard greens, and kohlrabi. J Am Soc Hortic Sci 1987;112(1):173–178

77. Fenwick GR, Heaney RK, Mullin WJ. Glucosinolates and their breakdown products in food and food plants. Crit Rev Food Sci Nutr 1983;18(2):123–201

78. Kushad MM, Brown AF, Kurilich AC, et al. Variation of glucosinolates in vegetable crops of Brassica oleracea. J Agric Food Chem 1999;47(4):1541–1548

79. McNaughton SA, Marks GC. Development of a food composition database for the estimation of dietary intakes of glucosinolates, the biologically active constituents of cruciferous vegetables. Br J Nutr 2003;90(3):687–697

80. Shapiro TA, Fahey JW, Wade KL, Stephenson KK, Talalay P. Chemoprotective glucosinolates and isothiocyanates of broccoli sprouts: metabolism and excretion in humans. Cancer Epidemiol Biomarkers Prev 2001;10(5):501–508

81. Conaway CC, Getahun SM, Liebes LL, et al. Disposition of glucosinolates and sulforaphane in humans after ingestion of steamed and fresh broccoli. Nutr Cancer 2000;38(2):168–178

82. Rouzaud G, Young SA, Duncan AJ. Hydrolysis of glucosinolates to isothiocyanates after ingestion of raw or microwaved cabbage by human volunteers. Cancer Epidemiol Biomarkers Prev 2004;13(1):125–131

83. Verkerk R, Dekker M. Glucosinolates and myrosinase activity in red cabbage (Brassica oleracea L. var. Capitata f. rubra DC.) after various microwave treatments. J Agric Food Chem 2004;52(24):7318–7323

84. He YH, Friesen MD, Ruch RJ, Schut HA. Indole-3-carbinol as a chemopreventive agent in 2-amino-1-methyl-6-phenylimidazo[4,5-b]pyridine (PhIP) carcinogenesis: inhibition of PhIP-DNA adduct formation, acceleration of PhIP metabolism, and induction of cytochrome P450 in female F344 rats. Food Chem Toxicol 2000;38(1):15–23

85. Lake BG, Tredger JM, Renwick AB, Barton PT, Price RJ. 3,3'-Diindolylmethane induces CYP1A2 in cultured precision-cut human liver slices. Xenobiotica 1998; 28(8):803–811

86. Leibelt DA, Hedstrom OR, Fischer KA, Pereira CB, Williams DE. Evaluation of chronic dietary exposure to indole-3-carbinol and absorption-enhanced 3,3'-diindolylmethane in sprague-dawley rats. Toxicol Sci 2003;74(1):10–21

17 Lignans

The mammalian lignans, enterodiol and enterolactone (**Fig. 17–1**), are formed by the activity of intestinal bacteria on lignan precursors found in plants.[1] Because enterodiol and enterolactone can mimic some of the effects of estrogens, their plant-derived precursors are classified as phytoestrogens. Lignan precursors (plant lignans) that have been identified in the human diet include secoisolariciresinol, matairesinol, pinoresinol, lariciresinol (**Fig. 17–2**), and others. Because secoisolariciresinol and matairesinol were among the first plant lignans identified in the human diet, they are thus the most extensively studied. Lignans are found in a wide variety of plant foods including flaxseeds, legumes, whole grains, fruits, and vegetables. Although most research on phytoestrogen-rich diets has focused on soy isoflavones, lignans are the principal source of dietary phytoestrogens in typical Western diets.[2,3]

Metabolism and Bioavailability

When plant lignans are ingested, they can be metabolized by intestinal bacteria to the mammalian lignans, enterodiol and enterolactone.[4] Enterodiol can also be converted to enterolactone by intestinal bacteria. Not surprisingly, antibiotic use in the past year was associated with lower serum enterolactone levels.[5] Thus, enterolactone levels measured in serum and urine reflect the activity of intestinal bacteria in addition to dietary intake of plant lignans. Because data on the lignan content of foods are limited, serum and urinary enterolactone levels are sometimes used as markers of dietary lignan intake in research. A pharmacokinetic study that measured plasma and urinary levels of enterodiol and enterolactone after a single dose (0.9 mg/kg of body weight) of secoisolariciresinol, the principal lignan in flaxseed, found that at least 40% was available to the body as enterodiol and enterolactone.[6] Plasma enterodiol concentrations peaked at 73 nmol/L an average of 15 hours after ingesting secoisolariciresinol, and plasma enterolactone concentrations peaked at 56 nmol/L an average of 20 hours after ingestion. Thus, substantial amounts of ingested plant lignans are available to humans in the form of enterodiol and enterolactone. Considerable variation between individuals in urinary and serum enterodiol:enterolactone ratios has been observed in flaxseed feeding studies, suggesting that some individuals convert most enterodiol to enterolactone, whereas others convert relatively little.[1] It is likely that individual differences in the metabolism of lignans influence the biological activities and health effects of these compounds.

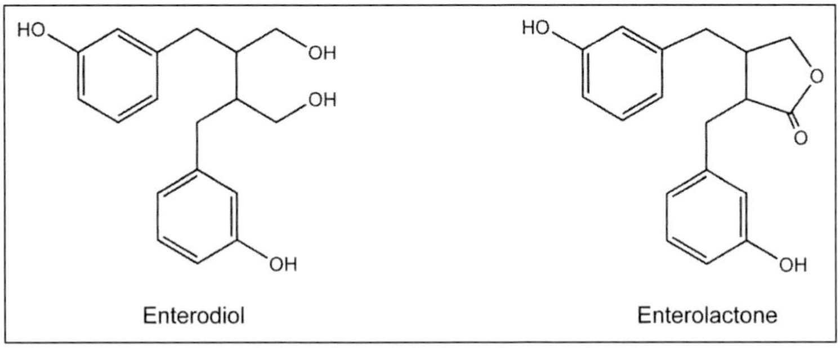

Figure 17–1 Chemical structures of the mammalian lignans, enterodiol and enterolactone.

Enterodiol

Enterolactone

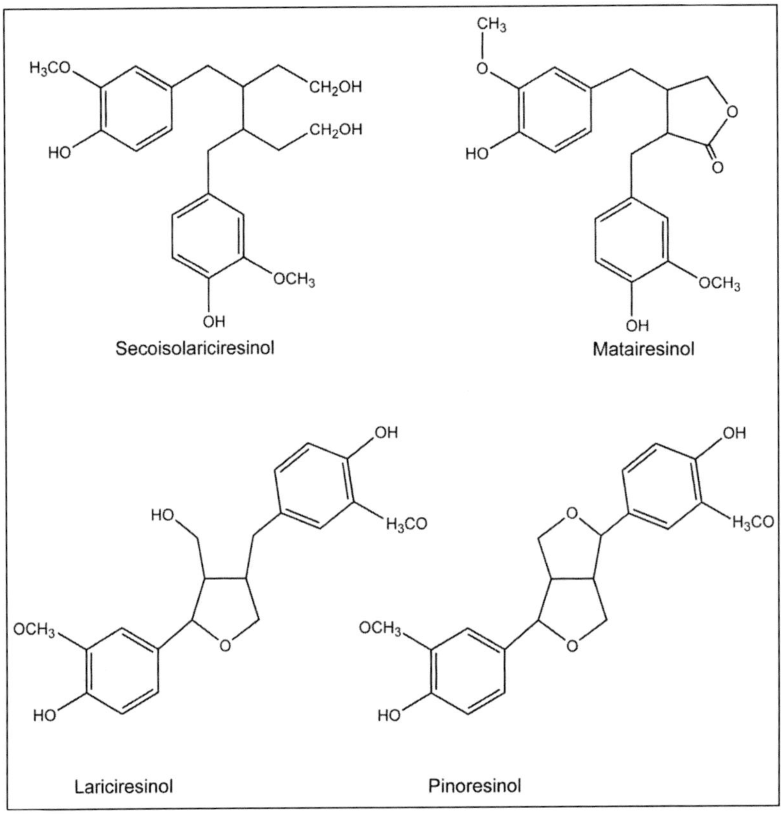

Figure 17–2
Chemical structures of secoisolariciresinol, matairesinol, lariciresinol, and pinoresinol, plant lignans that are precursors for mammalian lignans.

Biological Activities

Estrogenic and Anti-estrogenic Activities

Estrogens are signaling molecules (hormones) that exert their effects by binding to estrogen receptors within cells. The estrogen-receptor complex interacts with DNA to change the expression of estrogen-responsive genes. Estrogen receptors are present in numerous tissues other than those associated with reproduction, including bone, liver, heart, and brain.[7] Although phytoestrogens can also bind to estrogen receptors, their estrogenic activity is much weaker than endogenous estrogens, and they may actually block or antagonize the effects of estrogen in some tissues.[8] Scientists are interested in the tissue-selective activities of phytoestrogens because anti-estrogenic effects in re-productive tissue could help reduce the risk of hormone-associated cancers (breast, uterine, ovarian, and prostate), and estrogenic effects in bone could help maintain bone density. The mammalian lignans, enterodiol and enterolactone, are known to have weak estrogenic activity. At present, the extent to which mammalian lignans exert weak estrogenic and/or antiestrogenic effects in humans is not well understood.

Estrogen Receptor-Independent Activities

Mammalian lignans also have biological activities that are unrelated to their interactions with estrogen receptors. By inhibiting the activity of enzymes involved in estrogen metabolism, lignans may alter the biological activity of endogenous estrogens.[9] Lignans can act as antioxidants in the test tube, but the significance of such antioxidant activity in humans is not clear because lignans are rapidly and extensively metabolized.[4] Although one cross-sectional study found that a biomarker of oxidative damage was inversely associated with serum enterolactone levels in men,[10] it is not clear whether this effect was related to enterolactone or other antioxidants present in lignan-rich foods.

Prevention

Cardiovascular Disease

Diets rich in foods containing plant lignans (whole grains, nuts and seeds, legumes, fruits, and vegetables) are consistently associated with reductions in cardiovascular disease risk. However, it is likely that numerous nutrients and phytochemicals found in these foods contribute to their cardioprotective effects. In a prospective cohort study of 1889 Finnish men followed for an average of 12 years, those with the highest serum enterolactone levels (a marker of plant lignan intake) were significantly less likely to die from coronary heart disease or cardiovascular disease than those with the lowest levels.[11] Flaxseeds are among the richest sources of plant lignans in the human diet, but they are also good sources of other nutrients and phytochemicals with cardioprotective effects, such as omega-3 fatty acids and fiber. Three small clinical trials found that adding 38 to 50 g/d of flaxseed to the usual diet for 4 to 6 weeks resulted in modest 8 to 14% decreases in low-density lipoprotein (LDL) cholesterol levels;[12-14] although three other trials did not observe significant reductions in LDL cholesterol after adding 30 to 40 g/d of flaxseed to the diet.[15-17] Although the results of prospective cohort studies consistently indicate that diets rich in whole grains, nuts, fruits, and vegetables are associated with significant reductions in cardiovascular disease risk, it is not yet clear whether lignans themselves are cardioprotective.

Hormone-Associated Cancers

Breast Cancer

Presently, there is little evidence that dietary intake of plant lignans is significantly associated with breast cancer risk. Neither of the two prospective cohort studies that examined plant lignan intake and breast cancer risk found them to be related.[18,19] Although one retrospective case-control study found that German women with the highest dietary intakes of matairesinol were significantly less likely to have breast cancer than those with the lowest intakes,[20] two other case-control studies conducted in the United States did not observe significant relationships between dietary lignan intake and breast cancer risk.[21,22] Two retrospective case-control studies found breast cancer risk to be lower in those with higher rates of urinary enterolactone excretion,[23,24] but the only prospective study found no significant association between urinary enterolactone excretion and breast cancer risk.[25] Similarly, two case-control studies found breast cancer risk to be higher in those with very low serum enterolactone concentrations,[26,27] but two prospective studies found no significant association between serum enterolactone concentrations and breast cancer risk.[28,29] A recent prospective study in Denmark found that serum enterolactone concentrations were not associated with the risk of estrogen receptor α (ERα)-positive breast cancer, but the risk of ERα-negative breast cancer was significantly lower in women with higher serum enterolactone concentrations.[30] In general, ERα-negative breast tumors tend to be more aggressive and less responsive to treatment than ERα-positive breast tumors. At present, it is not clear whether high intakes of plant lignans or high circulating levels of mammalian lignans offer significant protective effects against breast cancer.

Endometrial and Ovarian Cancer

In the only case-control study of lignans and endometrial cancer, women in the United States with the highest intakes of plant lignans had the lowest risk of endometrial cancer, but the reduction in risk was statistically significant in postmenopausal women only.[31] Similarly, in the only U.S. case-control study of lignans and ovarian cancer, women with the highest intakes of plant lignans had the lowest risk of ovarian cancer.[32] However, high intakes of other phytochemicals associated with plant-based diets like fiber, carotenoids, and sitosterols were also associated with decreased ovarian cancer risk. Although these studies support the hypothesis that diets rich in plant foods may be helpful in decreasing the risk of hormone-associated cancers, they do not provide strong evidence that lignans are protective against endometrial or ovarian cancer.

Prostate Cancer

Although dietary lignans are the principal source of phytoestrogens in the typical Western diet, relationships between dietary lignan intake and prostate cancer risk have not been well studied. Three prospective case-control studies examined the relationship between circulating enterolactone concentrations, a marker of lignan intake, and the subsequent development of prostate cancer in Scandinavian men.[33,34] In all three studies, initial serum enterolactone concentrations in men who were diagnosed with prostate cancer 5 to 14 years later were not significantly different from serum enterolactone levels in matched control groups of men who did not develop prostate cancer. In a retrospective case-control study, recalled dietary lignan intake did not differ between men in the United States diagnosed with prostate cancer and a matched control group.[35] At present, limited data from epidemiological studies do not support a relationship between dietary lignan intake and prostate cancer risk.

Osteoporosis

Research on the effects of dietary lignan intake on osteoporosis risk is very limited. In two small observational studies, urinary enterolactone excretion was used as a marker of dietary lignan intake. One study of 75 postmenopausal Korean women, who were classified as osteoporotic, osteopenic, or normal on the basis of bone mineral density (BMD) measurements,

found that urinary enterolactone excretion was positively associated with BMD of the lumbar spine and hip.[36] However, a study of 50 postmenopausal Dutch women found that higher levels of urinary enterolactone excretion were associated with higher rates of bone loss.[37] In two separate placebo controlled trials, supplementation of postmenopausal women with 25 to 40 g/d of ground flaxseed for 3 to 4 months did not significantly alter biochemical markers of bone formation or bone resorption (loss).[17,38] More research is necessary to determine whether high dietary intakes of plant lignans can decrease the risk or severity of osteoporosis.

Sources

Food Sources

Lignans are present in a wide variety of plant foods, including seeds (flax, pumpkin, sunflower, poppy), whole grains (rye, oats, barley), bran (wheat, oat, rye), fruits (particularly berries), and vegetables.[39] Secoisolariciresinol and matairesinol were the first plant lignans identified in foods.[40] Pinoresinol and lariciresinol are more recently identified plant lignans that contribute substantially to total dietary lignan intakes. A survey of 4660 Dutch men and women during 1997 to 1998 found that the median total lignan intake was 979 µg/d.[41] Lariciresinol and pinoresinol contributed ~75% to the total lignan intake; secoisolariciresinol and matairesinol contributed only ~25%. Plant lignans are the principal source of phytoestrogens in the diets of people who do not typically consume soy foods. The daily phytoestrogen intake of postmenopausal women in the United States was estimated to be less than 1000 µg/d with 80% from lignans and 20% from isoflavones.[42]

Flaxseed is by far the richest dietary source of plant lignans.[43] Lignans are not associated with the oil fraction of foods so flaxseed oils do not typically provide lignans unless ground flaxseed has been added to the oil. A variety of factors may affect the lignan contents of plants, including geographic location, climate, maturity, and storage conditions. **Table 17–1** provides the total lignan (secoisolariciresinol,

Table 17–1 Total Lignan Content* of Selected Foods[44]

Food	Serving	Total Lignans (mg)
Flaxseeds	1 oz	85.5
Sesame seeds	1 oz	11.2
Curly kale	1/2 cup, chopped	0.8
Broccoli	1/2 cup, chopped	0.6
Apricots	1/2 cup, sliced	0.4
Cabbage	1/2 cup, chopped	0.3
Brussels sprouts	1/2 cup, chopped	0.3
Strawberries	1/2 cup	0.2
Tofu	1/4 block (4 oz)	0.2
Dark rye bread	1 slice	0.1

* Secoisolariciresinol, matairesinol, pinoresinol, and lariciresinol.

matairesinol, pinoresinol, and lariciresinol) contents of selected lignan-rich foods.[44]

Supplements

Dietary supplements containing lignans derived from flaxseed are available in the United States without a prescription. One such supplement provides 50 mg of secoisolariciresinol diglycoside per capsule.

Safety

Adverse Effects

Lignans in plant foods are not known to have any adverse effects. Flaxseeds, which are rich in lignans as well as fiber, may increase stool frequency or cause diarrhea in doses of 45 to 50 g/d in adults.[12,45] The safety of lignan supplements in pregnant or lactating women has not been established. Therefore, lignan supplements should be avoided by women who are pregnant, breastfeeding, or trying to conceive.

Summary

- Lignans are found in a wide variety of plant-based foods, including seeds, whole grains, legumes, fruits, and vegetables.
- Flaxseeds are the richest dietary source of plant lignans.
- When ingested, plant lignans are converted to the mammalian lignans, enterodiol and enterolactone, by bacteria that normally colonize the human intestine.
- Enterodiol and enterolactone have weak estrogenic activity but may also exert biological effects through nonestrogenic mechanisms.
- Lignan-rich foods are part of a healthy dietary pattern, but the role of lignans in the prevention of cardiovascular disease, hormone-associated cancers, and osteoporosis is not yet clear.

References

1. Lampe JW. Isoflavonoid and lignan phytoestrogens as dietary biomarkers. J Nutr 2003;133(Suppl 3):956S–964S
2. de Kleijn MJ, van der Schouw YT, Wilson PW, Grobbee DE, Jacques PF. Dietary intake of phytoestrogens is associated with a favorable metabolic cardiovascular risk profile in postmenopausal U.S. women: the Framingham study. J Nutr 2002;132(2):276–282
3. Valsta LM, Kilkkinen A, Mazur W, et al. Phyto-oestrogen database of foods and average intake in Finland. Br J Nutr 2003;89(Suppl 1):S31–S38
4. Rowland I, Faughnan M, Hoey L, Wahala K, Williamson G, Cassidy A. Bioavailability of phyto-oestrogens. Br J Nutr 2003;89(Suppl 1):S45–S58
5. Kilkkinen A, Pietinen P, Klaukka T, Virtamo J, Korhonen P, Adlercreutz H. Use of oral antimicrobials decreases serum enterolactone concentration. Am J Epidemiol 2002;155(5):472–477
6. Kuijsten A, Arts IC, Vree TB, Hollman PC. Pharmacokinetics of enterolignans in healthy men and women consuming a single dose of secoisolariciresinol diglucoside. J Nutr 2005;135(4):795–801
7. Kleinsmith LJ, Kerrigan D, Kelly J. Science behind the news: understanding estrogen receptors, tamoxifen and raloxifene. National Cancer Institute. 2003. Available at: http://press2.nci.nih.gov/sciencebehind/estrogen/estrogen01.htm
8. Wang LQ. Mammalian phytoestrogens: enterodiol and enterolactone. J Chromatogr B Analyt Technol Biomed Life Sci 2002;777(1–2):289–309
9. Brooks JD, Thompson LU. Mammalian lignans and genistein decrease the activities of aromatase and 17beta-hydroxysteroid dehydrogenase in MCF-7 cells. J Steroid Biochem Mol Biol 2005;94(5):461–467

10. Vanharanta M, Voutilainen S, Nurmi T, et al. Association between low serum enterolactone and increased plasma F2-isoprostanes, a measure of lipid peroxidation. Atherosclerosis 2002;160(2):465–469

11. Vanharanta M, Voutilainen S, Rissanen TH, Adlercreutz H, Salonen JT. Risk of cardiovascular disease-related and all-cause death according to serum concentrations of enterolactone: Kuopio Ischaemic Heart Disease Risk Factor Study. Arch Intern Med 2003; 163(9):1099–1104

12. Cunnane SC, Hamadeh MJ, Liede AC, Thompson LU, Wolever TM, Jenkins DJ. Nutritional attributes of traditional flaxseed in healthy young adults. Am J Clin Nutr 1995;61(1):62–68

13. Arjmandi BH, Khan DA, Jurna S. Whole flaxseed consumption lowers serum LDL-cholesterol and lipoprotein(a) concentrations in postmenopausal women. Nutr Res 1998;18:1203–1214

14. Jenkins DJ, Kendall CW, Vidgen E, et al. Health aspects of partially defatted flaxseed, including effects on serum lipids, oxidative measures, and ex vivo androgen and progestin activity: a controlled crossover trial. Am J Clin Nutr 1999;69(3):395–402

15. Clark WF, Kortas C, Heidenheim AP, Garland J, Spanner E, Parbtani A. Flaxseed in lupus nephritis: a two-year nonplacebo-controlled crossover study. J Am Coll Nutr 2001;20(2 Suppl):143–148

16. Lemay A, Dodin S, Kadri N, Jacques H, Forest JC. Flaxseed dietary supplement versus hormone replacement therapy in hypercholesterolemic menopausal women. Obstet Gynecol 2002;100(3):495–504

17. Lucas EA, Wild RD, Hammond LJ, et al. Flaxseed improves lipid profile without altering biomarkers of bone metabolism in postmenopausal women. J Clin Endocrinol Metab 2002;87(4):1527–1532

18. Horn-Ross PL, Hoggatt KJ, West DW, et al. Recent diet and breast cancer risk: the California Teachers Study (USA). Cancer Causes Control 2002;13(5):407–415

19. Keinan-Boker L, van Der Schouw YT, Grobbee DE, Peeters PH. Dietary phytoestrogens and breast cancer risk. Am J Clin Nutr 2004;79(2):282–288

20. Linseisen J, Piller R, Hermann S, Chang-Claude J. Dietary phytoestrogen intake and premenopausal breast cancer risk in a German case-control study. Int J Cancer 2004;110(2):284–290

21. McCann SE, Moysich KB, Freudenheim JL, Ambrosone CB, Shields PG. The risk of breast cancer associated with dietary lignans differs by CYP17 genotype in women. J Nutr 2002;132(10):3036–3041

22. Horn-Ross PL, John EM, Lee M, et al. Phytoestrogen consumption and breast cancer risk in a multiethnic population: the Bay Area Breast Cancer Study. Am J Epidemiol 2001;154(5):434–441

23. Ingram D, Sanders K, Kolybaba M, Lopez D. Case-control study of phyto-oestrogens and breast cancer. Lancet 1997;350(9083):990–994

24. Dai Q, Franke AA, Jin F, et al. Urinary excretion of phytoestrogens and risk of breast cancer among Chinese women in Shanghai. Cancer Epidemiol Biomarkers Prev 2002;11(9):815–821

25. den Tonkelaar I, Keinan-Boker L, Veer PV, et al. Urinary phytoestrogens and postmenopausal breast cancer risk. Cancer Epidemiol Biomarkers Prev 2001;10(3): 223–228

26. Hulten K, Winkvist A, Lenner P, Johansson R, Adlercreutz H, Hallmans G. An incident case-referent study on plasma enterolactone and breast cancer risk. Eur J Nutr 2002;41(4):168–176

27. Pietinen P, Stumpf K, Mannisto S, Kataja V, Uusitupa M, Adlercreutz H. Serum enterolactone and risk of breast cancer: a case-control study in eastern Finland. Cancer Epidemiol Biomarkers Prev 2001;10(4):339–344

28. Zeleniuch-Jacquotte A, Adlercreutz H, Shore RE, et al. Circulating enterolactone and risk of breast cancer: a prospective study in New York. Br J Cancer 2004; 91(1):99–105

29. Kilkkinen A, Virtamo J, Vartiainen E, et al. Serum enterolactone concentration is not associated with breast cancer risk in a nested case-control study. Int J Cancer 2004;108(2):277–280

30. Olsen A, Knudsen KE, Thomsen BL, et al. Plasma enterolactone and breast cancer incidence by estrogen receptor status. Cancer Epidemiol Biomarkers Prev 2004;13(12):2084–2089

31. Horn-Ross PL, John EM, Canchola AJ, Stewart SL, Lee MM. Phytoestrogen intake and endometrial cancer risk. J Natl Cancer Inst 2003;95(15):1158–1164

32. McCann SE, Freudenheim JL, Marshall JR, Graham S. Risk of human ovarian cancer is related to dietary intake of selected nutrients, phytochemicals and food groups. J Nutr 2003;133(6):1937–1942

33. Kilkkinen A, Virtamo J, Virtanen MJ, Adlercreutz H, Albanes D, Pietinen P. Serum enterolactone concentration is not associated with prostate cancer risk in a nested case-control study. Cancer Epidemiol Biomarkers Prev 2003;12(11 Pt 1):1209–1212

34. Stattin P, Adlercreutz H, Tenkanen L, et al. Circulating enterolactone and prostate cancer risk: a Nordic nested case-control study. Int J Cancer 2002;99(1): 124–129

35. Strom SS, Yamamura Y, Duphorne CM, et al. Phytoestrogen intake and prostate cancer: a case-control study using a new database. Nutr Cancer 1999;33(1): 20–25

36. Kim MK, Chung BC, Yu VY, et al. Relationships of urinary phyto-oestrogen excretion to BMD in postmenopausal women. Clin Endocrinol (Oxf) 2002; 56(3):321–328

37. Kardinaal AF, Morton MS, Bruggemann-Rotgans IE, van Beresteijn EC. Phyto-oestrogen excretion and rate of bone loss in postmenopausal women. Eur J Clin Nutr 1998;52(11):850–855

38. Brooks JD, Ward WE, Lewis JE, et al. Supplementation with flaxseed alters estrogen metabolism in postmenopausal women to a greater extent than does supplementation with an equal amount of soy. Am J Clin Nutr 2004;79(2):318–325

39. Meagher LP, Beecher GR. Assessment of data on the lignan content of foods. J Food Compos Anal. 2000; 13(6):935–947

40. Ososki AL, Kennelly EJ. Phytoestrogens: a review of the present state of research. Phytother Res 2003; 17(8):845–869

41. Milder IE, Feskens EJ, Arts IC, de Mesquita HB, Hollman PC, Kromhout D. Intake of the plant lignans secoisolariciresinol, matairesinol, lariciresinol, and pinoresinol in Dutch men and women. J Nutr 2005; 135(5):1202–1207

42. de Kleijn MJ, van der Schouw YT, Wilson PW, et al. Intake of dietary phytoestrogens is low in postmenopausal women in the United States: the

Framingham study(1–4). J Nutr 2001;131(6):1826–1832

43. Thompson LU. Experimental studies on lignans and cancer. Baillieres Clin Endocrinol Metab 1998;12(4): 691–705

44. Milder IE, Arts IC, van de Putte B, Venema DP, Hollman PC. Lignan contents of Dutch plant foods: a database including lariciresinol, pinoresinol, secoisolariciresinol and matairesinol. Br J Nutr 2005;93(3):393–402

45. Clark WF, Parbtani A, Huff MW, et al. Flaxseed: a potential treatment for lupus nephritis. Kidney Int 1995;48(2):475–480

18 Organosulfur Compounds from Garlic

Garlic (*Allium sativum* L.) has been used for culinary and medicinal purposes by many cultures for centuries.[1] Garlic is a particularly rich source of organosulfur compounds, which are thought to be responsible for its flavor and aroma, as well as its potential health benefits.[2] Consumer interest in the health benefits of garlic is strong enough to place it among the best-selling herbal supplements in the United States.[3] Scientists are interested in the potential for organosulfur compounds derived from garlic to prevent and treat chronic diseases, such as cancer and cardiovascular disease.[4]

Organosulfur Compounds from Garlic

Two classes of organosulfur compounds are found in whole garlic cloves: (1) γ-glutamyl-cysteines, and (2) cysteine sulfoxides. Allylcysteine sulfoxide (alliin) accounts for ~80% of the cysteine sulfoxides in garlic.[1] When raw garlic cloves are crushed, chopped, or chewed, enzymes known as allinase are released. Allinase catalyzes the formation of sulfenic acids from cysteine sulfoxides (**Fig. 18–1**). Sulfenic acids spontaneously react with each other to form unstable compounds called thiosulfinates. In the case of alliin, the resulting sulfenic acids react with each other to form a thiosulfinate known as allicin. The formation of thiosulfinates is very rapid and has been found to be complete within 10 to 60 seconds of crushing garlic. Allicin breaks down to form a variety of fat-soluble organosulfur compounds including diallyl sulfide (DAS), diallyl disulfide (DADS), and diallyl trisulfide (DATS), or, in the presence of oil, ajoene, and vinyl dithiins.[2] Crushing garlic does not change its γ-glutamylcysteine content. Water-soluble organosulfur compounds, such as S-allylcysteine are formed from γ-glutamylcysteines during long-term incubation of crushed garlic in aqueous solutions, as in the manufacture of aged garlic extracts (see the Sources section below).

Bioavailability and Metabolism

Allicin-Derived Compounds

The absorption and metabolism of allicin-derived compounds is only partially understood.[5] Although several biological activities have been attributed to various allicin-derived compounds, it is not yet clear which of these compounds or metabolites actually reach target tissues.[1] Animal studies using radiolabeled compounds indicate that allicin or its breakdown products are absorbed intestinally.[6,7] However, allicin and allicin-derived compounds, including diallylsufides, ajoene, and vinyldithiins, have never been detected in human blood, urine, or stool, even after the consumption of up to 25 g of fresh garlic or 60 mg of pure allicin.[1] These findings suggest that allicin and allicin-derived compounds are rapidly metabolized. The concentration of allyl methyl sulfide in the breath has been proposed as an indicator of the bioavailability of allicin and allicin-derived compounds.[5] Human consumption of crushed garlic and equivalent amounts of allicin, DADS, DATS, and ajoene resulted in similar increases in breath concentrations of allyl methyl sulfide, suggesting that allicin and allicin-derived compounds are metabolized to allyl methyl sulfide, a volatile compound that can measured in exhaled air.

γ-Glutamylcysteines and S-Allylcysteine

γ-Glutamylcysteines, are thought to be absorbed intact and hydrolyzed to *S*-allylcysteine and *S*-1-propenylcysteine because metabolites

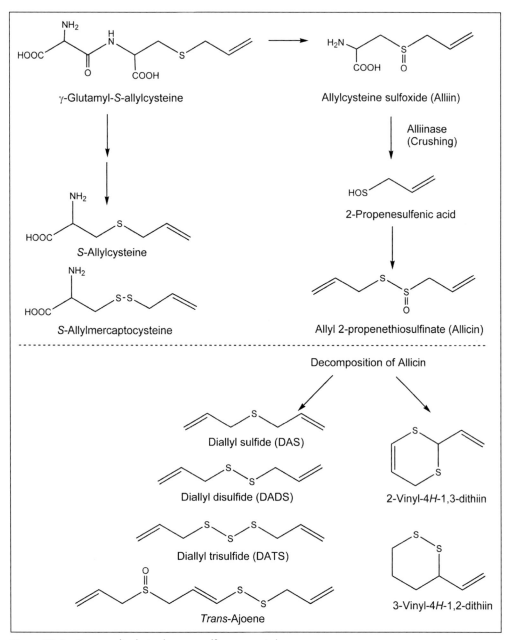

γ-Glutamyl-S-allylcysteine

Allylcysteine sulfoxide (Alliin)

Alliinase
(Crushing)

2-Propenesulfenic acid

S-Allylcysteine

S-Allylmercaptocysteine

Allyl 2-propenethiosulfinate (Allicin)

Decomposition of Allicin

Diallyl sulfide (DAS)

Diallyl disulfide (DADS)

2-Vinyl-4H-1,3-dithiin

Diallyl trisulfide (DATS)

3-Vinyl-4H-1,2-dithiin

Trans-Ajoene

Figure 18–1   Some garlic-derived organosulfur compounds.

of these compounds have been measured in human urine after garlic consumption.[8,9] The consumption of aged garlic extract, a commercial garlic preparation that contains S-allylcysteine, has been found to increase plasma S-allylcysteine concentrations in humans.[10,11]

Biological Activities

Related to Cardiovascular Disease Prevention

Inhibition of Cholesterol Synthesis

Garlic and garlic-derived organosulfur compounds have been found to decrease the synthesis of cholesterol by hepatocytes (liver cells).[12] Several garlic-derived organosulfur compounds, including S-allylcysteine and ajoene, have been found to inhibit 3-hydroxy-3-methyl-glutaryl coenzyme A reductase (HMG-CoA reductase), a critical enzyme in the cholesterol synthesis pathway.[13,14]

Inhibition of Platelet Aggregation

A variety of garlic-derived organosulfur compounds have been found to inhibit platelet aggregation in the test tube.[15,16]

Anti-inflammatory Activity

Inflammation appears to play an important role in the pathology of cardiovascular disease.[17] Garlic-derived organosulfur compounds have been found to inhibit the activity of the inflammatory enzymes, cyclooxygenase and lipoxygenase, in vitro (reviewed in Thomson and Afzal[18]) and to decrease the expression of inducible nitric oxide synthase (iNOS) in inflammatory white blood cells (macrophages).[19,20] Recently, organosulfur compounds have been found to decrease the production of inflammatory signaling molecules in cultured macrophages[21] and human whole blood.[22]

Inhibition of Arterial Smooth Muscle Proliferation

The proliferation and migration of normally quiescent arterial smooth muscle cells is a central feature of vascular diseases, including atherosclerosis and coronary restenosis.[23] Although the significance of these findings for human cardiovascular disease is not yet clear, limited cell culture research suggests that organosulfur compounds from garlic may inhibit the proliferation and migration of vascular smooth muscle cells.[13,24,25]

Antioxidant Activity

Several organosulfur compounds have been found to have antioxidant activity in the test tube, and there is some evidence that organosulfur compounds can stimulate the synthesis of glutathione, an important intracellular antioxidant.[26] Although garlic oil supplementation of hypertensive adults was reported to decrease a biomarker of in vivo lipid (fat) oxidation in a small uncontrolled trial,[27] it is not yet clear whether garlic-derived organosulfur compounds have clinically important antioxidant effects in vivo.

Biological Activities Related to Cancer

Effects on Carcinogen Metabolism

Inhibition of Phase I Biotransformation Enzymes

Some chemical carcinogens do not become active carcinogens until they have been metabolized by phase I biotransformation enzymes, such as those belonging to the cytochrome P450 (CYP) family. Inhibition of specific CYP enzymes involved in carcinogen activation inhibits the development of cancer in some animal models.[28] In particular, DAS and its metabolites have been found to inhibit CYP2E1 activity in vitro[29] and when administered orally at high doses to animals.[30,31] Oral administration of garlic oil and DAS to humans has also resulted in evidence of decreased CYP2E1 activity.[32,33]

Induction of Phase II Biotransformation Enzymes

Reactions catalyzed by phase II biotransformation enzymes generally promote the elimination of drugs, toxins, and carcinogens from the body. Consequently, increasing the activity of phase II enzymes, such as glutathione S-transferase and quinone reductase, may help prevent cancer by enhancing the elimination of potential carcinogens.[34] In animal studies, oral administration of garlic preparations and organosulfur compounds increases the activity of phase II enzymes in a variety of tissues.[35-37] The genes for several phase II enzymes contain a specific sequence of DNA called an antioxidant response element (ARE). Recent research suggests that allyl sulfides, particularly DATS, promote the translocation of a transcription factor known as Nrf2 to the nucleus where it binds to an ARE and increases the transcription of ARE-containing genes.[38] Although very high doses of organosulfur compounds were administered in most animal studies, at least one study found that quinone reductase activity increased in the gastrointestinal tracts of mice given a dose of DADS that might be achieved by human intake.[39]

Enhanced Cellular Glutathione Synthesis

Glutathione is an important intracellular antioxidant, and is also required for some phase II biotransformation reactions. There is some evidence from cell culture and animal studies that garlic-derived organosulfur compounds increase intracellular glutathione concentrations.[38,40] Like the genes for many phase II enzymes, the gene for a critical enzyme in glutathione synthesis also contains an ARE. Thus, organosulfur compounds may increase cellular glutathione synthesis by promoting the nuclear translocation and binding of the Nrf2 transcription factor to genes containing AREs (see the Induction of Phase II Biotransformation Enzymes section above).

Induction of Cell-Cycle Arrest

Unregulated cell division is a hallmark of human cancers.[41] In normal cells, the cell cycle is tightly regulated to ensure faithful DNA replication and chromosomal segregation prior to cell division. Following DNA damage, the cell cycle can be transiently arrested to allow for DNA repair or activation of pathways leading to cell death (apoptosis). Organosulfur compounds, including DADS, DATS, ajoene, and S-allylmercaptocysteine (SAMC), have been found to induce cell-cycle arrest when added to cancer cells in cell culture experiments.[42,43]

Induction of Apoptosis

Apoptosis is a normal physiological process for the self-destruction of cells that are genetically damaged or no longer necessary. Precancerous

and cancerous cells are resistant to signals that induce apoptosis.[44] Garlic-derived organosulfur compounds, including allicin, ajoene, DAS, DADS, DATS, and SAMC, have been found to induce apoptosis when added to various cancer cell lines grown in culture (reviewed in Herman-Antosiewicz and Singh[42] and Wu and Kassie[44]). Oral administration of aqueous garlic extract and S-allylcysteine has been reported to enhance apoptosis in an animal model of oral cancer.[45,46]

Antimicrobial Activity

Garlic extracts have been found to have antibacterial and antifungal properties in the laboratory.[47,48] Thiosulfinates, particularly allicin, are thought to play an important role in the antimicrobial activity of garlic.[48-50] Allicin-derived compounds, including DATS and ajoene, also have some antimicrobial activity in vitro, although generally less than allicin.[1] In contrast, randomized controlled trials have not provided strong evidence that oral garlic preparations have significant antibacterial activity in humans.[51] A small randomized controlled trial found that 1% ajoene cream applied to the skin twice daily was as effective in treating tinea pedis (athlete's foot) as 1% terbinafine (Lamisil) cream.[52]

Prevention

Cardiovascular Disease

Interest in garlic and its potential to prevent cardiovascular disease began with observations that people living near the Mediterranean had lower mortality from cardiovascular disease.[53] Garlic is a common ingredient in Mediterranean cuisine, but several characteristics of the Mediterranean diet have been proposed to explain its cardioprotective effects. Although few epidemiological studies have examined associations between garlic consumption and cardiovascular disease risk, numerous intervention trials have explored the effects of garlic supplementation on cardiovascular disease risk factors.

Serum Lipid Profiles

More than 40 randomized controlled trials have examined the effects of supplementation with various garlic preparations on serum lipid profiles in individuals with elevated and normal serum cholesterol levels.[54] Although many of these trials had methodological limitations, the results of several meta-analyses indicate that garlic supplementation results in modest (6 to 11%) reductions in serum total cholesterol, low-density lipoprotein (LDL) cholesterol, and triglyceride levels compared with placebo.[54–56] The most comprehensive meta-analysis to date found that the modest reductions in serum cholesterol levels evident up to 3 months after starting supplementation were no longer significant after 6 months of supplementation.[54] Clinical trials have not found that the use of garlic supplements results in statistically or clinically significant improvements in serum lipid profiles when compared with a placebo.[57–62] However, the results of these trials cannot be extrapolated to garlic itself because the products used in these trials have been shown to produce little allicin under simulated gastrointestinal conditions.[63] There is some evidence that the potential lipid-lowering effects of garlic are related to allicin, but decisive evidence is lacking. Different garlic preparations vary with respect to the type and bioavailability of the organosulfur compounds they provide (see the Supplements section below). Well-designed, long-term, randomized controlled trials that compare the efficacy of different types of garlic preparations at standardized doses are needed to determine which forms of garlic, if any, are effective in improving serum lipid profiles.

Platelet Aggregation

Platelet aggregation is one of the first steps in the formation of blood clots that can occlude coronary or cerebral arteries, leading to myocardial infarction or ischemic stroke. Most randomized controlled trials have found that garlic supplementation results in significant reductions in measures of ex vivo platelet aggregation. Four out of five trials found that supplementation with dehydrated garlic or garlic oil macerates significantly decreased spontaneous platelet aggregation compared with placebo.[54] Supplementation with aged garlic extract inhibited ex vivo platelet aggregation induced by physiological activators in two separate trials.[11,64]

Blood Pressure

The majority of controlled clinical trials have not found that garlic supplementation resulted in significant reductions in systolic or diastolic blood pressure in people with normal or high blood pressure.[54,65] Only 3 out of 23 randomized controlled trials identified in a systematic review[54] reported statistically significant reductions in diastolic blood pressure,[66–68] and only one reported a statistically significant reduction in systolic blood pressure.[66] At present, there is little evidence to support the use of garlic supplementation to treat hypertension.

Garlic and Atherosclerosis

Two studies have attempted to assess the effect of garlic supplementation on the progression of atherosclerosis in humans. One study in Germany used ultrasound imaging to assess the effect of 900 mg/d of dehydrated garlic on the progression of atherosclerotic plaque in the carotid and femoral arteries.[69] After 4 years, the increase in plaque volume was significantly greater in women taking the placebo than in women taking the garlic supplement, but there was no significant difference between men taking garlic or placebo.[70] In a smaller pilot study, investigators measured coronary artery calcium using electron beam tomography to assess the effect of supplementation with aged garlic extract on the progression of atherosclerosis in 19 adults already taking HMG-CoA reductase inhibitors (statins).[71] After one year, increases in coronary calcium were significantly lower in those taking aged garlic extract (4 mL/d) than in those taking a placebo. Although coronary calcium scores are correlated with the severity of coronary atherosclerosis, the predictive value of this technique is still under investigation.[72] Both studies were funded by companies that market garlic supplements.

Summary: Cardiovascular Disease

In summary, the results of randomized controlled trials suggest that garlic supplementation inhibits platelet aggregation and modestly improves serum lipid profiles for up to 3 months. It is not yet known whether garlic supplementation can reduce atherosclerosis or prevent cardiovascular events, such as myocardial infarction (heart attack) or stroke.

Cancer

Gastric Cancer

In China, an ecological study found that 82% of the men and 74% of the women who lived in an area with low mortality from gastric cancer consumed garlic at least 3 times weekly, while only 1% of men and women who lived in an area with high mortality from gastric cancer consumed garlic at least 3 times weekly.[73] Three out of four case-control studies in Europe and Asia found that past garlic consumption was significantly lower in people diagnosed with gastric cancer than in cancer-free control groups.[74-76] In contrast, a prospective cohort study in the Netherlands found no association between the use of garlic supplements and gastric cancer risk.[77] A meta-analysis that combined the results of the case-control studies found that those with the highest garlic intakes had a risk of gastric cancer that was ~50% lower than those with low garlic intakes.[78]

Helicobacter pylori Infection and Gastric Cancer

Infection with some strains of *Helicobacter pylori* (*H. pylori*) bacteria markedly increases the risk of gastric cancer. Although garlic preparations and organosulfur compounds have been found to inhibit the growth of *H. pylori* in the laboratory, there is little evidence that high garlic intakes or garlic supplementation can prevent or eradicate *H. pylori* infection in humans.[79,80] Higher intakes of garlic were not associated with significantly lower prevalence of *H. pylori* infection in China or Turkey.[81,82] Moreover, clinical trials using garlic cloves,[83] steam-distilled garlic oil,[84] garlic oil macerate,[85] or garlic powder[86] have not found gar-

lic supplementation to be effective in eradicating *H. pylori* infection in humans.

Colorectal Cancer

Three out of four case-control studies found that garlic intake was significantly lower in people diagnosed with colorectal cancer than in cancer-free control groups.[87-89] In contrast, three prospective cohort studies found no association between garlic consumption and colorectal cancer risk.[90-92] However, garlic consumption was generally low in these cohorts, and one assessed only garlic supplement use.[90] A meta-analysis that combined the results of those studies found that the risk of colorectal cancer that was ~30% lower in those with the highest garlic intakes compared with those with the lowest intakes.[78] Colorectal adenomas (polyps) are precancerous lesions. One case-control study of adults undergoing sigmoidoscopy found that those with colorectal adenomas consumed significantly less garlic than those in whom no colorectal adenomas were found.[93] A small preliminary intervention trial in Japan found that adenoma size and recurrence were slightly lower in those given a high dose of aged garlic extract (2.4 mL/d) compared with those given a lower dose (0.16 mL/d), but the differences were not statistically significant after one year.[94] Larger randomized controlled trials are needed to determine whether garlic or garlic extracts can substantially reduce adenoma recurrence.

Summary: Cancer

The results of epidemiological studies in human populations suggest that high intakes of garlic and other *Allium* vegetables may help protect against gastric and colorectal cancer, but evidence that high intakes of garlic can reduce the risk of other types of cancer in humans is limited or inconsistent.[78,95] Although garlic and organosulfur compounds have been found to inhibit the development of chemically induced cancers in animal models of oral, esophageal, gastric, colon, uterine, breast, and skin cancer,[44] it is not known whether garlic-derived organosulfur compounds can prevent or slow the development of cancer in humans.

Sources

Food Sources

Allium vegetables, including garlic and onions, are the richest sources of organosulfur compounds in the human diet.[95] To date, the majority of scientific research relating to the health effects of organosulfur compounds has focused on those derived from garlic. Fresh garlic cloves contain ~2 to 6 mg/g of γ-glutamyl-S-allylcysteine (0.2 to 0.6% fresh weight) and 6 to 14 mg/g of alliin (0.6 to 1.4% fresh weight). Garlic cloves yield ~2500 to 4500 mcg of allicin per gram of fresh weight when crushed. One fresh garlic clove weighs 2 to 4 g.[1]

Effects of Cooking

The enzyme alliinase can be inactivated by heat. In one study, microwave cooking of unpeeled, uncrushed garlic totally destroyed alliinase enzyme activity.[96] Administering raw garlic to rats significantly decreased the amount of DNA damage caused by a chemical carcinogen, but heating uncrushed garlic cloves for 60 seconds in a microwave oven or 45 minutes in a convection oven prior to administration blocked the protective effect of garlic.[97] Crushing garlic and allowing it to stand for 10 minutes prior to microwave heating for 60 seconds or cutting the tops off garlic cloves and allowing them to stand for 10 minutes before heating in a convection oven partially restored the protective effect of garlic against DNA damage. Because organosulfur compounds derived from alliinase-catalyzed reactions appear to play a role in some of the biological effects of garlic, some scientists recommend that crushed or chopped garlic be allowed to "stand" for at least 10 minutes prior to cooking.[96]

Supplements

Several different types of garlic preparations are available commercially, and each type provides a different profile of organosulfur compounds depending on how it was processed[1] (**Table 18–1**). Not all garlic preparations are standardized, and even standardized brands may vary with respect to the amount and the bioavailability of the organosulfur compounds they provide.

Table 18–1   Principal Organosulfur Compounds in Commercial Garlic Preparations[1]

Product	Principal Organosulfur Compounds	Delivers Allicin-Derived Compounds?
Fresh garlic cloves	Cysteine sulfoxides (Alliin)	Yes, when chopped, crushed, or chewed raw.
	γ-Glutamylcysteines	Minimally, when garlic cloves are cooked before crushing or chopping.
Powdered garlic (tablets)	Cysteine sulfoxides (Alliin) γ-Glutamylcysteines	Varies greatly among commercial products. Enteric-coated tablets that pass the USP allicin-release test are likely to provide the most.
Steam-distilled garlic oil (capsules)	Diallyl disulfide Diallyl trisulfide Allyl methyl trisulfide	Yes
Garlic oil macerate (capsules)	Vinyldithiins Ajoene Diallyl trisulfide	Yes
Aged garlic extract (tablets or capsules)	S-Allylcysteine S-Allylmercaptocysteine S-1-Propenylcysteine	Minimally

Powdered (Dehydrated) Garlic

Powdered or dehydrated garlic is made from garlic cloves that are usually sliced and dried at a low temperature (65°C or less) to prevent alliinase inactivation.[98] The dried garlic is pulverized and often made into tablets. To meet United States Pharmacopeia (USP) standards, powdered garlic supplements must contain no less than 0.1% γ-glutamyl-S-allyl-cysteine and no less than 0.3% alliin (dry weight).[99] Although powdered garlic supplements do not actually contain allicin, the manufacturer may provide a value for the "allicin potential" or "allicin yield" of a supplement on the label. These values represent the maximum achievable allicin yield of a supplement.[100] It is determined by dissolving powdered garlic in water at room temperature and measuring the allicin content after 30 minutes.[99] Because alliinase is inactivated at the acid pH of the stomach, most powdered garlic tablets are enteric-coated to keep them from dissolving before they reach the neutral pH of the intestine. It has been argued that it is more appropriate to measure "allicin release" using a USP method for assessing drug release from enteric-coated tablets under conditions that mimic those of the stomach and intestine.[99] Allicin release by this method has been shown to parallel true bioavailability.[100] Most tablet brands have been found to produce little allicin under these conditions, due mainly to low alliinase activity and prolonged disintegration times.[63,100] Many manufacturers provide information on the "allicin potential" of their powdered garlic supplements, but few provide information on the "allicin release." Several controlled clinical trials have examined the effect of powdered or dehydrated garlic supplements on cardiovascular risk factors (see the Cardiovascular Disease section above). The most commonly used doses ranged from of 600 to 900 mg/d and provided 3600 to 5400 μg/d of potential allicin.[54]

Garlic Fluid Extracts (Aged Garlic Extract™)

When garlic cloves are incubated in a solution of ethanol and water for up to 20 months, allicin is mainly converted to allyl sulfides, which are lost by evaporation or converted to other compounds.[98] The resulting extract contains primarily water-soluble organosulfur compounds, such as SAC and SAMC.[101] Garlic fluid extracts, including aged garlic extracts, are standardized to their S-allylcysteine content. In controlled clinical trials, aged garlic extract at doses of 2.4 to 7.2 g/d resulted in short-term reductions in ex vivo platelet aggregation[11] and reductions in serum cholesterol levels for as long as 12 weeks.[102]

Steam Distilled Garlic Oil

Steam distillation of crushed garlic cloves results in a product that contains mainly allyl sulfides, including DAS, DADS, and DATS.[98] These fat-soluble steam distillation products are usually dissolved in vegetable oil.

Garlic Oil Macerates

Incubation of crushed garlic cloves in oil at room temperature results in the formation of vinyldithiins and ajoene from allicin, in addition to allyl sulfides, such as DADS and DATS.[1] Ether extracts are similar in composition to garlic oil macerates, but more concentrated.[65]

Safety

Adverse Effects

The most commonly reported adverse effects of oral ingestion of garlic and garlic supplements are breath and body odors.[54] Gastrointestinal symptoms have also been reported, including heart burn, abdominal pain, nausea, vomiting, flatulence, and diarrhea.[103] The most serious adverse effects associated with oral garlic supplementation are related to uncontrolled bleeding. Several cases of serious postoperative or spontaneous bleeding associated with garlic supplementation have been reported in the medical literature.[104–107] Garlic may trigger allergic responses in some individuals, including asthma in people with occupational exposure to garlic powder or dust.[108] Exposure of the skin to garlic has been reported to cause contact dermatitis in some individuals.[109] More serious skin lesions, including blisters and burns, have also been reported with topical exposure to garlic for 6 or more hours.

Pregnancy and Lactation

No adverse effects on pregnancy outcomes have been reported when garlic is consumed in the mothers' diet. Although no adverse pregnancy outcomes were reported in a study of Iranian women who took dehydrated garlic tablets (800 mg/d) for 2 months during the third trimester of pregnancy,[110] the safety of garlic supplements in pregnancy has not been established. There is some evidence that garlic consumption alters the odor and possibly the flavor of breast milk. In a controlled crossover trial, oral consumption of 1.5 g of garlic extract by lactating women increased the perceived intensity of breast milk odor.[111] Infants spent more time breastfeeding after their mothers consumed the garlic extract compared with a placebo, but the amount of milk consumed and number of feedings were not significantly different.

Drug Interactions

Anticoagulant Medications

Garlic may enhance the anticoagulant effects of warfarin (Coumadin). There have been two case reports in which prothrombin time (INR; International Normalized Ratio) increased in patients who started taking garlic tablets or garlic oil without changing their warfarin dose or other habits.[112] Garlic supplements have been found to inhibit platelet aggregation;[54] therefore, there is a potential for additive effects when garlic supplements are taken together with other medications or supplements that inhibit platelet aggregation.[113]

Human Immunodeficiency Virus (HIV) Protease Inhibitors

Supplementation of healthy volunteers with garlic caplets twice daily (allicin yield 7200 μg/d) for 3 weeks resulted in a 50 % decrease in the bioavailability of the protease inhibitor, saquinavir (Fortovase).[114] Although saquinavir undergoes significant metabolism by CYP3A4, supplementation with garlic extract for 2 weeks did not significantly alter a measure of CYP3A4 activity in healthy volunteers.[115] Garlic extract supplementation (10 mg/d) for 4 days did not significantly alter single-dose pharmacokinetics of the protease inhibitor ritonavir (Norvir), but further research is needed to determine steady-state interactions between well-characterized garlic supplements and ritonavir.[116]

Summary

- Garlic (*Allium sativum* L.) is a particularly rich source of organosulfur compounds, which are currently under investigation for their potential to prevent and treat disease.
- Crushing or chopping garlic releases an enzyme called alliinase that catalyzes the formation of allicin. Allicin rapidly breaks down to form a variety of organosulfur compounds.
- Cooking can inactivate alliinase; some scientists recommend letting garlic stand for 10 minutes after chopping or crushing before cooking it.
- Several different types of garlic supplements are available commercially, and each type provides a different profile of organosulfur compounds depending on how it was processed.
- The results of randomized controlled trials suggest that garlic supplementation inhibits platelet aggregation and modestly improves serum lipid (cholesterol) profiles for up to 3 months, but it is not known whether garlic supplementation can prevent cardiovascular disease.
- The results of a few epidemiological studies suggest that high intakes of garlic and other *Allium* vegetables (e. g., onions and leeks) may help protect against gastric and colorectal cancer, but it is not known whether garlic-derived organosulfur compounds are effective in preventing or treating human cancers.

References

1. Lawson LD. Garlic: a review of its medicinal effects and indicated active compounds. In: Lawson LD, Bauer R, eds. Phytomedicines of Europe: Chemistry and Biological Activity. Washington, D.C.: American Chemical Society; 1998:177–209
2. Block E. The chemistry of garlic and onions. Sci Am 1985;252(3):114–119
3. Blumenthal M. Herb sales down 7.4 percent in mainstream market. HerbalGram: American Botanical Council; 2005:63.
4. Tapiero H, Townsend DM, Tew KD. Organosulfur compounds from alliaceae in the prevention of human pathologies. Biomed Pharmacother 2004; 58(3):183–193
5. Lawson LD, Wang ZJ. Allicin and allicin-derived garlic compounds increase breath acetone through allyl methyl sulfide: use in measuring allicin bioavailability. J Agric Food Chem 2005;53(6):1974–1983
6. Germain E, Auger J, Ginies C, Siess MH, Teyssier C. In vivo metabolism of diallyl disulphide in the rat: identification of two new metabolites. Xenobiotica 2002;32(12):1127–1138
7. Lachmann G, Lorenz D, Radeck W, Steiper M. [The pharmacokinetics of the S35 labeled labeled garlic constituents alliin, allicin and vinyldithiine] Arzneimittelforschung 1994;44(6):734–743. In German
8. de Rooij BM, Boogaard PJ, Rijksen DA, Commandeur JN, Vermeulen NP. Urinary excretion of N-acetyl-S-allyl-L-cysteine upon garlic consumption by human volunteers. Arch Toxicol 1996;70(10):635–639
9. Jandke J, Spiteller G. Unusual conjugates in biological profiles originating from consumption of onions and garlic. J Chromatogr 1987;421(1):1–8
10. Kodera Y, Suzuki A, Imada O, et al. Physical, chemical, and biological properties of s-allylcysteine, an amino acid derived from garlic. J Agric Food Chem 2002; 50(3):622–632
11. Steiner M, Li W. Aged garlic extract, a modulator of cardiovascular risk factors: a dose-finding study on the effects of AGE on platelet functions. J Nutr 2001; 131(3s):980S–984S
12. Gebhardt R, Beck H. Differential inhibitory effects of garlic-derived organosulfur compounds on cholesterol biosynthesis in primary rat hepatocyte cultures. Lipids 1996;31(12):1269–1276
13. Ferri N, Yokoyama K, Sadilek M, et al. Ajoene, a garlic compound, inhibits protein prenylation and arterial smooth muscle cell proliferation. Br J Pharmacol 2003;138(5):811–818
14. Liu L, Yeh YY. S-alk(en)yl cysteines of garlic inhibit cholesterol synthesis by deactivating HMG-CoA reductase in cultured rat hepatocytes. J Nutr 2002; 132(6):1129–1134
15. Chan KC, Hsu CC, Yin MC. Protective effect of three diallyl sulphides against glucose-induced erythrocyte and platelet oxidation, and ADP-induced platelet aggregation. Thromb Res 2002;108(5–6):317–322
16. Lawson LD, Ransom DK, Hughes BG. Inhibition of whole blood platelet-aggregation by compounds in garlic clove extracts and commercial garlic products. Thromb Res 1992;65(2):141–156
17. Blake GJ, Ridker PM. C-reactive protein and other inflammatory risk markers in acute coronary syn-
dromes. J Am Coll Cardiol 2003; 41(4, Suppl S)37S–42S
18. Ali M, Thomson M, Afzal M. Garlic and onions: their effect on eicosanoid metabolism and its clinical relevance. Prostaglandins Leukot Essent Fatty Acids 2000;62(2):55–73
19. Dirsch VM, Kiemer AK, Wagner H, Vollmar AM. Effect of allicin and ajoene, two compounds of garlic, on inducible nitric oxide synthase. Atherosclerosis 1998;139(2):333–339
20. Kim KM, Chun SB, Koo MS, et al. Differential regulation of NO availability from macrophages and endothelial cells by the garlic component S-allyl cysteine. Free Radic Biol Med 2001;30(7):747–756
21. Chang HP, Huang SY, Chen YH. Modulation of cytokine secretion by garlic oil derivatives is associated with suppressed nitric oxide production in stimulated macrophages. J Agric Food Chem 2005;53(7): 2530–2534
22. Keiss HP, Dirsch VM, Hartung T, et al. Garlic (Allium sativum L.) modulates cytokine expression in lipopolysaccharide-activated human blood thereby inhibiting NF-kappaB activity. J Nutr 2003;133(7): 2171–2175
23. Hedin U, Roy J, Tran PK. Control of smooth muscle cell proliferation in vascular disease. Curr Opin Lipidol 2004;15(5):559–565
24. Campbell JH, Efendy JL, Smith NJ, Campbell GR. Molecular basis by which garlic suppresses atherosclerosis. J Nutr 2001;131(3s):1006S–1009S
25. Golovchenko I, Yang CH, Goalstone ML, Draznin B. Garlic extract methylallyl thiosulfinate blocks insulin potentiation of platelet-derived growth factor-stimulated migration of vascular smooth muscle cells. Metabolism 2003;52(2):254–259
26. Banerjee SK, Mukherjee PK, Maulik SK. Garlic as an antioxidant: the good, the bad and the ugly. Phytother Res 2003;17(2):97–106
27. Dhawan V, Jain S. Effect of garlic supplementation on oxidized low density lipoproteins and lipid peroxidation in patients of essential hypertension. Mol Cell Biochem 2004;266(1–2):109–115
28. Yang CS, Chhabra SK, Hong JY, Smith TJ. Mechanisms of inhibition of chemical toxicity and carcinogenesis by diallyl sulfide (DAS) and related compounds from garlic. J Nutr 2001;131(3s):1041S–1045S
29. Brady JF, Ishizaki H, Fukuto JM, et al. Inhibition of cytochrome P-450 2E1 by diallyl sulfide and its metabolites. Chem Res Toxicol 1991;4(6):642–647
30. Jeong HG, Lee YW. Protective effects of diallyl sulfide on N-nitrosodimethylamine-induced immunosuppression in mice. Cancer Lett 1998;134(1):73–79
31. Park KA, Kweon S, Choi H. Anticarcinogenic effect and modification of cytochrome P450 2E1 by dietary garlic powder in diethylnitrosamine-initiated rat hepatocarcinogenesis. J Biochem Mol Biol 2002; 35(6):615–622
32. Gurley BJ, Gardner SF, Hubbard MA, et al. Cytochrome P450 phenotypic ratios for predicting herb-drug interactions in humans. Clin Pharmacol Ther 2002;72(3):276–287
33. Loizou GD, Cocker J. The effects of alcohol and diallyl sulphide on CYP2E1 activity in humans: a phenotyping study using chlorzoxazone. Hum Exp Toxicol 2001;20(7):321–327

34. Munday R, Munday CM. Induction of phase II enzymes by aliphatic sulfides derived from garlic and onions: an overview. Methods Enzymol 2004; 382:449–456

35. Andorfer JH, Tchaikovskaya T, Listowsky I. Selective expression of glutathione S-transferase genes in the murine gastrointestinal tract in response to dietary organosulfur compounds. Carcinogenesis 2004; 25(3):359–367

36. Hatono S, Jimenez A, Wargovich MJ. Chemopreventive effect of S-allylcysteine and its relationship to the detoxification enzyme glutathione S-transferase. Carcinogenesis 1996;17(5):1041–1044

37. Munday R, Munday CM. Relative activities of organosulfur compounds derived from onions and garlic in increasing tissue activities of quinone reductase and glutathione transferase in rat tissues. Nutr Cancer 2001;40(2):205–210

38. Chen C, Pung D, Leong V, et al. Induction of detoxifying enzymes by garlic organosulfur compounds through transcription factor Nrf2: effect of chemical structure and stress signals. Free Radic Biol Med 2004;37(10):1578–1590

39. Munday R, Munday CM. Low doses of diallyl disulfide, a compound derived from garlic, increase tissue activities of quinone reductase and glutathione transferase in the gastrointestinal tract of the rat. Nutr Cancer 1999;34(1):42–48

40. Kweon S, Park KA, Choi H. Chemopreventive effect of garlic powder diet in diethylnitrosamine-induced rat hepatocarcinogenesis. Life Sci 2003;73(19):2515–2526

41. Stewart ZA, Westfall MD, Pietenpol JA. Cell-cycle dysregulation and anticancer therapy. Trends Pharmacol Sci 2003;24(3):139–145

42. Herman-Antosiewicz A, Singh SV. Signal transduction pathways leading to cell cycle arrest and apoptosis induction in cancer cells by Allium vegetable-derived organosulfur compounds: a review. Mutat Res 2004;555(1–2):121–131

43. Knowles LM, Milner JA. Possible mechanism by which allyl sulfides suppress neoplastic cell proliferation. J Nutr 2001;131(3s):1061S–1066S

44. Wu X, Kassie F, Mersch-Sundermann V. Induction of apoptosis in tumor cells by naturally occurring sulfur-containing compounds. Mutat Res 2005;589(2):81–102

45. Balasenthil S, Rao KS, Nagini S. Apoptosis induction by S-allylcysteine, a garlic constituent, during 7,12-dimethylbenz[a]anthracene-induced hamster buccal pouch carcinogenesis. Cell Biochem Funct 2002; 20(3):263–268

46. Balasenthil S, Rao KS, Nagini S. Garlic induces apoptosis during 7,12-dimethylbenz[a]anthracene-induced hamster buccal pouch carcinogenesis. Oral Oncol 2002;38(5):431–436

47. Fenwick GR, Hanley AB. The genus Allium–Part 3. Crit Rev Food Sci Nutr 1985;23(1):1–73

48. Harris JC, Cottrell SL, Plummer S, Lloyd D. Antimicrobial properties of Allium sativum (garlic). Appl Microbiol Biotechnol 2001;57(3):282–286

49. Ankri S, Mirelman D. Antimicrobial properties of allicin from garlic. Microbes Infect 1999;1(2):125–129

50. Cavallito CJ, Bailey JH. Allicin, the antibacterial principle of Allium sativum. I. Isolation, physical properties and antibacterial action. J Am Chem Soc 1944; 66(11):1950–1951

51. Martin KW, Ernst E. Herbal medicines for treatment of bacterial infections: a review of controlled clinical trials. J Antimicrob Chemother 2003;51(2):241–246

52. Ledezma E, Marcano K, Jorquera A, et al. Efficacy of ajoene in the treatment of tinea pedis: a double-blind and comparative study with terbinafine. J Am Acad Dermatol 2000;43(5 Pt 1):829–832

53. Keys A. Wine, garlic, and CHD in seven countries. Lancet 1980;1(8160):145–146

54. Ackermann RT, Mulrow CD, Ramirez G, Gardner CD, Morbidoni L, Lawrence VA. Garlic shows promise for improving some cardiovascular risk factors. Arch Intern Med 2001;161(6):813–824

55. Alder R, Lookinland S, Berry JA, Williams M. A systematic review of the effectiveness of garlic as an anti-hyperlipidemic agent. J Am Acad Nurse Pract 2003;15(3):120–129

56. Stevinson C, Pittler MH, Ernst E. Garlic for treating hypercholesterolemia. A meta-analysis of randomized clinical trials. Ann Intern Med 2000; 133(6):420–429

57. Berthold HK, Sudhop T, von Bergmann K. Effect of a garlic oil preparation on serum lipoproteins and cholesterol metabolism: a randomized controlled trial. JAMA 1998;279(23):1900–1902

58. Gardner CD, Chatterjee LM, Carlson JJ. The effect of a garlic preparation on plasma lipid levels in moderately hypercholesterolemic adults. Atherosclerosis 2001;154(1):213–220

59. Kannar D, Wattanapenpaiboon N, Savige GS, Wahlqvist ML. Hypocholesterolemic effect of an enteric-coated garlic supplement. J Am Coll Nutr 2001; 20(3):225–231

60. McCrindle BW, Helden E, Conner WT. Garlic extract therapy in children with hypercholesterolemia. Arch Pediatr Adolesc Med 1998;152(11):1089–1094

61. Neil HA, Silagy CA, Lancaster T, et al. Garlic powder in the treatment of moderate hyperlipidaemia: a controlled trial and meta-analysis. J R Coll Physicians Lond 1996;30(4):329–334

62. Turner B, Molgaard C, Marckmann P. Effect of garlic (Allium sativum) powder tablets on serum lipids, blood pressure and arterial stiffness in normolipidaemic volunteers: a randomised, double-blind, placebo-controlled trial. Br J Nutr 2004;92(4):701–706

63. Lawson LD, Wang ZJ, Papadimitriou D. Allicin release under simulated gastrointestinal conditions from garlic powder tablets employed in clinical trials on serum cholesterol. Planta Med 2001;67(1):13–18

64. Rahman K, Billington D. Dietary supplementation with aged garlic extract inhibits ADP-induced platelet aggregation in humans. J Nutr 2000;130(11):2662–2665

65. Brace LD. Cardiovascular benefits of garlic (Allium sativum L). J Cardiovasc Nurs 2002;16(4):33–49

66. Adler AJ, Holub BJ. Effect of garlic and fish-oil supplementation on serum lipid and lipoprotein concentrations in hypercholesterolemic men. Am J Clin Nutr 1997;65(2):445–450

67. Auer W, Eiber A, Hertkorn E, et al. Hypertension and hyperlipidaemia: garlic helps in mild cases. Br J Clin Pract Suppl 1990;69:3–6

68. Vorberg G, Schneider B. Therapy with garlic: results of a placebo-controlled, double-blind study. Br J Clin Pract Suppl 1990;69:7–11

69. Koscielny J, Klussendorf D, Latza R, et al. The anti-atherosclerotic effect of Allium sativum. Atherosclerosis 1999;144(1):237–249

70. Siegel G, Klussendorf D. The anti-atheroslerotic effect of Allium sativum: statistics re-evaluated. Atherosclerosis 2000;150(2):437–438

71. Budoff MJ, Takasu J, Flores FR, et al. Inhibiting progression of coronary calcification using Aged Garlic Extract in patients receiving statin therapy: a preliminary study. Prev Med 2004;39(5):985–991

72. Vliegenthart R. Non-invasive assessment of coronary calcification. Eur J Epidemiol 2004;19(12):1063–1072

73. Takezaki T, Gao CM, Ding JH, Liu TK, Li MS, Tajima K. Comparative study of lifestyles of residents in high and low risk areas for gastric cancer in Jiangsu Province, China; with special reference to allium vegetables. J Epidemiol 1999;9(5):297–305

74. Buiatti E, Palli D, Decarli A, et al. A case-control study of gastric cancer and diet in Italy. Int J Cancer 1989; 44(4):611–616

75. Kim HJ, Chang WK, Kim MK, Lee SS, Choi BY. Dietary factors and gastric cancer in Korea: a case-control study. Int J Cancer 2002;97(4):531–535

76. You WC, Blot WJ, Chang YS, et al. Allium vegetables and reduced risk of stomach cancer. J Natl Cancer Inst 1989;81(2):162–164

77. Dorant E, van den Brandt PA, Goldbohm RA, Sturmans F. Consumption of onions and a reduced risk of stomach carcinoma. Gastroenterology 1996;110(1):12–20

78. Fleischauer AT, Poole C, Arab L. Garlic consumption and cancer prevention: meta-analyses of colorectal and stomach cancers. Am J Clin Nutr 2000;72(4):1047–1052

79. Canizares P, Gracia I, Gomez LA, et al. Allyl-thiosulfinates, the bacteriostatic compounds of garlic against Helicobacter pylori. Biotechnol Prog 2004;20(1):397–401

80. O'Gara EA, Hill DJ, Maslin DJ. Activities of garlic oil, garlic powder, and their diallyl constituents against Helicobacter pylori. Appl Environ Microbiol 2000;66(5):2269–2273

81. Salih BA, Abasiyanik FM. Does regular garlic intake affect the prevalence of Helicobacter pylori in asymptomatic subjects? Saudi Med J 2003;24(8):842–845

82. You WC, Zhang L, Gail MH, et al. Helicobacter pylori infection, garlic intake and precancerous lesions in a Chinese population at low risk of gastric cancer. Int J Epidemiol 1998;27(6):941–944

83. Graham DY, Anderson SY, Lang T. Garlic or jalapeno peppers for treatment of Helicobacter pylori infection. Am J Gastroenterol 1999;94(5):1200–1202

84. McNulty CA, Wilson MP, Havinga W, Johnston B, O'Gara EA, Maslin DJ. A pilot study to determine the effectiveness of garlic oil capsules in the treatment of dyspeptic patients with Helicobacter pylori. Helicobacter 2001;6(3):249–253

85. Aydin A, Ersoz G, Tekesin O, Akcicek E, Tuncyurek M. Garlic oil and Helicobacter pylori infection. Am J Gastroenterol 2000;95(2):563–564

86. Ernst E. Is garlic an effective treatment for Helicobacter pylori infection? Arch Intern Med 1999;159(20):2484–2485

87. Hu JF, Liu YY, Yu YK, Zhao TZ, Liu SD, Wang QQ. Diet and cancer of the colon and rectum: a case-control study in China. Int J Epidemiol 1991;20(2):362–367

88. Iscovich JM, L'Abbe KA, Castelleto R, et al. Colon cancer in Argentina. I: Risk from intake of dietary items. Int J Cancer 1992;51(6):851–857

89. Levi F, Pasche C, La Vecchia C, Lucchini F, Franceschi S. Food groups and colorectal cancer risk. Br J Cancer 1999;79(7–8):1283–1287

90. Dorant E, van den Brandt PA, Goldbohm RA. A prospective cohort study on the relationship between onion and leek consumption, garlic supplement use and the risk of colorectal carcinoma in The Netherlands. Carcinogenesis 1996;17(3):477–484

91. Giovannucci E, Rimm EB, Stampfer MJ, Colditz GA, Ascherio A, Willett WC. Intake of fat, meat, and fiber in relation to risk of colon cancer in men. Cancer Res 1994;54(9):2390–2397

92. Steinmetz KA, Kushi LH, Bostick RM, Folsom AR, Potter JD. Vegetables, fruit, and colon cancer in the Iowa Women's Health Study. Am J Epidemiol 1994;139(1):1–15

93. Witte JS, Longnecker MP, Bird CL, Lee ER, Frankl HD, Haile RW. Relation of vegetable, fruit, and grain consumption to colorectal adenomatous polyps. Am J Epidemiol 1996;144(11):1015–1025

94. Tanaka S, Haruma K, Kunihiro M, et al. Effects of aged garlic extract (AGE) on colorectal adenomas: a double-blinded study. Hiroshima J Med Sci 2004;53(3–4):39–45

95. Bianchini F, Vainio H. Allium vegetables and organosulfur compounds: do they help prevent cancer? Environ Health Perspect 2001;109(9):893–902

96. Song K, Milner JA. The influence of heating on the anticancer properties of garlic. J Nutr 2001;131(3s):1054S–1057S

97. Song K, Milner JA. Heating garlic inhibits its ability to suppress 7, 12-dimethylbenz(a)anthracene-induced DNA adduct formation in rat mammary tissue. J Nutr 1999;129(3):657–661

98. Staba EJ, Lash L, Staba JE. A commentary on the effects of garlic extraction and formulation on product composition. J Nutr 2001;131(3s):1118S–1119S

99. Dietary Supplements. Garlic. The United States Pharmacopeia. Vol 28. Rockville, MD: United States Pharmacopeial Convention, Inc.; 2005:2087–2092

100. Lawson LD, Wang ZJ. Low allicin release from garlic supplements: a major problem due to the sensitivities of alliinase activity. J Agric Food Chem 2001;49(5):2592–2599

101. Amagase H, Petesch BL, Matsuura H, Kasuga S, Itakura Y. Intake of garlic and its bioactive components. J Nutr 2001;131(3s):955S–962S

102. Steiner M, Khan AH, Holbert D, Lin RI. A double-blind crossover study in moderately hypercholesterolemic men that compared the effect of aged garlic extract and placebo administration on blood lipids. Am J Clin Nutr 1996;64(6):866–870

103. Mulrow C, Lawrence V, Ackermann R, et al. Garlic: effects on cardiovascular risks and disease, protective effects against cancer, and clinical adverse effects. Agency for Healthcare Research and Quality. 2000. Available at: http://www.ncbi.nlm.nih.gov/books/bv.fcgi?rid=hstat1.chapter.28361. Accessed 8/1/06

104. Burnham BE. Garlic as a possible risk for postoperative bleeding. Plast Reconstr Surg 1995;95(1):213

105. Carden SM, Good WV, Carden PA, Good RM. Garlic and the strabismus surgeon. Clin Experiment Ophthalmol 2002;30(4):303–304

106. German K, Kumar U, Blackford HN. Garlic and the risk of TURP bleeding. Br J Urol 1995;76(4):518

107. Rose KD, Croissant PD, Parliament CF, Levin MB. Spontaneous spinal epidural hematoma with associated platelet dysfunction from excessive garlic ingestion: a case report. Neurosurgery 1990;26(5): 880–882

108. Anibarro B, Fontela JL, De La Hoz F. Occupational asthma induced by garlic dust. J Allergy Clin Immunol 1997;100(6 Pt 1):734–738

109. Jappe U, Bonnekoh B, Hausen BM, Gollnick H. Garlic-related dermatoses: case report and review of the literature. Am J Contact Dermat 1999;10(1):37–39

110. Ziaei S, Hantoshzadeh S, Rezasoltani P, Lamyian M. The effect of garlic tablet on plasma lipids and platelet aggregation in nulliparous pregnants at high risk of preeclampsia. Eur J Obstet Gynecol Reprod Biol 2001;99(2):201–206

111. Mennella JA, Beauchamp GK. Maternal diet alters the sensory qualities of human milk and the nursling's behavior. Pediatrics 1991;88(4):737–744

112. Sunter WH. Warfarin and garlic. Pharm J. 1991;246: 722

113. Izzo AA, Ernst E. Interactions between herbal medicines and prescribed drugs: a systematic review. Drugs 2001;61(15):2163–2175

114. Piscitelli SC, Burstein AH, Welden N, Gallicano KD, Falloon J. The effect of garlic supplements on the pharmacokinetics of saquinavir. Clin Infect Dis 2002; 34(2):234–238

115. Markowitz JS, Devane CL, Chavin KD, Taylor RM, Ruan Y, Donovan JL. Effects of garlic (Allium sativum L.) supplementation on cytochrome P450 2D6 and 3A4 activity in healthy volunteers. Clin Pharmacol Ther 2003;74(2):170–177

116. Gallicano K, Foster B, Choudhri S. Effect of short-term administration of garlic supplements on single-dose ritonavir pharmacokinetics in healthy volunteers. Br J Clin Pharmacol 2003;55(2):199–202

19 Phytosterols

Throughout much of human evolution, it is likely that large amounts of plant foods were consumed.[1] In addition to being rich in fiber and plant protein, the diets of our ancestors were also rich in phytosterols—plant-derived sterols that are similar in structure and function to cholesterol. There is increasing evidence that the reintroduction of plant foods providing phytosterols into the modern diet can improve serum lipid profiles and reduce the risk of cardiovascular disease.[2]

Although in animals and humans cholesterol is the predominant sterol, a variety of phytosterols is found in plants.[3] Nutritionists recognize two classes of phytosterols: sterols, which have a double bond in the sterol ring, and stanols, which lack a double bond in the sterol ring (**Fig. 19–1**). The most abundant sterols in plants and the human diet are sitosterol and campesterol. Stanols are also present in plants, but they make up only ~10% of total dietary phytosterols. Cholesterol in

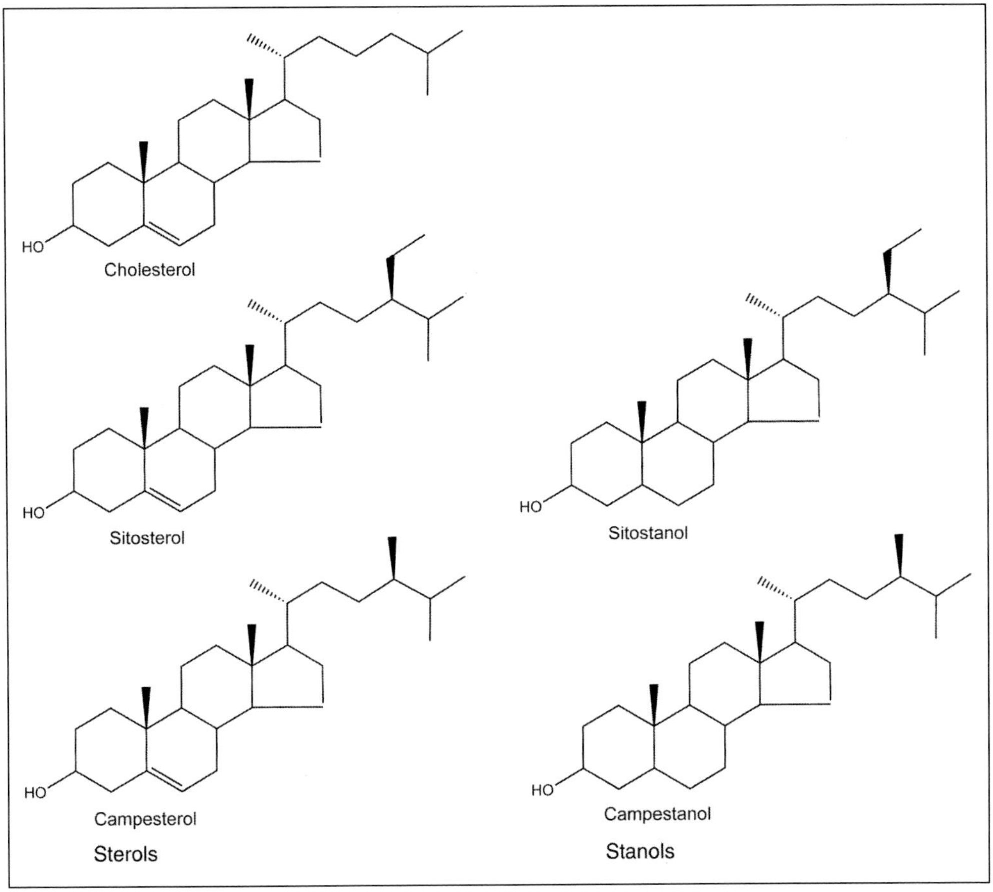

Figure 19–1 Chemical structure of cholesterol compared with plant sterols (sitosterol and campesterol) and plant stanols (sitostanol and campestanol).

human blood and tissues is derived from the diet as well as endogenous cholesterol synthesis. In contrast, all phytosterols in human blood and tissues are derived from the diet because humans cannot synthesize phytosterols.[4]

Definitions

Phytosterols–A collective term for plant-derived sterols and stanols.
Plant sterols or stanols–Terms that are generally applied to plant-derived sterols or stanols, which are added to foods or supplements.
Plant sterol or stanol esters–Plant sterols or stanols that have been esterified by creating an ester bond between a fatty acid and the sterol or stanol. Esterification makes plant sterols and stanols more fat-soluble so they are easily incorporated into fat-containing foods, such as margarines and salad dressings. In this chapter, the weights of plant sterol and stanol esters are expressed as the equivalent weights of free (unesterified) sterols and stanols.

Bioavailability and Metabolism

Absorption and Metabolism of Dietary Cholesterol

Dietary cholesterol must be incorporated into mixed micelles to be absorbed by the cells that line the intestine (enterocytes).[5] Mixed micelles are mixtures of bile salts, lipids, and sterols formed in the small intestine after a fat-containing meal is consumed. Inside the enterocyte, cholesterol is esterified and incorporated into triglyceride-rich lipoproteins known as chylomicrons, which enter the circulation.[6] As circulating chylomicrons become depleted of triglycerides, they become chylomicron remnants, which are taken up by the liver. In the liver, cholesterol from chylomicron remnants may be repackaged into other lipoproteins for transport or secreted into bile, which is released into the small intestine.

Absorption and Metabolism of Dietary Phytosterols

Although varied diets typically contain similar amounts of phytosterols and cholesterol, serum phytosterol concentrations are usually several hundred times lower than serum cholesterol concentrations in humans.[7] Less than 5% of dietary phytosterols are systemically absorbed, in contrast to ~50 to 60% of dietary cholesterol.[8] Like cholesterol, phytosterols must be incorporated into mixed micelles before they are taken up by enterocytes. Once inside the enterocyte, systemic absorption of phytosterols is inhibited by the activity of efflux transporters, consisting of a pair of ATP-binding cassette (ABC) proteins known as ABCG5 and ABCG8.[4] ABCG5 and ABCG8 each form one half of a transporter that secretes phytosterols and unesterified cholesterol from the enterocyte into the intestinal lumen. Phytosterols are secreted back into the intestine by ABCG5/G8 transporters at a much greater rate than cholesterol, resulting in much lower intestinal absorption of dietary phytosterols than cholesterol. Within the enterocyte, phytosterols are not as readily esterified as cholesterol, so they are incorporated into chylomicrons at much lower concentrations. Those phytosterols that are incorporated into chylomicrons enter the circulation and are taken up by the liver. Once inside the liver, phytosterols are rapidly secreted into bile by hepatic ABCG5/G8 transporters. Although cholesterol may also be secreted into bile, the rate of phytosterol secretion into bile is much greater than cholesterol secretion.[9] Thus, the low serum concentrations of phytosterols relative to cholesterol can be explained by decreased intestinal absorption and increased excretion of phytosterols into bile.

Biological Activities

Effects on Cholesterol Absorption and Lipoprotein Metabolism

It is well-established that high intakes of plant sterols or stanols can lower serum total and low-density lipoprotein (LDL) cholesterol concentrations in humans (see the Cardiovascular

Disease section below).[10,11] In the intestinal lumen, phytosterols displace cholesterol from mixed micelles and inhibit cholesterol absorption.[12] In humans, the consumption of 1.5 to 1.8 g/d of plant sterols or stanols reduced cholesterol absorption by 30 to 40%.[13,14] At higher doses (2.2 g/d of plant sterols), cholesterol absorption was reduced by 60%.[15] In response to decreased cholesterol absorption, tissue LDL-receptor expression is increased, resulting in increased clearance of circulating LDL.[16] Decreased cholesterol absorption is also associated with increased cholesterol synthesis, and increasing phytosterol intake has been found to increase endogenous cholesterol synthesis in humans.[13] Despite the increase in cholesterol synthesis induced by increasing phytosterol intake, the net result is a reduction in serum LDL cholesterol concentration.

Other Biological Activities

Experiments in cell culture and animal models suggest that phytosterols may have biological activities unrelated to cholesterol lowering. However, their significance in humans is not yet known.

Alterations in Cell Membrane Properties

Cholesterol is an important structural component of mammalian cell membranes.[17] Displacement of cholesterol with phytosterols has been found to alter the physical properties of cell membranes in vitro,[18] which could potentially affect signal transduction or membrane-bound enzyme activity.[19,20] Limited evidence from an animal model of hemorrhagic stroke suggested that very high intakes of plant sterols or stanols displaced cholesterol in red blood cell membranes, resulting in decreased deformability and potentially increased fragility.[21,22] However, daily phytosterol supplementation (1 g/1000 kcal) for 4 weeks did not alter red blood cell fragility in humans.[23]

Alterations in Testosterone Metabolism

Limited evidence from animal studies suggests that very high phytosterol intakes can alter testosterone metabolism by inhibiting 5-α-re-ductase, a membrane-bound enzyme that converts testosterone to dihydrotestosterone, a more potent metabolite.[24,25] It is not known whether human phytosterol consumption alters testosterone metabolism. No significant changes in free or total serum testosterone concentrations were observed in men who consumed 1.6 g/d of plant sterol esters for one year.[26]

Induction of Apoptosis in Cancer Cells

Unlike normal cells, cancerous cells lose their ability to respond to death signals by undergoing apoptosis (programmed cell death). Sitosterol has been found to induce apoptosis when added to cultured prostate,[27] breast,[28] and colon cancer cells.[29]

Anti-inflammatory Effects

Limited data from cell culture and animal studies suggest that phytosterols may attenuate the inflammatory activity of immune cells, including macrophages and neutrophils.[30,31]

Prevention

Cardiovascular Disease

Foods Enriched with Plant Sterols or Stanols

Low-Density Lipoprotein Cholesterol

Numerous clinical trials have found that daily consumption of foods enriched with plant sterols or stanols in free or esterified forms lowers serum total and LDL cholesterol concentrations.[10,32] A meta-analysis that combined the results of 18 controlled clinical trials found that the consumption of spreads providing an average of 2 g/d of plant sterols or stanols lowered serum LDL cholesterol concentrations by 9 to 14%.[33] A meta-analysis that combined the results of 23 controlled clinical trials found that the consumption of plant foods providing an average of 3.4 g/d of plant sterols or stanols decreased LDL cholesterol concentrations by ~ 11%.[34] The most extensive meta-analysis published to date analyzed the results of 23 clinical trials of plant sterol-enriched foods and 27 clinical trials of plant stanol-enriched foods separately.[11] At doses of at least 2 g/d, both plant sterols and stanols decreased LDL cholesterol concentrations by ~ 10%. Doses higher than 2 g/d did not substantially improve the cholesterol-lowering effects of plant sterols or stanols. The results of studies providing lower doses of plant sterols or stanols suggest that 0.8 to 1.0 g/d is the lowest dose that results in clinically significant LDL cholesterol reductions of at least 5%.[35-39] In general, trials that have compared the cholesterol-lowering efficacy of plant sterols with that of stanols have found them to be equivalent.[40-42] Few of these studies lasted longer than 4 weeks, but at least two studies have found that the cholesterol-lowering effects of plant sterols and stanols last for up to one year.[26,43] Recently, concerns have been raised that plant sterols are not as effective as stanols in maintaining long-term LDL-cholesterol reductions.[44,45] Long-term trials that directly compare the efficacy of plant sterols and plant stanols are needed to address these concerns.[11]

Coronary Heart Disease Risk

The effect of long-term use of foods enriched with plant sterols or stanols on coronary heart disease (CHD) risk is not known. The results of numerous intervention trials suggest that a 10% reduction in LDL cholesterol induced by medication or diet modification could decrease the risk of CHD by as much as 20%.[46] The National Cholesterol Education Program (NCEP) Adult Treatment Panel III has included the use of plant sterol or stanol esters (2 g/d) as a component of maximal dietary therapy for elevated LDL cholesterol.[47] The addition of plant sterol- or stanol-enriched foods to a heart healthy diet that is low in saturated fat and rich in fruits and vegetables, whole grains, and fiber offers the potential for additive effects in CHD risk reduction. For example, following a diet that substituted mono- and polyunsaturated fats for saturated fat resulted in a 9% reduction in serum LDL cholesterol after 30 days, but the addition of 1.7 g/d of plant sterols to the same diet resulted in a 24% reduction.[48] A diet that provided a portfolio of cholesterol-lowering foods, including plant sterols, soy protein, almonds, and viscous fibers, lowered serum LDL cholesterol concentrations by an average of 30%, a decrease that was not significantly different from that induced by statin therapy.[49] The U.S. Food and Drug Administration (FDA) has authorized the use of health claims on food labels indicating that regular consumption of foods enriched with plant sterol or stanol esters may reduce the risk of heart disease.[50]

Dietary Phytosterols

The results of clinical trials indicating that the daily consumption of foods enriched with plant sterols or stanols can significantly reduce LDL cholesterol concentrations do not account for naturally occurring phytosterols in the diet.[51] Relatively few studies have considered the effects of dietary phytosterol intakes on serum LDL cholesterol concentrations. Dietary phytosterol intakes have been estimated to range from ~ 150 to 450 mg/d in various populations.[52] Limited evidence suggests that dietary phytosterols may play an important role in decreasing cholesterol absorption. A recent cross-sectional study in the UK found that dietary phytosterol intakes were inversely related to serum total and LDL cholesterol concentrations even after adjusting for saturated fat and fiber intake.[53] In single meal tests, removal of 150 mg of phytosterols from corn oil increased cholesterol absorption by 38%,[54] and removal of 328 mg of phytosterols from wheat germ increased cholesterol absorption by 43%.[55] Although more research is needed, these findings suggest that dietary intakes of phytosterols from plant foods could have an important impact on cardiovascular health.

Cancer

Limited data from animal studies suggest that very high intakes of phytosterols, particularly sitosterol, may inhibit the growth of breast and prostate cancer.[56-58] Only a few epidemiological studies have examined associations between dietary phytosterol intakes and cancer risk in humans because databases providing information on the phytosterol content of commonly consumed foods have only been developed recently. A series of case-control studies in Uruguay found that dietary phytosterol intakes were lower in people diagnosed with gastric, lung, or breast cancer than in cancer-free control groups.[59-61] Case-control studies in the United States found that women diagnosed with breast or endometrial (uterine) cancer had lower dietary phytosterol intakes than women who did not have cancer.[62,63] In contrast, another case-control study in the United States found that men diagnosed with prostate cancer had higher dietary campesterol intakes than men who did not have cancer, but total phytosterol consumption was not associated with prostate cancer risk.[64] Although some epidemiological studies have found that higher intakes of plant foods containing phytosterols are associated with decreased cancer risk, it is not clear whether phytosterols or other compounds in plant foods are the protective factors.

Treatment

Benign Prostatic Hyperplasia

Benign prostatic hyperplasia (BPH) is the term used to describe a noncancerous enlargement of the prostate. The enlarged prostate may exert pressure on the urethra, resulting in difficulty urinating. Plant extracts that provide a mixture of phytosterols (marketed as β-sitosterol) are often included in herbal therapies for urinary symptoms related to BPH. However, relatively few controlled studies have examined the efficacy of phytosterol supplements in men with symptomatic BPH. In a 6-month study of 200 men with symptomatic BPH, 60 mg/d of a β-sitosterol preparation improved symptom scores, increased peak urinary flow, and decreased post-void residual urine volume compared with placebo.[65] A follow-up study reported that these improvements were maintained for up to 18 months in the 38 participants who continued β-sitosterol treatment after the study ended.[66] Similarly, in a 6-month study of 177 men with symptomatic BPH, 130 mg/d of a different β-sitosterol preparation improved urinary symptom scores, increased peak flow, and decreased post-void residual volume compared with placebo.[67] A systematic review that combined the results of

those and two other controlled clinical trials found that β-sitosterol extracts increased peak urinary flow by an average of 3.9 mL/second and decreased post-void residual volume by an average of 29 mL.[68] Although the results of a few clinical trials suggest that relatively low doses of phytosterols can improve lower urinary tract symptoms related to BPH, further research is needed to confirm these findings.[69]

Sources

Foods

Unlike the typical diet in most developed countries today, the diets of our ancestors were rich in phytosterols, likely providing as much as 1000 mg/d.[1] Present-day dietary phytosterol intakes have been estimated to vary from 150 to 450 mg/d in different populations.[3] Vegetarians, particularly vegans, generally have the highest intakes of dietary phytosterols.[70] Phytosterols are found in all plant foods, but the highest concentrations are found in unrefined plant oils, including vegetable, nut, and olive oils.[3] Nuts, seeds, whole grains, and legumes are also good dietary sources of phytosterols.[5] The phytosterol contents of selected foods are presented in **Table 19–1**.

Foods Enriched with Plant Sterols and Plant Stanols

The majority of clinical trials that demonstrated a cholesterol-lowering effect used plant sterol or stanol esters solubilized in fat-containing foods, such as margarine or mayonnaise.[11] More recent studies indicate that low-fat or even nonfat foods can effectively deliver plant sterols or stanols if they are adequately solubilized.[10,51] Plant sterols or stanols added to low-fat yogurt,[39,71] low-fat milk,[72,73] and orange juice[74] have been reported to lower LDL cholesterol in controlled clinical trials. A variety of foods containing added plant sterols or stanols are available in Europe, Asia, and the United States, including margarines, mayonnaises, vegetable oils, salad dressings, yogurt, milk, soy milk, orange juice, snack bars, and meats.[10] Available research indicates that the maximum effective dose for lowering LDL

Table 19–1   Total Phytosterol Content of Selected Foods[94–97]

Food	Serving	Phytosterols (mg)
Wheat germ	¹/₂ cup	197
Corn oil	1 Tbs	102
Canola oil	1 Tbs	91
Peanuts	1 oz	62
Wheat bran	¹/₂ cup	58
Almonds	1 oz	34
Brussels sprouts	¹/₂ cup	34
Rye bread	2 slices	33
Macadamia nuts	1 oz	33
Olive oil	1 Tbs	22
Take Control® spread	1 Tbs	1650 mg plant sterol esters (1000 mg free sterols)
Benecol® spread	1 Tbs	850 mg plant stanol esters (500 mg free stanols)

cholesterol is ~ 2 g/d[11] and the minimum effective dose is 0.8 to 1.0 g/d.[10] In the majority of clinical trials that demonstrated a cholesterol-lowering effect, the daily dose of plant sterols or stanols was divided among two or three meals. However, consumption of the daily dose of plant sterols or stanols with a single meal has been found to lower LDL cholesterol in a few clinical trials.[39,75,76]

Supplements

Phytosterol supplements marketed as β-sitosterol are available without a prescription in the United States. Doses of 60 to 130 mg/d of β-sitosterol have been found to alleviate the symptoms of BPH in a few clinical trials (see the Benign Prostatic Hyperplasia section above). Soft gel chews providing 0.5 g of plant stanols are being marketed for cholesterol lowering at a recommended dose of 2 g/d. Phytosterol supplements should be taken with meals that contain fat.

Safety

In the United States, plant sterols and stanols added to a variety of food products are generally recognized as safe (GRAS) by the FDA.[77] Additionally, the Scientific Committee on Foods of the European Union concluded that plant sterols and stanols added to various food products are safe for human use.[78] However, the Committee recommended that intakes of plant sterols and stanols from food products should not exceed 3 g/d.

Adverse Effects

Few adverse effects have been associated with regular consumption of plant sterols or stanols for up to one year. People who consumed a plant sterol-enriched spread providing 1.6 g/d did not report any more adverse effects than those consuming a control spread for up to one year,[26] and people consuming a plant stanol-enriched spread providing 1.8 to 2.6 g/d for one year did not report any adverse effects.[43] Consumption of up to 8.6 g/d of phytosterols in margarine for 3 to 4 weeks was well-tolerated by healthy men and women and did not adversely affect intestinal microflora or female hormone levels.[79] Although phytosterols are usually well-tolerated, nausea, indigestion, diarrhea, and constipation have occasionally been reported.[65,67]

Sitosterolemia (Phytosterolemia)

Sitosterolemia, also known as phytosterolemia, is a very rare autosomal recessive disease that results from inheriting a mutation in both copies of the *ABCG5* or *ABCG8* gene.[80] Individuals who are homozygous for a mutation in either half of the transporter protein have dramatically elevated serum phytosterol concentrations due to increased intestinal absorption and decreased biliary excretion of phytosterols. Although serum cholesterol concentrations may be normal or only mildly elevated, individuals with sitosterolemia are at high risk for premature atherosclerosis. People with sitosterolemia should avoid foods or supplements with added plant sterols.[10] Two studies have examined the effect of plant sterol consumption in heterozygous carriers of sitosterolemia, a more common condition. Consumption of 3 g/d of plant sterols for 4 weeks by two heterozygous carriers,[81] and consumption of 2.2 g/d of plant sterols for 6 to 12 weeks by 12 heterozygous carriers did not result in abnormally elevated serum phytosterols.[82]

Pregnancy and Lactation

Plant sterols or stanols added to foods or supplements are not recommended for pregnant or lactating women because their safety has not been studied.[10] At present, there is no evidence that high dietary intakes of naturally occurring phytosterols, such as those consumed by vegetarian women, adversely affect pregnancy or lactation.

Drug Interactions

The LDL-cholesterol-lowering effects of plant sterols or stanols may be additive to those of HMG-CoA reductase inhibitors (statins).[83,84] The results of controlled clinical trials suggest that consumption of 2 to 3 g/d of plant sterols or stanols by individuals on statin therapy may result in an additional 7 to 11% reduction in LDL cholesterol, an effect comparable to doubling the statin dose.[45,85–87] Consumption of 4.5 g/d of stanol esters for 8 weeks did not affect prothrombin times in patients on warfarin for anticoagulation.[88]

Nutrient Interactions

Fat-Soluble Vitamins (Vitamins A, D, E, and K)

Because plant sterols and stanols decrease cholesterol absorption and serum LDL cholesterol concentrations, their effects on fat-soluble vitamin status have also been studied in clinical trials. Plasma vitamin A (retinol) concentrations were not affected by plant stanol or sterol ester consumption for up to one year.[11,26] Although the majority of studies found no changes in plasma vitamin D (25-hydroxyvitamin D_3) concentrations, one study observed a small (7%) but statistically significant decrease in plasma 25-hydroxyvitamin D_3 concentrations at the end of one year in those who consumed 1.6 g/d of sterol esters compared with placebo.[26] There is little evidence that plant sterol or stanol consumption adversely affects vitamin K status. Consumption of 1.6 g/d of sterol esters for 6 months was associated with a nonsignificant 14% decrease in plasma vitamin K_1 concentrations, but carboxylated osteocalcin, a functional indicator of vitamin K status, was unaffected.[26] In other studies of shorter duration, consumption of plant sterol and stanol esters did not significantly change plasma concentrations of vitamin K_1[89] or vitamin K-dependent clotting factors.[90] Consumption of plant sterol- or stanol-enriched foods has been found to decrease plasma vitamin E (α-tocopherol) concentrations in several studies.[11] However, those decreases generally do not persist when plasma α-tocopherol concentrations are standardized to LDL cholesterol concentrations. This suggests that observed reductions in plasma α-tocopherol are due in part to reductions in its carrier lipoprotein, LDL. In general, consumption of plant sterol- and stanol-enriched foods at doses of 1.5 g/d or more has not been found to have adverse effects on fat-soluble vitamin status in well-nourished populations.

Carotenoids

Dietary carotenoids are fat-soluble phytochemicals that circulate in lipoproteins. Several studies have observed 10 to 20% reductions in plasma carotenoids after short-term and long-term consumption of plant sterol- or stanol-enriched foods.[11] Even when standardized to serum total or LDL cholesterol concentrations, decreases in β-carotene, α-carotene, and lycopene may persist, suggesting that phytosterols can inhibit the absorption of these carotenoids.[91] It is not clear whether reductions in plasma carotenoid concentrations confer any health risks, but several studies have found that increasing intakes of carotenoid-rich fruits and vegetables can prevent phytosterol-induced decreases in plasma carotenoids.[92] In one case, advice to consume 5 daily servings of fruits and vegetables, including 1 serving of carotenoid-rich vegetables, was enough to maintain plasma carotenoid levels in people consuming 2.5 g/d of plant sterol or stanol esters.[93]

Summary

- Phytosterols are plant-derived compounds that are similar in structure and function to cholesterol.
- Although early human diets were rich in phytosterols, providing as much as 1 g/d, the typical Western diet today is relatively low in phytosterols.
- Phytosterols inhibit the intestinal absorption of cholesterol.
- Numerous clinical trials have demonstrated that daily consumption of foods enriched with at least 0.8 g of plant sterols or stanols lowers serum LDL cholesterol.
- Although some epidemiological studies have found that higher intakes of plant foods containing phytosterols are associated with decreased cancer risk, it is not clear whether phytosterols or other compounds in plant foods are the protective factors.
- The results of a few clinical trials suggest that phytosterol supplementation at relatively low doses can improve urinary tract symptoms related to benign prostatic hyperplasia, but further research is needed to confirm these findings.
- Foods rich in phytosterols include unrefined vegetable oils, whole grains, nuts, and legumes.

- Foods and beverages with added plant sterols or stanols are now available in many countries throughout the world.

References

1. Jenkins DJ, Kendall CW, Marchie A, et al. The Garden of Eden–plant based diets, the genetic drive to conserve cholesterol and its implications for heart disease in the 21st century. Comp Biochem Physiol A Mol Integr Physiol 2003;136(1):141–151
2. Kendall CW, Jenkins DJ. A dietary portfolio: maximal reduction of low-density lipoprotein cholesterol with diet. Curr Atheroscler Rep 2004;6(6):492–498
3. Ostlund RE Jr. Phytosterols in human nutrition. Annu Rev Nutr 2002;22:533–549
4. Sudhop T, Lutjohann D, von Bergmann K. Sterol transporters: targets of natural sterols and new lipid lowering drugs. Pharmacol Ther 2005;105(3):333–341
5. de Jong A, Plat J, Mensink RP. Metabolic effects of plant sterols and stanols (Review). J Nutr Biochem 2003;14(7):362–369
6. Plat J, Mensink RP. Plant stanol and sterol esters in the control of blood cholesterol levels: mechanism and safety aspects. Am J Cardiol 2005;96(1 Suppl):15–22
7. von Bergmann K, Sudhop T, Lutjohann D. Cholesterol and plant sterol absorption: recent insights. Am J Cardiol 2005;96(1A):10D–14D
8. Ostlund RE Jr, McGill JB, Zeng CM, et al. Gastrointestinal absorption and plasma kinetics of soy Delta(5)-phytosterols and phytostanols in humans. Am J Physiol Endocrinol Metab 2002;282(4):E911–E916
9. Sudhop T, Sahin Y, Lindenthal B, et al. Comparison of the hepatic clearances of campesterol, sitosterol, and cholesterol in healthy subjects suggests that efflux transporters controlling intestinal sterol absorption also regulate biliary secretion. Gut 2002;51(6):860–863
10. Berger A, Jones PJ, Abumweis SS. Plant sterols: factors affecting their efficacy and safety as functional food ingredients. Lipids Health Dis 2004;3(1):5
11. Katan MB, Grundy SM, Jones P, Law M, Miettinen T, Paoletti R. Efficacy and safety of plant stanols and sterols in the management of blood cholesterol levels. Mayo Clin Proc 2003;78(8):965–978
12. Nissinen M, Gylling H, Vuoristo M, Miettinen TA. Micellar distribution of cholesterol and phytosterols after duodenal plant stanol ester infusion. Am J Physiol Gastrointest Liver Physiol 2002;282(6):G1009–G1015
13. Jones PJ, Raeini-Sarjaz M, Ntanios FY, Vanstone CA, Feng JY, Parsons WE. Modulation of plasma lipid levels and cholesterol kinetics by phytosterol versus phytostanol esters. J Lipid Res 2000;41(5):697–705
14. Normen L, Dutta P, Lia A, Andersson H. Soy sterol esters and beta-sitostanol ester as inhibitors of cholesterol absorption in human small bowel. Am J Clin Nutr 2000;71(4):908–913
15. Richelle M, Enslen M, Hager C, et al. Both free and esterified plant sterols reduce cholesterol absorption and the bioavailability of beta-carotene and alpha-tocopherol in normocholesterolemic humans. Am J Clin Nutr 2004;80(1):171–177
16. Plat J, Mensink RP. Effects of plant stanol esters on LDL receptor protein expression and on LDL receptor and

HMG-CoA reductase mRNA expression in mononuclear blood cells of healthy men and women. FASEB J 2002;16(2):258–260

17. Mouritsen OG, Zuckermann MJ. What's so special about cholesterol? Lipids 2004;39(11):1101–1113

18. Halling KK, Slotte JP. Membrane properties of plant sterols in phospholipid bilayers as determined by differential scanning calorimetry, resonance energy transfer and detergent-induced solubilization. Biochim Biophys Acta 2004;1664(2):161–171

19. Awad AB, Chen YC, Fink CS, Hennessey T. Beta-sitosterol inhibits HT-29 human colon cancer cell growth and alters membrane lipids. Anticancer Res 1996;16(5A):2797–2804

20. Leikin AI, Brenner RR. Fatty acid desaturase activities are modulated by phytosterol incorporation in microsomes. Biochim Biophys Acta 1989;1005(2):187–191

21. Ratnayake WM, L'Abbe MR, Mueller R, et al. Vegetable oils high in phytosterols make erythrocytes less deformable and shorten the life span of stroke-prone spontaneously hypertensive rats. J Nutr 2000;130(5):1166–1178

22. Ratnayake WM, Plouffe L, L'Abbe MR, Trick K, Mueller R, Hayward S. Comparative health effects of margarines fortified with plant sterols and stanols on a rat model for hemorrhagic stroke. Lipids 2003;38(12):1237–1247

23. Jones PJ, Raeini-Sarjaz M, Jenkins DJ, et al. Effects of a diet high in plant sterols, vegetable proteins, and viscous fibers (dietary portfolio) on circulating sterol levels and red cell fragility in hypercholesterolemic subjects. Lipids 2005;40(2):169–174

24. Awad AB, Hartati MS, Fink CS. Phytosterol feeding induces alteration in testosterone metabolism in rat tissues. J Nutr Biochem 1998;9(12):712–717

25. Cabeza M, Bratoeff E, Heuze I, Ramirez E, Sanchez M, Flores E. Effect of beta-sitosterol as inhibitor of 5 alpha-reductase in hamster prostate. Proc West Pharmacol Soc 2003;46:153–155

26. Hendriks HF, Brink EJ, Meijer GW, Princen HM, Ntanios FY. Safety of long-term consumption of plant sterol esters-enriched spread. Eur J Clin Nutr 2003;57(5):681–692

27. von Holtz RL, Fink CS, Awad AB. Beta-sitosterol activates the sphingomyelin cycle and induces apoptosis in LNCaP human prostate cancer cells. Nutr Cancer 1998;32(1):8–12

28. Awad AB, Roy R, Fink CS. Beta-sitosterol, a plant sterol, induces apoptosis and activates key caspases in MDA-MB-231 human breast cancer cells. Oncol Rep 2003;10(2):497–500

29. Choi YH, Kong KR, Kim YA, et al. Induction of Bax and activation of caspases during beta-sitosterol-mediated apoptosis in human colon cancer cells. Int J Oncol 2003;23(6):1657–1662

30. Awad AB, Toczek J, Fink CS. Phytosterols decrease prostaglandin release in cultured P388D1/MAB macrophages. Prostaglandins Leukot Essent Fatty Acids 2004;70(6):511–520

31. Navarro A, De las Heras B, Villar A. Anti-inflammatory and immunomodulating properties of a sterol fraction from Sideritis foetens Clem. Biol Pharm Bull 2001;24(5):470–473

32. St-Onge MP, Jones PJ. Phytosterols and human lipid metabolism: efficacy, safety, and novel foods. Lipids 2003;38(4):367–375

33. Law M. Plant sterol and stanol margarines and health. BMJ 2000;320(7238):861–864

34. Chen JT, Wesley R, Shamburek RD, Pucino F, Csako G. Meta-analysis of natural therapies for hyperlipidemia: plant sterols and stanols versus policosanol. Pharmacotherapy 2005;25(2):171–183

35. Hendriks HF, Weststrate JA, van Vliet T, Meijer GW. Spreads enriched with three different levels of vegetable oil sterols and the degree of cholesterol lowering in normocholesterolaemic and mildly hypercholesterolaemic subjects. Eur J Clin Nutr 1999;53(4):319–327

36. Miettinen TA, Vanhanen H. Dietary sitostanol related to absorption, synthesis and serum level of cholesterol in different apolipoprotein E phenotypes. Atherosclerosis 1994;105(2):217–226

37. Pelletier X, Belbraouet S, Mirabel D, et al. A diet moderately enriched in phytosterols lowers plasma cholesterol concentrations in normocholesterolemic humans. Ann Nutr Metab 1995;39(5):291–295

38. Sierksma A, Weststrate JA, Meijer GW. Spreads enriched with plant sterols, either esterified 4,4-dimethylsterols or free 4-desmethylsterols, and plasma total- and LDL-cholesterol concentrations. Br J Nutr 1999;82(4):273–282

39. Volpe R, Niittynen L, Korpela R, et al. Effects of yoghurt enriched with plant sterols on serum lipids in patients with moderate hypercholesterolaemia. Br J Nutr 2001;86(2):233–239

40. Hallikainen MA, Sarkkinen ES, Gylling H, Erkkila AT, Uusitupa MI. Comparison of the effects of plant sterol ester and plant stanol ester-enriched margarines in lowering serum cholesterol concentrations in hypercholesterolaemic subjects on a low-fat diet. Eur J Clin Nutr 2000;54(9):715–725

41. Vanstone CA, Raeini-Sarjaz M, Parsons WE, Jones PJ. Unesterified plant sterols and stanols lower LDL-cholesterol concentrations equivalently in hypercholesterolemic persons. Am J Clin Nutr 2002;76(6):1272–1278

42. Weststrate JA, Meijer GW. Plant sterol-enriched margarines and reduction of plasma total- and LDL-cholesterol concentrations in normocholesterolaemic and mildly hypercholesterolaemic subjects. Eur J Clin Nutr 1998;52(5):334–343

43. Miettinen TA, Puska P, Gylling H, Vanhanen H, Vartiainen E. Reduction of serum cholesterol with sitostanol-ester margarine in a mildly hypercholesterolemic population. N Engl J Med 1995;333(20):1308–1312

44. Miettinen TA, Gylling H. Plant stanol and sterol esters in prevention of cardiovascular diseases. Ann Med 2004;36(2):126–134

45. O'Neill FH, Brynes A, Mandeno R, et al. Comparison of the effects of dietary plant sterol and stanol esters on lipid metabolism. Nutr Metab Cardiovasc Dis 2004;14(3):133–142

46. National Cholesterol Education Program. Third Report of the National Cholesterol Education Program Expert Panel on Detection, Evaluation, and Treatment of High Blood Cholesterol in Adults (Adult Treatment Panel III). National Heart Lung and Blood Institute, National Institutes of Health. 2002. Available at: http://www.nhlbi.nih.gov/guidelines/cholesterol/atp3_rpt.htm. Accessed 7/26/06

47. Grundy SM. Stanol esters as a component of maximal dietary therapy in the National Cholesterol Education

Program Adult Treatment Panel III Report. Am J Cardiol 2005;96(1AI):47D–50D

48. Jones PJ, Ntanios FY, Raeini-Sarjaz M, Vanstone CA. Cholesterol-lowering efficacy of a sitostanol-containing phytosterol mixture with a prudent diet in hyperlipidemic men. Am J Clin Nutr 1999;69(6):1144–1150

49. Jenkins DJ, Kendall CW, Marchie A, et al. Direct comparison of a dietary portfolio of cholesterol-lowering foods with a statin in hypercholesterolemic participants. Am J Clin Nutr 2005;81(2):380–387

50. Food and Drug Administration. Health claims: plant sterol/stanol esters and risk of coronary heart disease (CHD). U. S. Government Printing Office. 2002. Available at: http://www.cfsan.fda.gov/~lrd/cf101-83.html. Accessed 7/26/06

51. Ostlund RE Jr. Phytosterols and cholesterol metabolism. Curr Opin Lipidol 2004;15(1):37–41

52. Ostlund RE Jr, Racette SB, Stenson WF. Effects of trace components of dietary fat on cholesterol metabolism: phytosterols, oxysterols, and squalene. Nutr Rev 2002;60(11):349–359

53. Andersson SW, Skinner J, Ellegard L, et al. Intake of dietary plant sterols is inversely related to serum cholesterol concentration in men and women in the EPIC Norfolk population: a cross-sectional study. Eur J Clin Nutr 2004;58(10):1378–1385

54. Ostlund RE Jr, Racette SB, Okeke A, Stenson WF. Phytosterols that are naturally present in commercial corn oil significantly reduce cholesterol absorption in humans. Am J Clin Nutr 2002;75(6):1000–1004

55. Ostlund RE Jr, Racette SB, Stenson WF. Inhibition of cholesterol absorption by phytosterol-replete wheat germ compared with phytosterol-depleted wheat germ. Am J Clin Nutr 2003;77(6):1385–1389

56. Ju YH, Clausen LM, Allred KF, Almada AL, Helferich WG. Beta-sitosterol, beta-sitosterol glucoside, and a mixture of beta-sitosterol and beta-sitosterol glucoside modulate the growth of estrogen-responsive breast cancer cells in vitro and in ovariectomized athymic mice. J Nutr 2004;134(5):1145–1151

57. Awad AB, Fink CS, Williams H, Kim U. In vitro and in vivo (SCID mice) effects of phytosterols on the growth and dissemination of human prostate cancer PC-3 cells. Eur J Cancer Prev 2001;10(6):507–513

58. Awad AB, Downie A, Fink CS, Kim U. Dietary phytosterol inhibits the growth and metastasis of MDA-MB-231 human breast cancer cells grown in SCID mice. Anticancer Res 2000;20(2A):821–824

59. De Stefani E, Boffetta P, Ronco A, et al. Plant sterols and risk of stomach cancer: a case-control study in Uruguay. Nutr Cancer 2000;37(2):140–144

60. Mendilaharsu M, De Stefani E, Deneo-Pellegrini H, Carzoglio J, Ronco A. Phytosterols and risk of lung cancer: a case-control study in Uruguay. Lung Cancer 1998;21(1):37–45

61. Ronco A, De Stefani E, Boffetta P, Deneo-Pellegrini H, Mendilaharsu M, Leborgne F. Vegetables, fruits, and related nutrients and risk of breast cancer: a case-control study in Uruguay. Nutr Cancer 1999;35(2):111–119

62. McCann SE, Freudenheim JL, Marshall JR, Brasure JR, Swanson MK, Graham S. Diet in the epidemiology of endometrial cancer in western New York (United States). Cancer Causes Control 2000;11(10):965–974

63. McCann SE, Freudenheim JL, Marshall JR, Graham S. Risk of human ovarian cancer is related to dietary intake of selected nutrients, phytochemicals and food groups. J Nutr 2003;133(6):1937–1942

64. Strom SS, Yamamura Y, Duphorne CM, et al. Phytoestrogen intake and prostate cancer: a case-control study using a new database. Nutr Cancer 1999;33(1):20–25

65. Berges RR, Windeler J, Trampisch HJ, Senge T. Randomised, placebo-controlled, double-blind clinical trial of beta-sitosterol in patients with benign prostatic hyperplasia. Beta-sitosterol Study Group. Lancet 1995;345(8964):1529–1532

66. Berges RR, Kassen A, Senge T. Treatment of symptomatic benign prostate hyperplasia with beta-sitosterol: an 18-month follow-up. BJU Int 2000;85(7):842–846

67. Klippel KF, Hiltl DM, Schipp B. A multicentric, placebo-controlled, double-blind clinical trial of beta-sitosterol (phytosterol) for the treatment of benign prostatic hyperplasia. German BPH-Phyto Study group. Br J Urol 1997;80(3):427–432

68. Wilt TJ, MacDonald R, Ishani A. beta-sitosterol for the treatment of benign prostatic hyperplasia: a systematic review. BJU Int 1999;83(9):976–983

69. Dreikorn K. The role of phytotherapy in treating lower urinary tract symptoms and benign prostatic hyperplasia. World J Urol 2002;19(6):426–435

70. Nair PP, Turjman N, Kessie G, et al. Diet, nutrition intake, and metabolism in populations at high and low risk for colon cancer. Dietary cholesterol, beta-sitosterol, and stigmasterol. Am J Clin Nutr 1984;40(4 Suppl):927–930

71. Mensink RP, Ebbing S, Lindhout M, Plat J, van Heugten MM. Effects of plant stanol esters supplied in low-fat yoghurt on serum lipids and lipoproteins, non-cholesterol sterols and fat soluble antioxidant concentrations. Atherosclerosis 2002;160(1):205–213

72. Noakes M, Clifton PM, Doornbos AM, Trautwein EA. Plant sterol ester-enriched milk and yoghurt effectively reduce serum cholesterol in modestly hypercholesterolemic subjects. Eur J Clin Nutr 2005;44(4):214–222

73. Thomsen AB, Hansen HB, Christiansen C, Green H, Berger A. Effect of free plant sterols in low-fat milk on serum lipid profile in hypercholesterolemic subjects. Eur J Clin Nutr 2004;58(6):860–870

74. Devaraj S, Jialal I, Vega-Lopez S. Plant sterol-fortified orange juice effectively lowers cholesterol levels in mildly hypercholesterolemic healthy individuals. Arterioscler Thromb Vasc Biol 2004;24(3):e25–e28

75. Matvienko OA, Lewis DS, Swanson M, et al. A single daily dose of soybean phytosterols in ground beef decreases serum total cholesterol and LDL cholesterol in young, mildly hypercholesterolemic men. Am J Clin Nutr 2002;76(1):57–64

76. Plat J, van Onselen EN, van Heugten MM, Mensink RP. Effects on serum lipids, lipoproteins and fat soluble antioxidant concentrations of consumption frequency of margarines and shortenings enriched with plant stanol esters. Eur J Clin Nutr 2000;54(9):671–677

77. Food and Drug Administration. GRAS Notice No. GRN 000112. 2003. Available at: http://www.cfsan.fda.gov/~rdb/opa-g112.html. Accessed 7/26/06

78. Scientific Committee on Food. Opinion on applications for approval of a variety of plant sterol-enriched foods. 2003. Available at: http://europa.eu.int/comm/food/fs/sc/scf/out174_en.pdf. Accessed 7/26/06

79. Ayesh R, Weststrate JA, Drewitt PN, Hepburn PA. Safety evaluation of phytosterol esters. Part 5. Faecal short-chain fatty acid and microflora content, faecal bacterial enzyme activity and serum female sex hormones in healthy normolipidaemic volunteers consuming a controlled diet either with or without a phytosterol ester-enriched margarine. Food Chem Toxicol 1999;37(12):1127–1138

80. Berge KE. Sitosterolemia: a gateway to new knowledge about cholesterol metabolism. Ann Med 2003; 35(7):502–511

81. Stalenhoef AF, Hectors M, Demacker PN. Effect of plant sterol-enriched margarine on plasma lipids and sterols in subjects heterozygous for phytosterolaemia. J Intern Med 2001;249(2):163–166

82. Kwiterovich PO Jr, Chen SC, Virgil DG, Schweitzer A, Arnold DR, Kratz LE. Response of obligate heterozygotes for phytosterolemia to a low-fat diet and to a plant sterol ester dietary challenge. J Lipid Res 2003; 44(6):1143–1155

83. Normen L, Holmes D, Frohlich J. Plant sterols and their role in combined use with statins for lipid lowering. Curr Opin Investig Drugs 2005;6(3):307–316

84. Thompson GR. Additive effects of plant sterol and stanol esters to statin therapy. Am J Cardiol 2005; 96(1A):37D–39D

85. Blair SN, Capuzzi DM, Gottlieb SO, Nguyen T, Morgan JM, Cater NB. Incremental reduction of serum total cholesterol and low-density lipoprotein cholesterol with the addition of plant sterol ester-containing spread to statin therapy. Am J Cardiol 2000;86(1):46–52

86. Neil HA, Meijer GW, Roe LS. Randomised controlled trial of use by hypercholesterolaemic patients of a vegetable oil sterol-enriched fat spread. Atherosclerosis 2001;156(2):329–337

87. Simons LA. Additive effect of plant sterol-ester margarine and cerivastatin in lowering low-density lipoprotein cholesterol in primary hypercholesterolemia. Am J Cardiol 2002;90(7):737–740

88. Nguyen TT, Dale LC. Plant stanol esters and vitamin K. Mayo Clin Proc 1999;74(6):642–643

89. Raeini-Sarjaz M, Ntanios FY, Vanstone CA, Jones PJ. No changes in serum fat-soluble vitamin and carotenoid concentrations with the intake of plant sterol/stanol esters in the context of a controlled diet. Metabolism 2002;51(5):652–656

90. Plat J, Mensink RP. Vegetable oil based versus wood based stanol ester mixtures: effects on serum lipids and hemostatic factors in non-hypercholesterolemic subjects. Atherosclerosis 2000;148(1):101–112

91. Plat J, Mensink RP. Effects of diets enriched with two different plant stanol ester mixtures on plasma ubiquinol-10 and fat-soluble antioxidant concentrations. Metabolism 2001;50(5):520–529

92. Ntanios FY, Duchateau GS. A healthy diet rich in carotenoids is effective in maintaining normal blood carotenoid levels during the daily use of plant sterol-enriched spreads. Int J Vitam Nutr Res 2002;72(1):32–39

93. Noakes M, Clifton P, Ntanios F, Shrapnel W, Record I, McInerney J. An increase in dietary carotenoids when consuming plant sterols or stanols is effective in maintaining plasma carotenoid concentrations. Am J Clin Nutr 2002;75(1):79–86

94. Normen L, Bryngelsson S, Johnsson M, et al. The phytosterol content of some cereal foods commonly consumed in Sweden and in the Netherlands. J Food Compos Anal. 2002;15(6):693–704

95. Normen L, Johnsson M, Andersson H, van Gameren Y, Dutta P. Plant sterols in vegetables and fruits commonly consumed in Sweden. Eur J Nutr 1999;38(2): 84–89

96. Phillips KM, Ruggio DM, Toivo JI, Swank MA, Simpkins AH. Free and esterified sterol composition of edible oils and fats. J Food Compos Anal. 2002;15(2):123–142

97. U.S. Department of Agriculture, Agricultural Research Service. USDA Nutrient Database for Standard Reference, Release 17. 2004. Available at: http://www.nal.usda.gov/fnic/foodcomp. Accessed 7/26/06

20 Resveratrol

Resveratrol (3,4′,5-trihydroxystilbene) belongs to a class of polyphenolic compounds called stilbenes.[1] Some types of plants produce resveratrol and other stilbenes in response to stress, injury, fungal infection, and ultraviolet (UV) radiation.[2] Resveratrol is a fat-soluble compound that occurs in a *trans* and a *cis* configuration (**Fig. 20–1**). Both *cis*- and *trans*-resveratrol also occur as glucosides (bound to a glucose molecule). Resveratrol-3-O-β-glucoside is also called piceid.[3] Scientists became interested in exploring potential health benefits of resveratrol in 1992 when its presence was first reported in red wine,[4] leading to speculation that resveratrol might help explain the "French Paradox" (see the Cardiovascular Disease section below). Reports on the potential for resveratrol to inhibit the development of cancer[5] and extend lifespan[6] in cell culture and animal models have continued to generate scientific interest. At present, relatively little is known about the effects of resveratrol in humans.

Metabolism and Bioavailability

Although *trans*-resveratrol appears to be well-absorbed by humans when taken orally, its bioavailability is relatively low due to its rapid

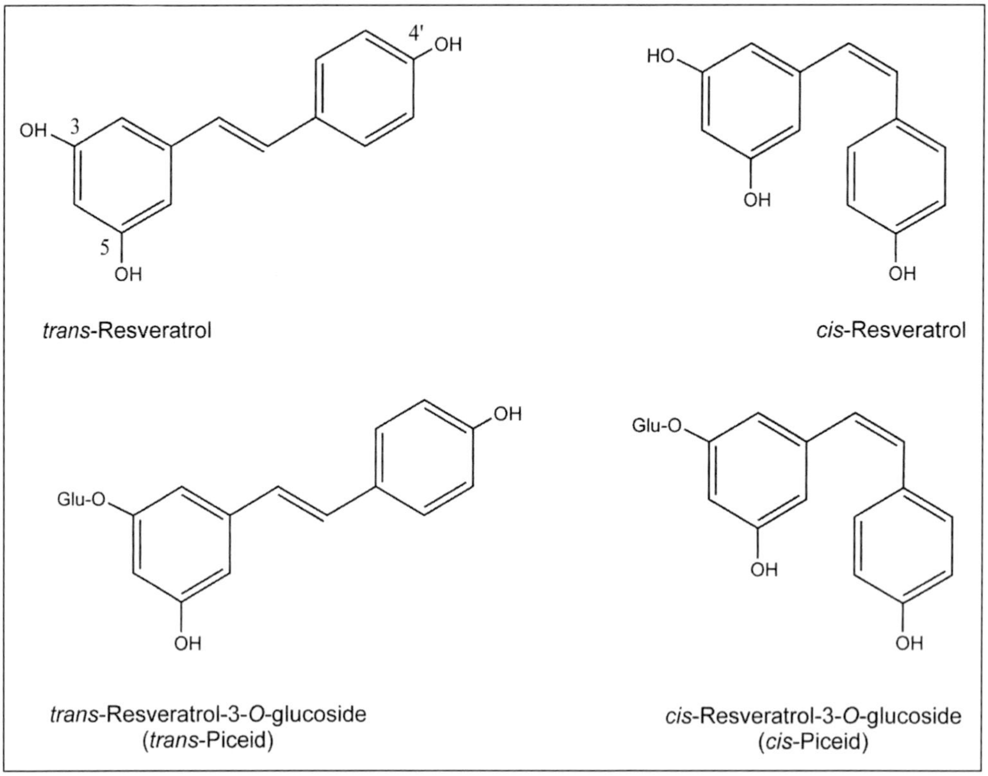

Figure 20–1 Chemical structures of *trans*-resveratrol, *cis*-resveratrol, *trans*-resveratrol-3-O-glucoside (*trans*-piceid), and *cis*-3-O-glucoside (*cis*-piceid).

metabolism and elimination.[7] When healthy men and women took an oral dose of 25 mg of *trans*-resveratrol, only traces of the unchanged resveratrol were detected in plasma; however, plasma concentrations of resveratrol metabolites peaked 30 to 60 minutes later at concentrations around 2 μmol/L.[7,8] The bioavailability of resveratrol from grape juice, which contains mostly glucosides of resveratrol (piceid), may be even lower than that of *trans*-resveratrol.[9] Information about the bioavailability, of resveratrol in humans is important because much of the basic research on resveratrol has been conducted in cultured cells exposed to unmetabolized resveratrol at concentrations that are often 10 to 100 times greater than peak concentrations observed in human plasma after oral consumption.[10] Although cells that line the digestive tract are exposed to unmetabolized resveratrol, research in humans suggests that other tissues are exposed primarily to resveratrol metabolites. Little is known about the biological activity of resveratrol metabolites, and it is not known whether some tissues are capable of converting resveratrol metabolites back to resveratrol.[7]

Biological Activities

Direct Antioxidant Activity

In the test tube, resveratrol effectively scavenges (neutralizes) free radicals and other oxidants[11] and inhibits low-density lipoprotein (LDL) oxidation.[12,13] However, there is little evidence that resveratrol is an important antioxidant in vivo.[14] After oral consumption of resveratrol, circulating and intracellular levels of resveratrol in humans are likely to be much lower than those of other important antioxidants, such as vitamin C, vitamin E, and glutathione. Moreover, the antioxidant activity of resveratrol metabolites, which make up most of the circulating resveratrol, may be lower than that of resveratrol.

Estrogenic and Anti-estrogenic Activities

Endogenous estrogens are steroid hormones synthesized by humans and other mammals that bind to estrogen receptors within cells. The estrogen-receptor complex interacts with unique sequences in DNA to modulate the expression of estrogen-responsive genes.[15] A compound that binds to estrogen receptors and elicits similar responses to endogenous estrogens is considered an estrogen agonist, whereas a compound that binds estrogen receptors, but prevents or inhibits the response elicited by endogenous estrogens, is considered an estrogen antagonist. The chemical structure of resveratrol is very similar to that of the synthetic estrogen agonist, diethylstilbestrol (**Fig. 20–2**), suggesting that resveratrol might also function as an estrogen agonist. However, in cell culture experiments resveratrol acts as an estrogen agonist under some conditions and as an estrogen antagonist under other conditions.[16,17] In estrogen receptor (ER)-positive breast cancer cells, resveratrol acted as an estrogen agonist in the absence of the endogenous estrogen, 17β-estradiol, but acted as an estrogen antagonist in the presence of 17β-estradiol.[18,19] At present, it appears that resveratrol has the potential to act as an estrogen agonist or antagonist depending on such factors as cell type, ER isoform (ERα or ERβ), and the presence of endogenous estrogens.[15]

Biological Activities Related to Cancer Prevention

Effects on Biotransformation Enzymes

Some compounds, such as polycyclic aromatic hydrocarbons, are not carcinogenic until they have been metabolized by cytochrome P450 enzymes.[2] By inhibiting the expression and activity of certain cytochrome P450 enzymes,[20,21] resveratrol could help prevent cancer by decreasing exposure to these activated carcinogens. In contrast, increasing the activity of phase II biotransformation enzymes generally promotes the excretion of potentially toxic or carcinogenic chemicals. Resveratrol has been found to increase the expression and activity of the phase II enzyme NAD(P)H:quinone reductase in cultured cells.[5,22]

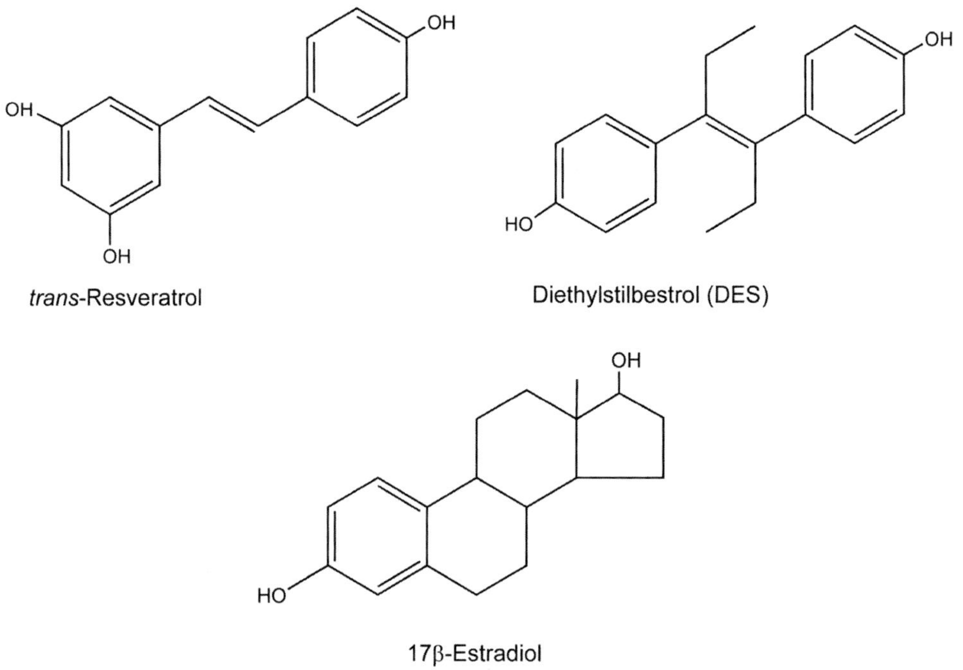

Figure 20–2   Chemical structures of *trans*-resveratrol; diethylstilbestrol, a synthetic estrogen agonist and 17β-estradiol, an endogenous estrogen.

Preservation of Normal Cell-Cycle Regulation

Following DNA damage, the cell cycle can be transiently arrested to allow for DNA repair or activation of pathways leading to cell death (apoptosis) if the damage is irreparable.[23] Defective cell-cycle regulation may result in the propagation of mutations that contribute to the development of cancer. Resveratrol has been found to induce cell-cycle arrest when added to cancer cells grown in culture.[24]

Inhibition of Proliferation and Induction of Apoptosis

Unlike normal cells, cancer cells proliferate rapidly and lose the ability to respond to cell death signals by undergoing apoptosis. Resveratrol has been found to inhibit proliferation and induce apoptosis in several cancer cell lines.[2]

Inhibition of Tumor Invasion and Angiogenesis

Cancerous cells invade normal tissue aided by enzymes called matrix metalloproteinases. Resveratrol has been found to inhibit the activity of at least one type of matrix metalloproteinase.[25] Invasive tumors must also develop new blood vessels to fuel their rapid growth by a process known as angiogenesis. Resveratrol has been found to inhibit angiogenesis in vitro.[26,27]

Anti-inflammatory Effects

Inflammation promotes cellular proliferation and angiogenesis and inhibits apoptosis.[28] Resveratrol has been found to inhibit the activity of several inflammatory enzymes in vitro, including cyclooxygenase and lipoxygenase.[29,30]

Biological Activities Related to Cardiovascular Disease Prevention

Inhibition of Vascular Cell Adhesion Molecule Expression

Atherosclerosis is now recognized as an inflammatory disease, and several measures of inflammation are associated with increased risk of myocardial infarction.[31] One of the earliest events in the development of atherosclerosis is the recruitment of inflammatory white blood cells from the blood to the artery wall by vascular cell adhesion molecules.[32] Resveratrol has been found to inhibit the expression of adhesion molecules in cultured endothelial cells.[33,34]

Inhibition of Vascular Smooth Muscle Cell Proliferation

The proliferation of vascular smooth muscle cells plays an important role in the progression of atherosclerosis.[35] Resveratrol has been found to inhibit the proliferation of vascular smooth muscle cells in culture.[36,37]

Stimulation of Endothelial Nitric Oxide Synthase Activity

Endothelial nitric oxide synthase (eNOS) is an enzyme that catalyzes the formation of nitric oxide (NO) by vascular endothelial cells. NO is needed to maintain arterial relaxation (vasodilation), and impaired NO-dependent vasodilation is associated with increased risk of cardiovascular disease.[38] Resveratrol has been found to stimulate eNOS activity in cultured endothelial cells.[39,40]

Inhibition of Platelet Aggregation

Platelet aggregation is one of the first steps in the formation of a blood clot that can occlude a coronary or cerebral artery, resulting in myocardial infarction or stroke. Resveratrol has been found to inhibit platelet aggregation in the test tube.[41,42]

It is important to keep in mind that that many of the biological activities discussed above were observed in cells cultured in the presence of resveratrol at higher concentrations than are likely to be achieved in humans consuming resveratrol orally (see the Metabolism and Bioavailability section above).

Prevention

Cardiovascular Disease

Red Wine Polyphenols

Significant reductions in cardiovascular disease risk have been associated with moderate consumption of alcoholic beverages.[43] The "French Paradox"—the observation that mortality from coronary heart disease is relatively low in France despite relatively high levels of dietary saturated fat and cigarette smoking—led to the idea that the regular consumption of red wine might provide additional protection from cardiovascular disease.[44,45] Red wine contains resveratrol and even higher levels of flavonoids. These polyphenolic compounds have antioxidant, antiinflammatory, and other potentially antiatherogenic effects in the test tube and in some animal models of atherosclerosis.[46] However, it is not yet known whether increased consumption of polyphenols from red wine provides any additional protection from cardiovascular disease beyond that associated with its alcohol content. The results of epidemiological studies addressing this question have been inconsistent. Although some large prospective studies found that wine drinkers were at lower risk of cardiovascular disease than beer or liquor drinkers,[47-49] others found no difference.[50-52] Socioeconomic and lifestyle differences between people who prefer wine and those who prefer beer or liquor may explain part of the additional benefit observed in some studies. Several studies have found that people who prefer wine tend to have higher incomes, and more education, smoke less, and eat more fruits and vegetables and less saturated fat than people who prefer other alcoholic beverages.[53-55] Although moderate alcohol consumption has been consistently associated with 20 to 30% reductions in coronary heart disease risk, it is not yet clear whether red wine polyphenols confer any additional risk reduction.

Resveratrol

Resveratrol has been found to exert several potentially cardioprotective effects in vitro, including the inhibition of platelet aggregation,[41,42,56] promotion of vasodilation by enhancing the production of NO,[40,57] and inhibition of inflammatory enzymes.[30,58,59] However, the concentrations of resveratrol required to produce these effects are often higher than those that have been measured in human plasma after oral consumption of resveratrol.[7] The results of some animal studies suggest that high oral doses of resveratrol could decrease the risk of thrombosis and atherosclerosis,[60,61] but at least one study found increased atherosclerosis in animals fed resveratrol.[62] Although its presence in red wine has stimulated a great deal of interest in the potential for resveratrol to prevent cardiovascular disease, there is currently no convincing evidence that resveratrol has cardioprotective effects in humans, particularly in the amounts present in 1 to 2 glasses of red wine (see the Sources section).

Cancer

When added to cells cultured outside the body, resveratrol has been found to inhibit the proliferation of a variety of human cancer cell lines, including those from breast, prostate, stomach, colon, pancreatic, and thyroid cancers.[2] In animal models, oral administration of resveratrol inhibited the development of esophageal,[63] intestinal,[64] and mammary (breast) cancer[18,65] induced by chemical carcinogens. However, oral resveratrol was not effective in inhibiting the development of lung cancer induced by cigarette smoke carcinogens,[66,67] and the effects of oral resveratrol administration on mice that are genetically predisposed to colon cancer have been mixed.[68,69] It is not known whether high intakes of resveratrol can help prevent cancer in humans. Studies on human metabolism of resveratrol suggest that even very high dietary intakes of resveratrol may not result in tissue levels that are high enough to realize most of the protective effects demonstrated in cell culture studies.[7,10]

Longevity

Caloric restriction is known to extend the lifespan of several species, including mammals.[70] In yeast, caloric restriction stimulates the activity of an enzyme known as Sir2.[71] Providing resveratrol to yeast increased Sir2 activity in the absence of caloric restriction and extended the replicative lifespan of yeast by 70%.[6] Resveratrol feeding also extended the lifespan of worms (*C. elegans*) and fruit flies (*D. melanogaster*) by a similar mechanism,[72] but it is not known whether resveratrol will have similar effects in higher animals. Although resveratrol increased the activity of the homologous human enzyme (Sirt1) in the test tube,[6] it is not known whether resveratrol can extend the human lifespan. Moreover, the resveratrol concentrations required to increase human Sirt1 activity were considerably higher than concentrations that have been measured in human plasma after oral consumption.

Sources

Food Sources

Resveratrol is found in grapes, wine, grape juice, peanuts, and berries of *Vaccinum* species, including blueberries, bilberries, and cranberries.[73–75] In grapes, resveratrol is found only in the skins.[76] The amount of resveratrol in grape skins varies with the grape cultivar, its geographic origin, and exposure to fungal infection.[77] The amount of fermentation time a wine spends in contact with grape skins is an important determinant of its resveratrol content. Consequently, white and rosé wines generally contain less resveratrol than red wines.[4] Red or purple grape juices may also be good sources of resveratrol.[3] The predominant form of resveratrol in grapes and grape juice is *trans*-resveratrol glucoside (*trans*-piceid), but wines also contain significant amounts of resveratrol aglycones, thought to be the result of sugar cleavage during fermentation.[73] Many wines also contain significant amounts of *cis*-resveratrol (**Fig. 20–1**), which may also be produced during fermentation or released from viniferins (resveratrol polymers).[78] Red wine is a relatively rich source of resveratrol, but other

Table 20–1   Total Resveratrol Content of Some White, Rosé, and Red Wines and Red (Purple) Grape Juice[3,87,88]

Beverage	Total Resveratrol (mg/L)	Total Resveratrol in a 5-oz Glass (mg)
White wines (Spanish)	0.05–1.80	0.01–0.27
Rosé wines (Spanish)	0.43–3.52	0.06–0.53
Red wines (Spanish)	1.92–12.59	0.29–1.89
Red wines (global)	1.98–7.13	0.30–1.07
Red grape juice (Spanish)	1.14–8.69	0.17–1.30

polyphenols are present in red wine at considerably higher concentrations than resveratrol (see Chapter 13).[79] The total resveratrol content of some beverages and foods are listed in **Tables 20–1** and **20–2**, respectively. These values should be considered approximate because the resveratrol content of foods and beverages can vary considerably.

Supplements

Most resveratrol supplements available in the United States contain extracts of the root of *Polygonum cuspidatum*, also known as Hu Zhang or kojo-kon.[80] Red wine extracts and red grape extracts containing resveratrol and other polyphenols are also available in the United States as dietary supplements. Resveratrol supplements may contain anywhere from 10 to 50 mg of resveratrol, but the effective doses for chronic disease prevention in humans are not known.

Safety

Adverse Effects

Resveratrol is not known to be toxic or cause adverse effects in humans, but there have been few controlled clinical trials. In rats, daily oral administration of *trans*-resveratrol at doses up to 300 mg/kg of body weight for 4 weeks resulted in no apparent adverse effects.[81,82]

Table 20–2   Total Resveratrol Content of Selected Foods[73,75,89]

Food	Serving	Total Resveratrol (mg)
Peanuts (raw)	1 cup	0.01–0.26
Peanuts (boiled)	1 cup	0.32–1.28
Peanut butter	1 cup	0.04–0.13
Red grapes	1 cup	0.24–1.25

Pregnancy and Lactation

The safety of resveratrol-containing supplements during pregnancy and lactation has not been established.[80] No safe level of alcohol consumption has been established at any stage of pregnancy;[83] therefore, pregnant women should avoid consuming wine as a source of resveratrol.

Estrogen-Sensitive Cancers

Until more is known about the estrogenic activity of resveratrol in humans, women with a history of estrogen-sensitive cancers, such as breast, ovarian, and uterine cancers, should avoid resveratrol supplements (see the Estrogenic and Antiestrogenic Activities section above).

Drug Interactions

Anticoagulant and Antiplatelet Drugs

Resveratrol has been found to inhibit human platelet aggregation in vitro.[42,84] Theoretically, high intakes of resveratrol (e.g., from supplements) could increase the risk of bleeding when taken with anticoagulant drugs, such as warfarin (Coumadin), and antiplatelet drugs, such as clopidogrel (Plavix), dipyridamole (Persantine), nonsteroidal anti-inflammatory drugs (NSAIDs), and aspirin.

Drugs Metabolized by Cytochrome P450 3A4

Resveratrol has been reported to inhibit the activity of cytochrome P450 3A4 (CYP3A4) in vitro.[85,86] Although this interaction has not been reported in humans, high intakes of resveratrol (e.g., from supplements) could theoretically increase the bioavailability and the risk of toxicity of drugs that undergo extensive first-pass metabolism by CYP3A4. Drugs known to be metabolized by CYP3A4 include, but are not limited to, HMG-CoA reductase inhibitors (atorvastatin, lovastatin, and simvastatin), calcium channel antagonists (felodipine, nicardipine, nifedipine, nisoldipine, nitrendipine, nimodipine, and verapamil), anti-arrhythmic agents (amiodarone), human immunodeficiency virus (HIV) protease inhibitors (saquinavir), immunosuppressants (cyclosporine and tacrolimus), antihistamines (terfenadine), benzodiazepines (midazolam and triazolam), and drugs used to treat erectile dysfunction (sildenafil).

Summary

- Resveratrol is a polyphenolic compound found in grapes, red wine, purple grape juice, peanuts, and some berries.
- When taken orally, resveratrol appears to be well-absorbed by humans, but its bioavailability is relatively low because it is rapidly metabolized and eliminated.
- Scientists became interested in exploring potential health benefits of resveratrol when its presence was reported in red wine, leading to speculation that resveratrol might help explain the "French Paradox."
- Moderate alcohol consumption has been consistently associated with 20 to 30% reductions in coronary heart disease risk, but it is not yet clear whether red wine polyphenols, such as resveratrol, confer any additional risk reduction.
- Although resveratrol can inhibit the growth of cancer cells in culture and some animal models, it is not known whether high intakes of resveratrol can prevent cancer in humans.
- Resveratrol administration increased the lifespan of yeast, worms, and fruit flies, but it is not known whether resveratrol will have similar effects in higher animal species or in humans.
- At present, relatively little is known about the effects of resveratrol in humans.

References

1. Soleas GJ, Diamandis EP, Goldberg DM. Resveratrol: a molecule whose time has come? And gone? Clin Biochem 1997;30(2):91–113
2. Aggarwal BB, Bhardwaj A, Aggarwal RS, Seeram NP, Shishodia S, Takada Y. Role of resveratrol in prevention and therapy of cancer: preclinical and clinical studies. Anticancer Res 2004;24(5A):2783–2840
3. Romero-Perez AI, Ibern-Gomez M, Lamuela-Raventos RM, de La Torre-Boronat MC. Piceid, the major resveratrol derivative in grape juices. J Agric Food Chem 1999;47(4):1533–1536
4. Siemann EH, Creasey LL. Concentration of the phytoalexin resveratrol in wine. Am J Enol Vitic 1992; 43(1):49–52
5. Jang M, Cai L, Udeani GO, et al. Cancer chemopreventive activity of resveratrol, a natural product derived from grapes. Science 1997;275(5297):218–220
6. Howitz KT, Bitterman KJ, Cohen HY, et al. Small molecule activators of sirtuins extend Saccharomyces cerevisiae lifespan. Nature 2003;425(6954):191–196
7. Walle T, Hsieh F, Delegge MH, Oatis JE Jr, Walle UK. High absorption but very low bioavailability of oral resveratrol in humans. Drug Metab Dispos 2004; 32(12):1377–1382
8. Goldberg DM, Yan J, Soleas GJ. Absorption of three wine-related polyphenols in three different matrices by healthy subjects. Clin Biochem 2003; 36(1):79–87
9. Meng X, Maliakal P, Lu H, Lee MJ, Yang CS. Urinary and plasma levels of resveratrol and quercetin in humans, mice, and rats after ingestion of pure compounds and grape juice. J Agric Food Chem 2004;52(4):935–942
10. Gescher AJ, Steward WP. Relationship between mechanisms, bioavailibility, and preclinical chemopreventive efficacy of resveratrol: a conundrum. Cancer Epidemiol Biomarkers Prev 2003;12(10):953–957
11. Stojanovic S, Sprinz H, Brede O. Efficiency and mechanism of the antioxidant action of trans-resveratrol and its analogues in the radical liposome oxidation. Arch Biochem Biophys 2001;391(1):79–89
12. Brito P, Almeida LM, Dinis TC. The interaction of resveratrol with ferrylmyoglobin and peroxynitrite; pro-

tection against LDL oxidation. Free Radic Res 2002; 36(6):621–631

13. Frankel EN, Waterhouse AL, Kinsella JE. Inhibition of human LDL oxidation by resveratrol. Lancet 1993; 341(8852):1103–1104

14. Bradamante S, Barenghi L, Villa A. Cardiovascular protective effects of resveratrol. Cardiovasc Drug Rev 2004;22(3):169–188

15. Tangkeangsirisin W, Serrero G. Resveratrol in the chemoprevention and chemotherapy of breast cancer. In: Bagchi D, Preuss HG, eds. Phytopharmaceuticals in Cancer Chemoprevention. Boca Raton: CRC Press; 2005:449–463

16. Bowers JL, Tyulmenkov VV, Jernigan SC, Klinge CM. Resveratrol acts as a mixed agonist/antagonist for estrogen receptors alpha and beta. Endocrinology 2000;141(10):3657–3667

17. Gehm BD, McAndrews JM, Chien PY, Jameson JL. Resveratrol, a polyphenolic compound found in grapes and wine, is an agonist for the estrogen receptor. Proc Natl Acad Sci U S A 1997;94(25):14138–14143

18. Bhat KP, Lantvit D, Christov K, Mehta RG, Moon RC, Pezzuto JM. Estrogenic and antiestrogenic properties of resveratrol in mammary tumor models. Cancer Res 2001;61(20):7456–7463

19. Lu R, Serrero G. Resveratrol, a natural product derived from grape, exhibits antiestrogenic activity and inhibits the growth of human breast cancer cells. J Cell Physiol 1999;179(3):297–304

20. Chen ZH, Hurh YJ, Na HK, et al. Resveratrol inhibits TCDD-induced expression of CYP1A1 and CYP1B1 and catechol estrogen-mediated oxidative DNA damage in cultured human mammary epithelial cells. Carcinogenesis 2004;25(10):2005–2013

21. Ciolino HP, Yeh GC. Inhibition of aryl hydrocarbon-induced cytochrome P-450 1A1 enzyme activity and CYP1A1 expression by resveratrol. Mol Pharmacol 1999;56(4):760–767

22. Yang SH, Kim JS, Oh TJ, et al. Genome-scale analysis of resveratrol-induced gene expression profile in human ovarian cancer cells using a cDNA microarray. Int J Oncol 2003;22(4):741–750

23. Stewart ZA, Westfall MD, Pietenpol JA. Cell-cycle dysregulation and anticancer therapy. Trends Pharmacol Sci 2003;24(3):139–145

24. Joe AK, Liu H, Suzui M, Vural ME, Xiao D, Weinstein IB. Resveratrol induces growth inhibition, S-phase arrest, apoptosis, and changes in biomarker expression in several human cancer cell lines. Clin Cancer Res 2002; 8(3):893–903

25. Woo JH, Lim JH, Kim YH, et al. Resveratrol inhibits phorbol myristate acetate-induced matrix metalloproteinase-9 expression by inhibiting JNK and PKC delta signal transduction. Oncogene 2004;23(10): 1845–1853

26. Igura K, Ohta T, Kuroda Y, Kaji K. Resveratrol and quercetin inhibit angiogenesis in vitro. Cancer Lett 2001; 171(1):11–16

27. Lin MT, Yen ML, Lin CY, Kuo ML. Inhibition of vascular endothelial growth factor-induced angiogenesis by resveratrol through interruption of Src-dependent vascular endothelial cadherin tyrosine phosphorylation. Mol Pharmacol 2003;64(5):1029–1036

28. Steele VE, Hawk ET, Viner JL, Lubet RA. Mechanisms and applications of non-steroidal anti-inflammatory drugs in the chemoprevention of cancer. Mutat Res 2003;523-524:137–144

29. Donnelly LE, Newton R, Kennedy GE, et al. Anti-inflammatory effects of resveratrol in lung epithelial cells: molecular mechanisms. Am J Physiol Lung Cell Mol Physiol 2004;287(4):L774–L783

30. Pinto MC, Garcia-Barrado JA, Macias P. Resveratrol is a potent inhibitor of the dioxygenase activity of lipoxygenase. J Agric Food Chem 1999;47(12):4842–4846

31. Blake GJ, Ridker PM. C-reactive protein and other inflammatory risk markers in acute coronary syndromes. J Am Coll Cardiol 2003; 41(4, Suppl S)37S–42S

32. Stocker R, Keaney JF Jr. Role of oxidative modifications in atherosclerosis. Physiol Rev 2004;84(4):1381–1478

33. Carluccio MA, Siculella L, Ancora MA, et al. Olive oil and red wine antioxidant polyphenols inhibit endothelial activation: antiatherogenic properties of Mediterranean diet phytochemicals. Arterioscler Thromb Vasc Biol 2003;23(4):622–629

34. Ferrero ME, Bertelli AE, Fulgenzi A, et al. Activity in vitro of resveratrol on granulocyte and monocyte adhesion to endothelium. Am J Clin Nutr 1998;68(6): 1208–1214

35. Faxon DP, Fuster V, Libby P, et al. Atherosclerotic Vascular Disease Conference: Writing Group III: pathophysiology. Circulation 2004;109(21):2617–2625

36. Mnjoyan ZH, Fujise K. Profound negative regulatory effects by resveratrol on vascular smooth muscle cells: a role of p53-p21(WAF1/CIP1) pathway. Biochem Biophys Res Commun 2003;311(2):546–552

37. Haider UG, Sorescu D, Griendling KK, Vollmar AM, Dirsch VM. Resveratrol increases serine15-phosphorylated but transcriptionally impaired p53 and induces a reversible DNA replication block in serum-activated vascular smooth muscle cells. Mol Pharmacol 2003;63(4):925–932

38. Duffy SJ, Vita JA. Effects of phenolics on vascular endothelial function. Curr Opin Lipidol 2003;14(1):21–27

39. Klinge CM, Blankenship KA, Risinger KE, et al. Resveratrol and estradiol rapidly activate MAPK signaling through estrogen receptors alpha and beta in endothelial cells. J Biol Chem 2004;280(9):7460–7468

40. Wallerath T, Deckert G, Ternes T, et al. Resveratrol, a polyphenolic phytoalexin present in red wine, enhances expression and activity of endothelial nitric oxide synthase. Circulation 2002;106(13):1652–1658

41. Kirk RI, Deitch JA, Wu JM, Lerea KM. Resveratrol decreases early signaling events in washed platelets but has little effect on platelets in whole blood. Blood Cells Mol Dis 2000;26(2):144–150

42. Pace-Asciak CR, Hahn S, Diamandis EP, Soleas G, Goldberg DM. The red wine phenolics trans-resveratrol and quercetin block human platelet aggregation and eicosanoid synthesis: implications for protection against coronary heart disease. Clin Chim Acta 1995; 235(2):207–219

43. Klatsky AL. Drink to your health? Sci Am 2003;288(2): 74–81

44. Criqui MH, Ringel BL. Does diet or alcohol explain the French paradox? Lancet. 1994;344(8939-8940):1719–1723

45. St Leger AS, Cochrane AL, Moore F. Factors associated with cardiac mortality in developed countries with particular reference to the consumption of wine. Lancet 1979;1(8124):1017–1020

46. German JB, Walzem RL. The health benefits of wine. Annu Rev Nutr 2000;20:561–593

47. Gronbaek M, Becker U, Johansen D, et al. Type of alcohol consumed and mortality from all causes, coronary heart disease, and cancer. Ann Intern Med 2000; 133(6):411–419

48. Klatsky AL, Friedman GD, Armstrong MA, Kipp H. Wine, liquor, beer, and mortality. Am J Epidemiol 2003;158(6):585–595

49. Renaud SC, Gueguen R, Siest G, Salamon R. Wine, beer, and mortality in middle-aged men from eastern France. Arch Intern Med 1999;159(16):1865–1870

50. Mukamal KJ, Conigrave KM, Mittleman MA, et al. Roles of drinking pattern and type of alcohol consumed in coronary heart disease in men. N Engl J Med 2003;348(2):109–118

51. Rimm EB, Klatsky A, Grobbee D, Stampfer MJ. Review of moderate alcohol consumption and reduced risk of coronary heart disease: is the effect due to beer, wine, or spirits. BMJ 1996;312(7033):731–736

52. Wannamethee SG, Shaper AG. Type of alcoholic drink and risk of major coronary heart disease events and all-cause mortality. Am J Public Health 1999;89(5): 685–690

53. Barefoot JC, Gronbaek M, Feaganes JR, McPherson RS, Williams RB, Siegler IC. Alcoholic beverage preference, diet, and health habits in the UNC Alumni Heart Study. Am J Clin Nutr 2002;76(2):466–472

54. McCann SE, Sempos C, Freudenheim JL, et al. Alcoholic beverage preference and characteristics of drinkers and nondrinkers in western New York (United States). Nutr Metab Cardiovasc Dis 2003;13(1):2–11

55. Mortensen EL, Jensen HH, Sanders SA, Reinisch JM. Better psychological functioning and higher social status may largely explain the apparent health benefits of wine: a study of wine and beer drinking in young Danish adults. Arch Intern Med 2001;161(15): 1844–1848

56. Wang Z, Huang Y, Zou J, Cao K, Xu Y, Wu JM. Effects of red wine and wine polyphenol resveratrol on platelet aggregation in vivo and in vitro. Int J Mol Med 2002; 9(1):77–79

57. Chen CK, Pace-Asciak CR. Vasorelaxing activity of resveratrol and quercetin in isolated rat aorta. Gen Pharmacol 1996;27(2):363–366

58. Szewczuk LM, Forti L, Stivala LA, Penning TM. Resveratrol is a peroxidase-mediated inactivator of COX-1 but not COX-2: a mechanistic approach to the design of COX-1 selective agents. J Biol Chem 2004;279(21): 22727–22737

59. Tsai SH, Lin-Shiau SY, Lin JK. Suppression of nitric oxide synthase and the down-regulation of the activation of NFkappaB in macrophages by resveratrol. Br J Pharmacol 1999;126(3):673–680

60. Fukao H, Ijiri Y, Miura M, et al. Effect of trans-resveratrol on the thrombogenicity and atherogenicity in apolipoprotein E-deficient and low-density lipoprotein receptor-deficient mice. Blood Coagul Fibrinolysis 2004;15(6):441–446

61. Wang Z, Zou J, Huang Y, Cao K, Xu Y, Wu JM. Effect of resveratrol on platelet aggregation in vivo and in vitro. Chin Med J (Engl) 2002;115(3):378–380

62. Wilson T, Knight TJ, Beitz DC, Lewis DS, Engen RL. Resveratrol promotes atherosclerosis in hypercholesterolemic rabbits. Life Sci 1996;59(1):PL15–PL21

63. Li ZG, Hong T, Shimada Y, et al. Suppression of N-nitrosomethylbenzylamine (NMBA)-induced esophageal tumorigenesis in F344 rats by resveratrol. Carcinogenesis 2002;23(9):1531–1536

64. Tessitore L, Davit A, Sarotto I, Caderni G. Resveratrol depresses the growth of colorectal aberrant crypt foci by affecting bax and p21(CIP) expression. Carcinogenesis 2000;21(8):1619–1622

65. Banerjee S, Bueso-Ramos C, Aggarwal BB. Suppression of 7,12-dimethylbenz(a)anthracene-induced mammary carcinogenesis in rats by resveratrol: role of nuclear factor-kappaB, cyclooxygenase 2, and matrix metalloprotease 9. Cancer Res 2002;62(17):4945–4954

66. Hecht SS, Kenney PM, Wang M, et al. Evaluation of butylated hydroxyanisole, myo-inositol, curcumin, esculetin, resveratrol and lycopene as inhibitors of benzo[a]pyrene plus 4-(methylnitrosamino)-1-(3-pyridyl)-1-butanone-induced lung tumorigenesis in A/J mice. Cancer Lett 1999;137(2):123–130

67. Berge G, Ovrebo S, Eilertsen E, Haugen A, Mollerup S. Analysis of resveratrol as a lung cancer chemopreventive agent in A/J mice exposed to benzo[a]pyrene. Br J Cancer 2004;91(7):1380–1383

68. Schneider Y, Duranton B, Gosse F, Schleiffer R, Seiler N, Raul F. Resveratrol inhibits intestinal tumorigenesis and modulates host-defense-related gene expression in an animal model of human familial adenomatous polyposis. Nutr Cancer 2001;39(1):102–107

69. Ziegler CC, Rainwater L, Whelan J, McEntee MF. Dietary resveratrol does not affect intestinal tumorigenesis in Apc(Min/+) mice. J Nutr 2004;134(1): 5–10

70. Heilbronn LK, Ravussin E. Calorie restriction and aging: review of the literature and implications for studies in humans. Am J Clin Nutr 2003;78(3):361–369

71. Lin SJ, Defossez PA, Guarente L. Requirement of NAD and SIR2 for life-span extension by calorie restriction in Saccharomyces cerevisiae. Science 2000;289 (5487):2126–2128

72. Wood JG, Rogina B, Lavu S, et al. Sirtuin activators mimic caloric restriction and delay ageing in metazoans. Nature 2004;430(7000):686–689

73. Burns J, Yokota T, Ashihara H, Lean ME, Crozier A. Plant foods and herbal sources of resveratrol. J Agric Food Chem 2002;50(11):3337–3340

74. Rimando AM, Kalt W, Magee JB, Dewey J, Ballington JR. Resveratrol, pterostilbene, and piceatannol in vaccinium berries. J Agric Food Chem 2004;52(15):4713–4719

75. Sanders TH, McMichael RW Jr, Hendrix KW. Occurrence of resveratrol in edible peanuts. J Agric Food Chem 2000;48(4):1243–1246

76. Creasey LL, Coffee M. Phytoalexin production potential of grape berries. J Am Soc Hortic Sci 1988;113(2): 230–234

77. Fremont L. Biological effects of resveratrol. Life Sci 2000;66(8):663–673

78. Goldberg DM, Karumanchiri A, Ng E, Yan J, Eleftherios P, Soleas G. Direct gas chromatographic-mass spectrometric method to assay cis-resveratrol in wines: preliminary survey of its concentration in commercial wines. J Agric Food Chem 1995;43(5):1245–1250

79. Burns J, Gardner PT, Matthews D, Duthie GG, Lean ME, Crozier A. Extraction of phenolics and changes in antioxidant activity of red wines during vinification. J Agric Food Chem 2001;49(12):5797–5808

80. Hendler SS, Rorvik DR, eds. PDR for Nutritional Supplements. Montvale: Medical Economics Company, Inc; 2001

81. Crowell JA, Korytko PJ, Morrissey RL, Booth TD, Levine BS. Resveratrol-associated renal toxicity. Toxicol Sci 2004;82(2):614–619

82. Juan ME, Vinardell MP, Planas JM. The daily oral administration of high doses of trans-resveratrol to rats for 28 days is not harmful. J Nutr 2002;132(2):257–260

83. American Academy of Pediatrics. Committee on Substance Abuse and Committee on Children with Disabilities. Fetal alcohol syndrome and alcohol-related neurodevelopmental disorders. Pediatrics 2000; 106(2 Pt 1):358–361

84. Bertelli AA, Giovannini L, Giannessi D, et al. Antiplatelet activity of synthetic and natural resveratrol in red wine. Int J Tissue React 1995;17(1):1–3

85. Piver B, Berthou F, Dreano Y, Lucas D. Inhibition of CYP3A, CYP1A and CYP2E1 activities by resveratrol and other non volatile red wine components. Toxicol Lett 2001;125(1–3):83–91

86. Regev-Shoshani G, Shoseyov O, Kerem Z. Influence of lipophilicity on the interactions of hydroxy stilbenes with cytochrome P450 3A4. Biochem Biophys Res Commun 2004;323(2):668–673

87. Moreno-Labanda JF, Mallavia R, Perez-Fons L, Lizama V, Saura D, Micol V. Determination of piceid and resveratrol in Spanish wines deriving from Monastrell (Vitis vinifera L.) grape variety. J Agric Food Chem 2004;52(17):5396–5403

88. Romero-Perez AI, Lamuela-Raventos RM, Waterhouse AL, de la Torre-Boronat MC. Levels of cis- and trans-resveratrol and their glucosides in white and rosé Vitis vinifera wines from Spain. J Agric Food Chem 1996;44(8):2124–2128

89. Sobolev VS, Cole RJ. Trans-resveratrol content in commercial peanuts and peanut products. J Agric Food Chem 1999;47(4):1435–1439

Appendix 1 Glycemic Index and Glycemic Load

Glycemic Index

In the past, carbohydrates were classified as simple or complex based on the number of simple sugars in the molecule. Carbohydrates composed of one or two simple sugars, such as fructose or sucrose, were labeled simple, whereas starchy foods were labeled complex because starch is composed of long chains of the simple sugar, glucose. Advice to eat less simple and more complex carbohydrates was based on the assumption that consuming starchy foods would lead to smaller increases in blood glucose than sugary foods.[1] This assumption turned out to be too simplistic because the blood glucose (glycemic) response to "complex" carbohydrates has been found to vary considerably. A more accurate indicator of the relative glycemic response to dietary carbohydrates is the glycemic index.

Measuring the Glycemic Index of Foods

To determine the glycemic index of a food, volunteers are typically given a test food that provides 50 g of carbohydrate and a control food (white bread or pure glucose) that provides the same amount of carbohydrate on different days.[2] Blood samples for the determination of glucose are taken prior to eating and at regular intervals after eating over the next several hours. The changes in blood glucose over time are plotted as a curve. The glycemic index is calculated as the area under the glucose curve after the test food is eaten, divided by the corresponding area after the control food is eaten. The value is multiplied by 100 to represent a percentage of the control food. For example, a baked russet potato has a glycemic index of 76 relative to glucose (**Table A1–1**) and 108 relative to white bread, which means that the blood glucose response to the carbohydrate in a baked potato is 76% of the blood glucose response to the same amount of carbohydrate in pure glucose and 108% of the blood glucose response to the same amount of carbohydrate in white bread.[3] In contrast, cooked brown rice has a glycemic index of 55 relative to glucose and 79 relative to white bread.[4] In the traditional system of classifying carbohydrates, both brown rice and potato would be classified as complex carbohydrates despite the difference in their effects on blood glucose levels.

Physiological Responses to Foods with High-Glycemic Index Values

By definition, the consumption of high-glycemic index foods results in higher and more rapid increases in blood glucose levels than the consumption of low-glycemic index foods. Rapid increases in blood glucose are potent signals to the β-cells of the pancreas to increase insulin secretion.[2] Over the next few hours, the high insulin levels induced by consumption of high-glycemic index foods may cause a sharp decrease in blood glucose levels (hypoglycemia). In contrast, the consumption of low-glycemic index foods results in lower, but more sustained increases in blood glucose and lower insulin demands on pancreatic β-cells.[5]

Glycemic Load

The glycemic index compares the potential of foods containing the same amount of carbohydrate to raise blood glucose. However, the amount of carbohydrate consumed also affects blood glucose levels and insulin responses. The glycemic load of a food is calculated by multiplying the glycemic index by the amount of carbohydrate in grams provided by a food and dividing the total by 100 (**Table A1–1**). In essence, each unit of the glycemic load represents the equivalent blood glucose-raising effect of 1 g of pure glucose or white bread.[1] Di-

Table A1–1   Glycemic Index (Relative to Glucose) and Glycemic-Load Values for Selected Foods[3,4]

Food	Glycemic Index (Glucose = 100)	Serving Size	Carbohydrate/ Serving (g)	Glycemic Load/ Serving
Dates, dried	103	~2 oz	40	42
Cornflakes	81	1 cup	26	21
Jelly beans	78	1 oz	28	22
Puffed rice cakes	78	~3 cakes	21	17
Russet potato, baked	76	1 medium	30	23
Doughnut	76	1 medium	23	17
White bread	73	1 large slice	14	10
White rice, boiled	64	1 cup	36	23
Brown rice	55	1 cup	33	18
Spaghetti, boiled	44	1 cup	40	18
Rye, bread	41	1 large slice	12	5
100% Bran cereal	38	1 cup	23	9
Apple, raw	38	1 medium	15	6
Lentils, boiled	29	1 cup	18	5
Pearled barley, boiled	25	1 cup	42	11
Cashews	22	1 oz	9	2
Peanuts	14	1 oz	6	1

etary glycemic load is the sum of the glycemic loads for all foods consumed in the diet. The concept of glycemic load was developed by scientists to simultaneously describe the quality (glycemic index) and quantity of carbohydrate in a meal or diet.

Prevention

Type 2 Diabetes Mellitus

After a high-glycemic-load meal, blood glucose levels rise more rapidly and insulin demand is greater than after a low-glycemic-load meal. High blood glucose levels and excessive insulin secretion are thought to contribute to the loss of the insulin-secreting function of the pancreatic β-cells that leads to irreversible diabetes.[6] High dietary glycemic-loads have been associated with an increased risk of developing type 2 diabetes mellitus (DM) in several large prospective studies. In the Nurses' Health Study (NHS), women with

the highest dietary glycemic loads were 37% more likely to develop type 2 DM over the next 6 years than women with the lowest dietary glycemic loads.[7] Additionally, women with high-glycemic-load diets that were low in cereal fiber were more than twice as likely to develop type 2 DM than women with low-glycemic-load diets that were high in cereal fiber. The results of the Health Professionals Follow-up Study (HPFS), which followed male health professionals over 6 years were similar.[8] In the NHS II study, a prospective study of younger and middle-aged women, those who consumed foods with the highest glycemic index values and the least cereal fiber were also at significantly higher risk of developing type 2 DM over the next 8 years.[9] The foods that were most consistently associated with increased risk of type 2 DM in the NHS and HPFS cohorts were potatoes (cooked or French-fried), white rice, white bread, and carbonated beverages.[6]

Cardiovascular Disease

Impaired glucose tolerance and insulin resistance are known to be risk factors for cardiovascular disease as well as type 2 DM. In addition to increased blood glucose and insulin concentrations, high dietary glycemic loads are associated with increased serum triglyceride concentrations and decreased HDL cholesterol concentrations, both cardiovascular disease risk factors.[10,11] High dietary glycemic loads have also been associated with increased serum levels of C-reactive protein (CRP), a marker of systemic inflammation that is also a sensitive predictor of cardiovascular disease risk.[12] In the NHS cohort, women with the highest dietary glycemic loads had a risk of developing coronary heart disease over the next 10 years that was almost twice as high as those with the lowest dietary glycemic loads.[13] The relationship between dietary glycemic load and coronary heart disease risk was more pronounced in overweight women, suggesting that people who are insulin resistant may be most susceptible to the adverse cardiovascular effects of high dietary glycemic loads.[1]

Obesity

In the first 2 hours after a meal, blood glucose and insulin levels rise higher after a high-glycemic-load meal than they do after a low-glycemic-load meal containing equal calories. However, in response to the excess insulin secretion, blood glucose levels drop lower over the next few hours after a high-glycemic-load meal than they do after a low-glycemic-load meal. This may explain why 15 out of 16 published studies found that the consumption of low-glycemic-index foods delayed the return of hunger, decreased subsequent food intake, and increased satiety (feeling full) when compared with high-glycemic-index foods.[14] The results of several small short-term trials (1 to 4 months) suggest that low-glycemic-load diets result in significantly more weight or fat loss than high-glycemic-load diets.[15–17] Although long-term randomized controlled trials of low-glycemic-load diets in the treatment of obesity are lacking, the results of short-term studies on appetite regulation and weight loss suggest that low-glycemic-load diets may be useful in promoting long-term weight loss and decreasing the prevalence of obesity.

Cancer

Evidence that high overall dietary glycemic index or high dietary glycemic loads are related to cancer risk is somewhat inconsistent. Prospective cohort studies in the United States and Denmark found no association between overall dietary glycemic index or dietary glycemic load and breast cancer risk.[18,19] In contrast, a prospective cohort study in Canada found that postmenopausal but not premenopausal women with high overall dietary glycemic index values were at increased risk of breast cancer, particularly those who reported no vigorous physical activity, whereas a prospective study in the United States found that premenopausal but not postmenopausal women with high overall dietary glycemic index values and low levels of physical activity were at increased risk of breast cancer.[20] Higher dietary glycemic loads were associated with moderately increased risk of colorectal cancer in a prospective study of American men, but no association between dietary glycemic load and colorectal cancer risk was observed in a prospective study of American women.[21] In contrast, another prospective cohort study of American women found that higher dietary glycemic loads were associated with increased risk of colorectal cancer.[22] Although there is some evidence that hyperinsulinemia may promote the growth of some types of cancer,[23] more research is needed to determine the effects of dietary glycemic load and/or glycemic index on cancer risk.

Treatment

Diabetes Mellitus

Low-glycemic index diets appear to improve the overall blood glucose control in people with type 1 and type 2 DM. A meta-analysis of 14 randomized controlled trials that included 356 diabetic patients found that low-glycemic index diets improved short-term and long-term control of blood glucose levels, reflected by clinically significant decreases in fructosamine and hemoglobin A_{1C} levels.[24] Episodes of serious hypoglycemia are a significant problem in people with type 1 DM. In a study of 63 men and women with type 1 DM, those randomized to a high-fiber, low-glycemic index diet had significantly fewer episodes of hypoglycemia than those on a low-fiber, high-glycemic index diet.[25]

Lowering Dietary Glycemic Load or Overall Dietary Glycemic Index

Some strategies for lowering dietary glycemic load or overall dietary glycemic index include:

- Increasing the consumption of whole grains, nuts, legumes, fruits, and nonstarchy vegetables
- Decreasing the consumption of starchy, high-glycemic index foods like potatoes, white rice, and white bread
- Decreasing the consumption of sugary foods such as cookies, cakes, candy, and soft drinks.

References

1. Liu S, Willett WC. Dietary glycemic load and atherothrombotic risk. Curr Atheroscler Rep 2002; 4(6):454–461
2. Ludwig DS. The glycemic index: physiological mechanisms relating to obesity, diabetes, and cardiovascular disease. JAMA 2002;287(18):2414–2423
3. Fernandes G, Velangi A, Wolever TM. Glycemic index of potatoes commonly consumed in North America. J Am Diet Assoc 2005;105(4):557–562
4. Foster-Powell K, Holt SH, Brand-Miller JC. International table of glycemic index and glycemic load values: 2002. Am J Clin Nutr 2002;76(1):5–56
5. Willett WC. Eat, Drink, and be Healthy: The Harvard Medical School Guide to Healthy Eating. New York: Simon & Schuster; 2001
6. Willett W, Manson J, Liu S. Glycemic index, glycemic load, and risk of type 2 diabetes. Am J Clin Nutr 2002; 76(1):274S–280S
7. Salmeron J, Manson JE, Stampfer MJ, Colditz GA, Wing AL, Willett WC. Dietary fiber, glycemic load, and risk of non-insulin-dependent diabetes mellitus in women. JAMA 1997;277(6):472–477
8. Salmeron J, Ascherio A, Rimm EB, et al. Dietary fiber, glycemic load, and risk of NIDDM in men. Diabetes Care 1997;20(4):545–550
9. Schulze MB, Liu S, Rimm EB, Manson JE, Willett WC, Hu FB. Glycemic index, glycemic load, and dietary fiber intake and incidence of type 2 diabetes in younger and middle-aged women. Am J Clin Nutr 2004;80(2):348–356
10. Ford ES, Liu S. Glycemic index and serum high-density lipoprotein cholesterol concentration among us adults. Arch Intern Med 2001;161(4):572–576
11. Liu S, Manson JE, Stampfer MJ, et al. Dietary glycemic load assessed by food-frequency questionnaire in relation to plasma high-density-lipoprotein cholesterol and fasting plasma triacylglycerols in postmenopausal women. Am J Clin Nutr 2001;73(3):560–566
12. Liu S, Manson JE, Buring JE, Stampfer MJ, Willett WC, Ridker PM. Relation between a diet with a high glycemic load and plasma concentrations of high-sensitivity C-reactive protein in middle-aged women. Am J Clin Nutr 2002;75(3):492–498
13. Liu S, Willett WC, Stampfer MJ, et al. A prospective study of dietary glycemic load, carbohydrate intake, and risk of coronary heart disease in US women. Am J Clin Nutr 2000;71(6):1455–1461
14. Ludwig DS. Dietary glycemic index and the regulation of body weight. Lipids 2003;38(2):117–121
15. Slabber M, Barnard HC, Kuyl JM, Dannhauser A, Schall R. Effects of a low-insulin-response, energy-restricted diet on weight loss and plasma insulin concentrations in hyperinsulinemic obese females. Am J Clin Nutr 1994;60(1):48–53
16. Bouche C, Rizkalla SW, Luo J, et al. Five-week, low-glycemic index diet decreases total fat mass and improves plasma lipid profile in moderately overweight nondiabetic men. Diabetes Care 2002;25(5):822–828
17. Spieth LE, Harnish JD, Lenders CM, et al. A low-glycemic index diet in the treatment of pediatric obesity. Arch Pediatr Adolesc Med 2000;154(9):947–951
18. Jonas CR, McCullough ML, Teras LR, Walker-Thurmond KA, Thun MJ, Calle EE. Dietary glycemic index, glycemic load, and risk of incident breast cancer in postmenopausal women. Cancer Epidemiol Biomarkers Prev 2003;12(6):573–577
19. Nielsen TG, Olsen A, Christensen J, Overvad K, Tjonneland A. Dietary carbohydrate intake is not associated with the breast cancer incidence rate ratio in postmenopausal Danish women. J Nutr 2005;135(1):124–128
20. Higginbotham S, Zhang ZF, Lee IM, Cook NR, Buring JE, Liu S. Dietary glycemic load and breast cancer risk in the Women's Health Study. Cancer Epidemiol Biomarkers Prev 2004;13(1):65–70
21. Michaud DS, Fuchs CS, Liu S, Willett WC, Colditz GA, Giovannucci E. Dietary glycemic load, carbohydrate, sugar, and colorectal cancer risk in men and women. Cancer Epidemiol Biomarkers Prev 2005;14(1):138–147
22. Higginbotham S, Zhang ZF, Lee IM, et al. Dietary glycemic load and risk of colorectal cancer in the Women's Health Study. J Natl Cancer Inst 2004;96(3):229–233
23. Boyd DB. Insulin and cancer. Integr Cancer Ther 2003;2(4):315–329
24. Brand-Miller J, Hayne S, Petocz P, Colagiuri S. Low-Glycemic Index Diets in the Management of Diabetes: A meta-analysis of randomized controlled trials. Diabetes Care 2003;26(8):2261–2267
25. Giacco R, Parillo M, Rivellese AA, et al. Long-term dietary treatment with increased amounts of fiber-rich low-glycemic index natural foods improves blood glucose control and reduces the number of hypoglycemic events in type 1 diabetic patients. Diabetes Care 2000;23(10):1461–1466

Appendix 2 Quick Reference to Diseases

Disease or Condition	Chapter Section	Food or Phytochemical	Page(s)
Asthma	Treatment	Essential fatty acids	86–87
Alzheimer's disease	Prevention	Curcumin	72
		Flavonoids	118
Benign prostatic hyperplasia	Treatment	Phytosterols	179
Cancer (general)	Prevention	Fruits and vegetables	2
	Treatment	Cruciferous vegetables	72
		Whole grains	23–24
		Tea	41–42
		Curcumin	71–72
		Flavonoids	118
		Isothiocyanates	140–141
		Indole-3-carbinol	149
		Phytosterols	178–179
		Resveratrol	190
Breast cancer	Prevention	Cruciferous vegetables	8–9
		Legumes	15
		Fiber	104
		Soy isoflavones	129
		Lignans	157
Colorectal cancer	Prevention	Cruciferous vegetables	8
		Coffee	29–30
		Fiber	104
		Organosulfur compounds (garlic)	167
Endometrial cancer	Prevention	Soy isoflavones	129
		Lignans	157
Gastric cancer	Prevention	Organosulfur compounds (garlic)	167
Liver cancer	Prevention	Coffee	31–32
		Chlorophyll and chlorophyllin	63–64
Lung cancer	Prevention	Cruciferous vegetables	7–8
		Carotenoids	49–50
Prostate cancer	Prevention	Cruciferous vegetables	9
		Legumes	15
		Carotenoids	50
		Soy isoflavones	130
		Lignans	158

Disease or Condition	Chapter Section	Food or Phytochemical	Page(s)
Cardiovascular disease	Prevention Treatment	Fruits and vegetables	1
		Legumes	13–14
		Nuts	18–19
		Whole grains	22–23
		Tea	41
		Carotenoids	50–51
		Essential fatty acids	82–83
		Fiber	103–104
		Flavonoids	116–118
		Soy isoflavones	129
		Lignans	157
		Organosulfur compounds (garlic)	164, 165–167
		Phytosterols	177–178
		Resveratrol	189, 190
Cataracts	Prevention	Fruits and vegetables	3
		Carotenoids	52
Cognitive decline	Prevention	Soy isoflavones	130–131
Cystic fibrosis	Treatment	Curcumin	73
Dental caries	Prevention	Tea	42
Depression	Treatment	Essential fatty acids	87–88
Chronic obstructive pulmonary disease	Prevention	Fruits and vegetables	3
Diabetes mellitus, type 2	Prevention Treatment	Fruits and vegetables	2
		Legumes	13
		Nuts	19–20
		Whole grains	22
		Coffee	29
		Fiber	103, 105
		Essential fatty acids	85–86
Diverticular disease	Prevention	Whole grains	24
		Fiber	104
IgA nephropathy	Treatment	Essential fatty acids	87
Infant development	Prevention	Essential fatty acids	91
Inflammatory bowel disease	Treatment	Essential fatty acids	86
Irritable bowel syndrome	Treatment	Fiber	105–106
Human papilloma virus infection	Treatment	Indole-3-carbinol	149–150
Kidney stones	Prevention	Tea	43
Macular degeneration, age-related	Prevention	Fruits and vegetables	3
		Carotenoids	51–52

Disease or Condition	Chapter Section	Food or Phytochemical	Page(s)
Menopausal symptoms	Treatment	Soy isoflavones	131
Osteoporosis	Prevention	Fruits and vegetables	2–3
		Tea	42
		Soy isoflavones	130
		Lignans	158
Parkinson's disease	Prevention	Coffee	29
Pregnancy	Prevention	Essential fatty acids	82
Rheumatoid arthritis	Treatment	Essential fatty acids	86
Schizophrenia	Treatment	Essential fatty acids	88
Systemic lupus erythematosus	Treatment	Indole-3-carbinol	150

Appendix 3 Drug Interactions

Drug classes are listed first, alphabetically, followed by specific drugs known to interact with dietary phytochemicals. Specific drugs are listed alphabetically by their generic name. A common U.S. brand name is usually listed in parentheses after the generic name. Because there may be drug-phytochemical interactions that are not listed in the table below, it is important to review the prescribing or patient information of any medication prior to its use for the possibility of clinically significant drug-phytochemical interactions. This table does not address the potential for multiple drug-phytochemical interactions in individuals taking more than one medication or phytochemical.

Drug Class	Phytochemical	Interaction	Page(s)
Anticoagulants and platelet inhibitors	Curcumin	Curcumin inhibits platelet aggregation in vitro, potentially increasing the risk of bleeding in people on anticoagulant therapy.	74
	Borage oil or evening primrose oil (omega-6 fatty acids)	High intakes of γ-linolenic acid may inhibit platelet aggregation, potentially increasing the risk of bleeding in people on anticoagulant therapy.	92
	Flaxseed oil, fish oil, or EPA/DHA supplements (omega-3 fatty acids)	High intakes of omega-3 fatty acids, particularly fish oil (EPA/DHA), may inhibit platelet aggregation and increase the risk of bleeding in people on anticoagulant therapy.	92
	Flavonoids	High intakes of flavonoids from grape juice and dark chocolate may inhibit platelet aggregation, potentially increasing the risk of bleeding in people on anticoagulant therapy.	121–122
	Garlic	Garlic supplements may inhibit platelet aggregation, potentially increasing the risk of bleeding in people on anticoagulant therapy.	170
	Resveratrol	Resveratrol inhibits platelet aggregation in vitro, potentially increasing the risk of bleeding in people on anticoagulant therapy.	191–192

Drug Class	Phytochemical	Interaction	Page(s)
Adrenergic agonists	Caffeine (coffee and tea)	Caffeine may enhance adrenergic effects and side effects.	33
Antibiotics	Soy isoflavones	Because soy isoflavones are metabolized by colonic bacteria, antibiotic therapy could decrease their biological activity.	133
Antibiotics (quinolones)	Caffeine (coffee and tea)	Quinolone class antibiotics impair hepatic caffeine metabolism, increasing the risk of caffeine-related side effects.	33
Benzodiazepines	Grapefruit juice (flavonoids)	Flavonoids and other compounds in grapefruit juice inhibit cytochrome P450 3A4, increasing the bioavailability and risk of toxicity from benzodiazepines.	121
Calcium channel antagonists	Grapefruit juice (flavonoids)	Flavonoids and other compounds in grapefruit juice inhibit cytochrome P450 3A4, increasing the bioavailability and risk of toxicity from calcium channel antagonists.	121
Estrogens	Caffeine (coffee and tea)	Estrogens impair hepatic caffeine metabolism, increasing the risk of caffeine-related side effects.	33
HMG-CoA reductase inhibitors (statins)	Grapefruit juice (flavonoids)	Flavonoids and other compounds in grapefruit juice inhibit cytochrome P450 3A4, increasing the bioavailability and risk of toxicity from HMG-CoA reductase inhibitors (statins).	121
	Phytosterols	The LDL cholesterol-lowering effect of plant sterols or stanols may be additive to that of HMG-CoA reductase inhibitors (statins).	181
Phenothiazines	Borage oil or evening primrose oil (omega-6 fatty acids)	High doses of γ-linolenic acid may increase the risk of seizure in people on phenothiazines.	92

Specific Drug	Phytochemical	Interaction	Page(s)
Acetaminophen (Tylenol)	Caffeine (coffee and tea)	Caffeine may decrease the elimination of acetaminophen and enhance its analgesic effect.	33
	Guar gum (fiber)	Guar gum may slow the absorption of acetaminophen when taken at the same time.	108
Amiodarone (Cordarone, Pacerone)	Grapefruit juice (flavonoids)	Flavonoids and other compounds in grapefruit juice inhibit cytochrome P450 3A4, increasing the bioavailability and risk of toxicity from amiodarone.	121
Aspirin	Caffeine (coffee and tea)	Caffeine may decrease the elimination of aspirin and enhance its analgesic effect.	33
Bumetanide (Bumex)	Guar gum (fiber)	Guar gum may slow the absorption of bumetanide when taken at the same time.	108
Buspirone (BuSpar)	Grapefruit juice (flavonoids)	Flavonoids and other compounds in grapefruit juice inhibit cytochrome P450 3A4, increasing the bioavailability and risk of toxicity from buspirone.	121
Carbamazepine (Tegretol)	Psyllium (fiber)	Psyllium may decrease the absorption of carbamazepine when taken at the same time.	108
	Grapefruit juice (flavonoids)	Flavonoids and other compounds in grapefruit juice inhibit cytochrome P450 3A4, increasing the bioavailability and risk of toxicity from carbamazepine.	121
Cholestyramine (Questran)	Carotenoids	Cholestyramine may inhibit carotenoid absorption.	56
Cimetidine (Tagamet)	Caffeine (coffee and tea)	Cimetidine impairs hepatic caffeine metabolism, increasing the risk of caffeine-related side effects.	33
Cisapride (Propulsid)	Grapefruit juice (flavonoids)	Flavonoids and other compounds in grapefruit juice inhibit cytochrome P450 3A4, increasing the bioavailability and risk of toxicity from cisapride.	121
Clozapine (Clozaril)	Caffeine (coffee and tea)	Caffeine may inhibit the hepatic metabolism of clozapine and increase the risk of toxicity.	33
Colestipol (Colestid)	Carotenoids	Colestipol may inhibit carotenoid absorption.	56

Specific Drug	Phytochemical	Interaction	Page(s)
Cyclophosphamide (Cytoxan)	Curcumin	Oral curcumin administration inhibited cyclophosphamide-induced tumor regression in an animal model of breast cancer.	74
Cyclosporine (Neoral)	Grapefruit juice (flavonoids)	Flavonoids and other compounds in grapefruit juice inhibit cytochrome P450 3A4, increasing the bioavailability and risk of toxicity from cyclosporine.	121
Digoxin (Lanoxin)	Psyllium (fiber)	Psyllium may decrease the absorption of digoxin when taken at the same time.	108
	Guar gum (fiber)	Guar gum may slow the absorption of digoxin when taken at the same time.	108
Disulfiram (Antabuse)	Caffeine (coffee and tea)	Disulfiram impairs hepatic caffeine metabolism, increasing the risk of caffeine-related side effects.	33
Glyburide (Glynase)	Guar gum (fiber)	Guar gum may decrease the absorption of glyburide when taken at the same time.	108
Fluconazole (Diflucan)	Caffeine (coffee and tea)	Fluconazole impairs hepatic caffeine metabolism, increasing the risk of caffeine-related side effects.	33
Fluvoxamine (Luvox)	Caffeine (coffee and tea)	Fluvoxamine impairs hepatic caffeine metabolism increasing the risk of caffeine-related side effects.	33
Levothyroxine	Soy protein (soy isoflavones)	Soy protein may decrease the bioavailability of levothyroxine when consumed at the same time.	133–134
Lithium	Caffeine (coffee and tea)	Caffeine may enhance the elimination of lithium and decrease plasma lithium concentrations.	33
	Psyllium (fiber)	Psyllium may decrease the absorption of lithium when taken at the same time.	108
Losartan (Cozaar)	Grapefruit juice (flavonoids)	Flavonoids and other compounds in grapefruit juice inhibit cytochrome P450 3A4, potentially decreasing the therapeutic effect of losartan.	121
Lovastatin (Mevacor)	Pectin (pectin)	Pectin may decrease the absorption of lovastatin when taken at the same time.	108

Specific Drug	Phytochemical	Interaction	Page(s)
Metformin (Glucophage)	Guar gum (fiber)	Guar gum may decrease the absorption of metformin when taken at the same time.	108
Mexiletine (Mexitil)	Caffeine (coffee and tea)	Mexiletine impairs hepatic caffeine metabolism, increasing the risk of caffeine-related side effects.	33
Orlistat (Xenical) Lipase inhibitor, obesity	Carotenoids	Orlistat may inhibit carotenoid absorption.	56
Penicillin	Guar gum (fiber)	Guar gum may decrease the absorption of penicillin when taken at the same time.	108
Phenytoin (Dilantin)	Caffeine (coffee and tea)	Increases hepatic caffeine metabolism.	33
	Piperine (in some curcumin supplements)	Piperine may slow the elimination of phenytoin.	74
Propranolol (Inderal)	Piperine (in some curcumin supplements)	Piperine may slow the elimination of propranolol.	74
Saquinavir (Fortovase)	Grapefruit juice (flavonoids)	Flavonoids and other compounds in grapefruit juice inhibit cytochrome P450 3A4, increasing the bioavailability and risk of toxicity from saquinavir.	121
	Garlic	Garlic supplements may decrease the bioavailability of saquinavir.	170
Sildenafil (Viagra)	Grapefruit juice (flavonoids)	Flavonoids and other compounds in grapefruit juice inhibit cytochrome P450 3A4, increasing the bioavailability and risk of toxicity from sildenafil.	121
Sertraline (Zoloft)	Grapefruit juice (flavonoids)	Flavonoids and other compounds in grapefruit juice inhibit cytochrome P450 3A4, increasing the bioavailability and risk of toxicity from sertraline.	121
Tamoxifen (Nolvadex)	Soy isoflavones	Some evidence from animal studies suggests that high intakes of soy isoflavones, particularly genistein, can interfere with the antitumor effects of tamoxifen.	133
Terbinafine (Lamisil)	Caffeine (coffee and tea)	Terbinafine impairs hepatic caffeine metabolism, increasing the risk of caffeine-related side effects.	33

Specific Drug	Phytochemical	Interaction	Page(s)
Terfenadine (Seldane)*	Grapefruit juice (flavonoids)	Flavonoids and other compounds in grapefruit juice inhibit cytochrome P450 3A4, increasing the bioavailability and risk of toxicity from terfenadine.*	121
Theophylline	Caffeine (coffee and tea)	Caffeine may decrease the elimination of theophylline and increase plasma theophylline levels.	33
	Piperine (in some curcumin supplements)	Piperine may slow the elimination of theophylline.	74
Warfarin (Coumadin)	Green tea	Excessive green tea intake may decrease the efficacy of warfarin.	43
	Psyllium (fiber)	Psyllium may decrease the absorption of warfarin when taken at the same time.	108
	Soy protein	High intakes of soy protein may decrease the efficacy of warfarin.	133
	Garlic	Garlic supplements may increase the anticoagulant activity of warfarin.	170

* Not available in the United States.

Abbreviations: EPA, eicosapentaenoic acid; DHA, docosahexaenoic acid; LDL, low-density lipoprotein.

Appendix 4 Nutrient Interactions

Nutrient	Phytochemical	Interaction	Page(s)
Calcium	Caffeine (coffee and tea)	Caffeine may decrease the absorption of calcium slightly.	33–34
Iron	Flavonoids and phenolic compounds (coffee and tea)	Flavonoids and other phenolic compounds in coffee, tea, and cocoa inhibit the absorption of nonheme iron when consumed at the same time.	122
Vitamin E	Omega-3 fatty acids	People on high doses of omega-3 fatty acids (EPA/DHA) may require additional vitamin E.	92
Calcium	Inulin and oligofructose (fiber)	Limited evidence suggests inulin and oligofructose may enhance calcium absorption.	108
β-Carotene and other carotenoids	Pectin and guar gum (fiber)	Pectin and guar gum may decrease the absorption of β-carotene, lutein, and lycopene consumed at the same time.	108
	Phytosterols	At doses used to lower LDL cholesterol, plant sterols or stanols may decrease plasma α-carotene, β-carotene, and lycopene concentrations.	181–182

Abbreviations: EPA, eicosapentaenoic acid; DHA, docosahexaenoic acid; LDL, low-density lipoprotein.

Appendix 5 Quick Reference to Phytochemical-Rich Foods

Some foods that are rich in the phytochemicals discussed in this book are listed in the table below. Information about the food sources of a specific phytochemical may be found in the chapter on that phytochemical under "Sources."

Plant Food	Class or Color	Examples	Phytochemicals
Vegetables	Dark green vegetables	Chard, spinach	Carotenoids (lutein and zeaxanthin), chlorophyll, fiber
	Yellow and orange vegetables	Carrots, pumpkin, squash, sweet potato	Carotenoids (α-carotene, β-carotene, β-cryptoxanthin), fiber
	Cruciferous vegetables	Brussels sprouts, broccoli, garden cress, kale, mustard greens	Carotenoids (lutein and zeaxanthin), chlorophyll, fiber, indoles, isothiocyanates, lignans, phytosterols
	Legumes	Soy and dried beans, peas, lentils	Fiber, flavonoids (isoflavones), phytosterols
	Allium vegetables	Onions, leeks, chives, garlic	Fiber, flavonoids (flavonols), organosulfur compounds
Fruits	Berries	Strawberries, raspberries, blueberries	Fiber, flavonoids (anthocyanins, flavanols, flavonols), lignans, resveratrol
	Grapes	Red and purple grapes	Fiber, flavonoids (anthocyanins, flavanols, flavonols), resveratrol
	Citrus fruits	Grapefruits, oranges, lemons	Fiber, flavonoids (flavanones)
	Red fruits	Apples	Fiber, flavonoids (flavanols, flavonols)
		Tomatoes, watermelon	Carotenoids (lycopene), fiber
Nuts and seeds	Nuts	Almonds, pine nuts, walnuts	Essential fatty acids, fiber, phytosterols
	Legumes	Peanuts	Essential fatty acids, fiber, phytosterols, resveratrol
	Seeds	Flaxseeds, sesame seeds	Essential fatty acids, fiber, lignans, phytosterols

Plant Food	Class or Color	Examples	Phytochemicals
Whole grains		Brown rice, barley, oats, rye, whole wheat	Fiber, lignans, phytosterols
Spices		Turmeric	Curcumin
		Parsley	Chlorophyll, flavonoids (flavones)
		Garlic	Organosulfur compounds

Appendix 6 Glossary

Acetylation The addition of an acetyl group ($-COCH_3$) group to a molecule.

Acidic Having a pH less than 7.

Adjunct therapy A treatment or therapy used in addition to another, not alone.

Aglycone The nonsugar component of a glycoside. Cleavage of the glycosidic bond of a glycoside results in the formation of a sugar and an aglycone.

AI Adequate intake. Established by the Food and Nutrition Board of the U.S. Institute of Medicine, the AI is a recommended intake value based on observed or experimentally determined estimates of nutrient intake by a group of healthy people that are assumed to be adequate. An AI is established when an RDA cannot be determined.

Alkaline Basic; having a pH greater than 7.

Alkaloid A plant-derived compound that is biologically active, contains a nitrogen in a heterocyclic ring, is alkaline, has a complex structure, and is of limited distribution in the plant kingdom.

Alzheimer's disease The most common cause of dementia in older adults. Alzheimer's disease is characterized by the formation of amyloid plaque in the brain and nerve cell degeneration. Symptoms include memory loss and confusion, which worsen over time.

Amino acids Organic (carbon-containing) molecules that serve as the building blocks of proteins.

Amyloid plaque Aggregates of a peptide called amyloid β (Aβ), which accumulate and form deposits in the brain in Alzheimer's disease.

Anaphylaxis A rapidly developing and severe systemic allergic reaction. Symptoms may include swelling of the tongue, throat, and trachea, which can result in difficulty breathing, shock, and loss of consciousness. If not treated rapidly, anaphylaxis can be fatal.

Angiogenesis The development of new blood vessels.

Angiography (coronary) Imaging of the coronary arteries used to identify the location and severity of any obstructions. Coronary angiography typically involves the administration of a contrast medium and imaging of the coronary arteries using an X-ray based technique.

Antagonist A substance that counteracts or nullifies the biological effects of another, such as a compound that binds to a receptor but does not elicit a biological response.

Antibodies Specialized proteins produced by white blood cells (lymphocytes) that recognize and bind to foreign proteins or pathogens to neutralize them or mark them for destruction.

Anticoagulant A class of compounds that inhibit blood clotting.

Anticonvulsant A class of medication used to prevent seizures.

Antigen A substance that is capable of eliciting an immune response.

Antioxidant Any substance that prevents or reduces damage caused by reactive oxygen species (ROS) or reactive nitrogen species (RNS).

Apoptosis Gene-directed cell death or programmed cell death that occurs when age, condition, or state of cell health dictates. Cells that die by apoptosis do not usually elicit the inflammatory responses that are associated with necrosis. Cancer cells are resistant to apoptosis.

Arrhythmia An abnormal heart rhythm. The heart rhythm may be too fast (tachycardia), too slow (bradycardia), or irregular. Some arrhythmias, such as ventricular fibrillation, may lead to cardiac arrest if not treated promptly.

Asthma A chronic inflammatory disease of the airways, characterized by recurrent episodes of reversible airflow obstruction.

Atherosclerosis An inflammatory disease resulting in the accumulation of cholesterol-laden plaque in artery walls. Rupture of atherosclerotic plaque results in clot formation, which may result in myocardial infarction or ischemic stroke.

ATP   Adenosine triphosphate. ATP is an important compound for the storage of energy in cells, as well as the synthesis of nucleic acids.

Atria   The two upper chambers of the heart.

Atrial fibrillation   A cardiac arrhythmia, characterized by rapid, uncoordinated beating of the atria, which results in ineffective atrial contractions. Atrial fibrillation is known as a supraventricular arrhythmia because it originates above the ventricles.

Atrophy   Decrease in size or wasting away of a body part or tissue.

Autoimmune disease   A condition in which the body's immune system reacts against its own tissues.

Autosomal   Refers to a trait or gene that is not located on the X or Y chromosome (not sex-linked).

Bacteria   Single-celled organisms that can exist independently, symbiotically (in cooperation with another organism), or parasitically (dependent upon another organism, sometimes to the detriment of the other organism).

Benign prostatic hyperplasia (BPH)   Noncancerous enlargement of the prostate. The enlarged prostate may exert pressure on the urethra, resulting in difficulty urinating.

Bias   Any systematic error in an epidemiological study that results in an incorrect estimate of the association between an exposure and disease risk.

Bile   A yellow-green fluid made in the liver and stored in the gallbladder. Bile may then pass through the common bile duct into the small intestine where some of its components aid in the digestion of fat.

Bile acids   Components of bile, which are formed by the metabolism of cholesterol, and aid in the digestion of fats.

Bioavailability   The fraction of an administered compound that reaches the systemic circulation and is transported to site of action (target tissue).

Biomarker   A physical, functional, or biochemical indicator of a physiological or disease process.

Biotransformation enzymes (Phase I and Phase II)   Enzymes involved in the metabolism and elimination of a variety of exogenous (drugs, toxins and carcinogens) and endogenous compounds (steroid hormones). In general, phase I biotransformation enzymes, including those of the cytochrome P450 family, catalyze reactions that increase the reactivity of fat-soluble compounds and prepare them for reactions catalyzed by phase II biotransformation enzymes. Reactions catalyzed by phase II enzymes generally increase water solubility and promote the elimination of these compounds.

Bipolar disorder   A mood previously called manic-depressive illness. Bipolar disorder is characterized by severe alterations in mood. During "manic" episodes, a person may experience extreme elevation in energy level and mood (euphoria) or extreme agitation and irritability. Episodes of depressed mood are also common in bipolar disorder.

Bone mineral density (BMD)   The amount of mineral in a given area of bone. BMD is positively associated with bone strength and resistance to fracture, and measurements of BMD are used to diagnose osteoporosis.

Bronchitis, chronic   Long-standing inflammation of the airways, characterized by excess production of sputum, leading to a chronic cough and obstruction of air flow. Cigarette smoking is the most common cause of chronic bronchitis.

Buffer   A substance that maintains or stabilizes the pH of a solution.

C-reactive protein (CRP)   A protein that is produced in the liver in response to inflammation. CRP is a biomarker of inflammation that is strongly associated with the risk of cardiovascular events, such as myocardial infarction and stroke.

Cancer   Refers to abnormal cells, that have a tendency to grow uncontrollably and metastasize or spread to other areas of the body. Cancer can involve any tissue of the body and can have different forms in one tissue. Cancer is a group of more than 100 different diseases.

Carcinogen   A cancer-causing agent; adjective; carcinogenic.

Carcinogenesis   The transformation of normal cells into cancer cells.

Cardiovascular disease   Literally, a disease affecting the heart and blood vessels. The term encompasses a number of conditions that result from atherosclerosis, including coronary heart disease, congestive heart failure, and stroke.

Carotid arteries The left and right common carotid arteries are the principal blood vessels that supply oxygenated blood to the head and neck. Each has two main branches, the external and internal carotid artery.

Case-control study A study with in which exposures of people who have been diagnosed with a disease (cases) are compared with those of people without the disease (controls). The results of case-control studies are more likely to be distorted by bias in the selection of cases and controls (selection bias) and dietary recall (recall bias) than prospective cohort studies.

Catalyze Increase the speed of a chemical reaction without being changed in the overall reaction process (see Enzyme below).

Cataract Clouding of the lens of the eye. As cataracts progress they can impair vision.

Cell adhesion molecules Molecules on the outside surfaces of cells that bind to other cells or to the extracellular matrix (material surrounding cells). Cell adhesion molecules influence many important functions, including the entry of immune cells into the arterial wall.

Cell cycle The orderly sequence of stages that a cell passes through between one cell division (mitosis) and the next. The cell cycle can be divided into four stages: the M (mitosis) phase, in which nuclear and cytoplasmic division occurs; the G1 phase or interphase; the S (synthesis) phase, in which DNA replication occurs; and the G2 phase, a quiescent period prior to the next M phase.

Cell membrane Also called a plasma membrane, the barrier that separates the contents of a cell from its outside environment and controls what moves in and out of the cell. A mammalian cell membrane consists of a phospholipid bilayer with embedded proteins and cholesterol.

Cell signaling Communication among individual cells so as to coordinate their behavior to benefit the organism as a whole. Cell-signaling systems elucidated in animal cells include cell-surface and intracellular receptor proteins, GTP-binding proteins, and protein kinases and protein phosphatases (enzymes that phosphorylate and dephosphorylate proteins).

Cervical intraepithelial neoplasia (CIN) A term used to describe abnormal growth of cells on the surface of the uterine cervix. CIN1 is also known as low-grade squamous intraepithelial lesion (LSIL). CIN2 and CIN3 are also known as high-grade squamous intraepithelial lesions (HSIL). Although these abnormal cells are not cancerous, they may progress to cervical cancer.

Chelate The combination of a metal with an organic molecule to form a ring-like structure known as a chelate. Chelation of a metal may inhibit or enhance its bioavailability.

Chemotherapy Literally, treatment with drugs. The term is commonly used to describe the systemic use of drugs to kill cancer cells, as a form of cancer treatment.

Cholesterol A compound that is an integral structural component of cell membranes and a precursor in the synthesis of steroid hormones. Dietary cholesterol is obtained from animal sources, but is also synthesized by the liver. Cholesterol is carried in the blood by lipoproteins. In atherosclerosis, cholesterol accumulates in plaques on the walls of some arteries.

Chromosome A structure in the nucleus of a cell that contains genes. Chromosomes are composed of DNA and associated proteins. Normal human cells contain 46 chromosomes (22 pairs of autosomes and 2 sex chromosomes).

Chronic obstructive pulmonary disease (COPD) A term that includes emphysema and chronic bronchitis, two chronic lung diseases that are characterized by airway obstruction.

Chylomicrons Triglyceride-rich lipoproteins that deliver dietary triglycerides from the intestine to the tissues immediately after a meal. Chylomicrons release their triglycerides to tissue through the activity of lipoprotein lipase enzymes in tissue capillary beds. When they are depleted of most of their triglycerides, chylomicron remnants are taken up by the liver, where the lipids and cholesterol that remain are excreted in bile or incorporated into other lipoproteins.

Cirrhosis A condition characterized by irreversible scarring of the liver, leading to abnormal liver function. Cirrhosis has a number of different causes, including chronic alcohol use and viral hepatitis B and C.

Clinical trial An intervention trial generally used to evaluate the efficacy and/or safety of a treatment or intervention in human participants.

Coagulation The process involved in blood clot formation.

Cohort A group of people who are followed over time as part of an epidemiological study.

Colon The portion of the large intestine that extends from the end of the small intestine to the rectum. The colon removes water from digested food after it has passed through the small intestine and stores the remaining stool until it can be evacuated.

Colorectal adenoma A polyp or growth in the lining of the colon or rectum. Although they are not cancerous, colorectal adenomas may develop into colorectal cancer over time.

Colorectal cancer Cancer of the colon and/or rectum.

Congenital malformations Birth defects.

Congestive heart failure (CHF) A condition in which the heart loses the ability to pump blood efficiently enough to meet the demands of the body. Symptoms may include edema (swelling), shortness of breath, weakness, and exercise intolerance.

Conjugation The formation of a water-soluble derivative of a chemical by its combination with another compound, such as glutathione, glucuronate, or sulfate.

Coronary artery The vessels that supply oxygenated blood to the heart muscle itself, so named because they encircle the heart in the form of a crown.

Coronary artery bypass graft (CABG) A surgical procedure used to create new routes around obstructions in coronary arteries and restore adequate blood flow to the heart muscle.

Coronary heart disease (CHD) Also known as coronary artery disease and coronary disease, coronary heart disease is the result of atherosclerosis of the coronary arteries. Atherosclerosis may result in narrowing or obstruction of one or more coronary arteries and is the underlying cause of myocardial infarction.

Crohn's disease An inflammatory bowel disease that usually affects the lower part of the small intestine or upper part of the colon, but may affect any part of the gastrointestinal tract.

Cross-sectional study A study of a group of people at one point in time to determine whether an exposure is associated with the occurrence of a disease. Because the disease outcome and the exposure (e.g., nutrient intake) are measured at the same time, a cross-sectional study provides a "snapshot" view of their relationship. Cross-sectional studies cannot provide information about causality.

Cystic fibrosis A hereditary disease caused by mutations in the cystic fibrosis transmembrane conductance regulator (*CFTCR*) gene. Cystic fibrosis is characterized by the production of abnormal secretions, leading to the accumulation of mucus in the lungs, pancreas, and intestine. This build-up of mucus causes difficulty breathing and recurrent lung infections, as well as problems with nutrient absorption due to problems in the pancreas and intestines.

Cytochrome P450 A family of phase I biotransformation enzymes that play an important role in the metabolism and elimination of drugs, toxins, carcinogens, and endogenous compounds, such as steroid hormones.

Cytoplasm The contents of a cell, excluding the nucleus.

De novo synthesis The formation of an essential molecule from simple precursor molecules.

Debridement The removal of necrotic or infected tissue or foreign material from a wound.

Dementia Significant impairment of intellectual abilities such as attention, orientation, memory, judgment, or language. By definition, dementia is not due to major depression or psychosis. Alzheimer's disease is the most common cause of dementia in older adults.

Dental caries Cavities or holes in the outer two layers of a tooth—the enamel and the dentin. Dental caries are caused by bacteria that metabolize carbohydrates (sugars) to form organic acids which dissolve tooth enamel.

Diabetes mellitus   A chronic metabolic disease characterized by abnormally high blood glucose (sugar) levels, resulting from the inability of the body to produce or respond to insulin. Type 1 diabetes mellitus, formerly known as insulin-dependent or juvenile-onset diabetes, is usually the result of autoimmune destruction of the insulin secreting β-cells of the pancreas. The most common form of diabetes is type 2 diabetes mellitus, formerly known as noninsulin-dependent or adult-onset diabetes, which develops when the tissues of the body become less sensitive to insulin secreted by the pancreas.

Diastolic blood pressure   The lowest arterial blood pressure during the heart beat cycle, and the second number in a blood pressure reading (e.g., 120/80).

Differentiation   Changes in a cell resulting in its specialization for specific functions, such as those of a nerve cell. In general, differentiation of cells leads to a decrease in proliferation.

Diffusion   A passive process in which particles in solution move from a region of higher concentration to one of lower concentration.

Dimer   A complex of two protein molecules. Heterodimers are complexes of two different proteins, whereas homodimers are complexes of two of the same protein.

Diuretic   An agent that increases the formation of urine by the kidneys, resulting in water loss from the individual using the diuretic.

Diverticulosis   A condition characterized by the formation of small pouches (diverticula) in the colon. Although most people with diverticulosis experience no symptoms, about 15 to 20% may develop pain or inflammation, known as diverticulitis.

Diverticulitis   Inflammation or infection of diverticula in the colon (see diverticulosis above), characterized by abdominal pain, fever, and constipation.

DNA   Deoxyribonucleic acid; a double-stranded nucleic acid composed of many nucleotides. The nucleotides in DNA are each composed of a nitrogen-containing base (adenine, guanine, cytosine, or thymine), a 5-carbon sugar (deoxyribose), and a phosphate group. The sequence of bases in DNA encodes the genetic information required to synthesize proteins.

Dominant trait   A trait that is expressed when only one copy of the gene responsible for the trait is present.

Ecological study   An epidemiological study that examines the relationships between exposures and disease rates in a series of populations (e.g., different countries). Ecological studies often rely on published statistics, such as food disappearance data or disease-specific death rates.

Eicosanoids   Chemical messengers derived from 20-carbon polyunsaturated fatty acids, such as arachidonic acid and eicosapentaenoic acid. Eicosanoids play critical roles in immune and inflammatory responses.

Electrolytes   Ionized (dissociated into positive and negative ions) salts in the body fluids. Major electrolytes in the body include sodium, potassium, magnesium, calcium, chloride, bicarbonate, and phosphate.

Emphysema   A chronic obstructive pulmonary (lung) disease, characterized by damage to the small air sacs (alveoli) and difficulty breathing. Damage to the alveoli decreases their elasticity and results in hyperinflation of the lungs, which impairs gas exchange. Smoking is the most common cause of emphysema.

Endogenous   Arising from within the body. Endogenous synthesis refers to the synthesis of a compound by the body.

Endometrium   The inner lining of the uterus.

Endothelium-dependent vasodilation   Arterial vasodilation resulting from the production of nitric oxide in the vascular endothelium.

Enterocytes   Cells that line the luminal surface of the intestine.

Enzyme   A biological catalyst. Enzymes increase the speed of a chemical reaction without being changed in the overall process.

Epidemiological study   A study examining disease occurrence in a human population.

Esophagus   The portion of the gastrointestinal tract that connects the throat (pharynx) to the stomach.

Ester   The product of a reaction between a carboxylic acid and an alcohol that involves the elimination of water. For example, a cholesterol ester is the product of a reaction between a fatty acid and cholesterol.

Estrogens   Hormones that bind to estrogen receptors (ERα or ERβ) in the nuclei of cells and promote the transcription of estrogen-responsive genes. Endogenous estrogens are steroid hormones produced by the body. Exogenous estrogens are synthetic or natural compounds that have estrogenic activity (i.e., bind the estrogen receptor and promote estrogen-responsive gene transcription).

Etiology   The cause or origin of a disease.

Excretion   The elimination of wastes from blood or tissues.

Familial adenomatous polyposis (FAP)   A hereditary syndrome characterized by the formation of many polyps in the colon and rectum, some of which may develop into colorectal cancer.

Fatty acid   An organic acid molecule consisting of a chain of carbon molecules and a carboxylic acid (COOH) group. Fatty acids are found in fats, oils, and as components of a number of essential lipids, such as phospholipids and triglycerides. Fatty acids can be oxidized by the body for energy.

Femoral neck   A portion of the femur (thigh bone) near the hip at the base of the head of femur, which makes up the ball of the hip joint. Fractures of the femoral neck may occur in individuals with osteoporosis.

Food Frequency Questionnaire (FFQ)   A type of dietary assessment in which participants are asked to report how frequently various foods are consumed over a specified period of time.

Forced expiratory volume (FEV$_1$)   The volume of air that can be expelled during the first second of a forced expiration. FEV$_1$ is used to assess pulmonary (lung) function.

Free radical   A very reactive atom or molecule typically possessing a single unpaired electron.

Gallbladder   A small sac adjacent to the liver. The gallbladder stores bile, which is secreted by the liver, and releases it into the small intestine through the common bile duct.

Gallstones   Crystals formed by the precipitation of cholesterol or bilirubin in the gallbladder. Gallstones may be asymptomatic (without symptoms) or they may result in inflammation and infection of the gallbladder.

Gastrointestinal   Referring to or affecting the digestive tract, which includes the mouth, pharynx (throat), esophagus, stomach, and intestines.

Gene expression   The process by which the information coded in genes (DNA) is converted to proteins and other cellular structures. Expressed genes include those that are transcribed to mRNA and translated to protein, as well as those that are only transcribed to RNA (e.g., ribosomal and transfer RNAs).

Genome   All of the genetic information (encoded in DNA) possessed by an organism.

Gestation   The period of time between fertilization and birth. In humans, normal gestation is usually about 40 weeks.

Glucose   A 6-carbon sugar, which plays a major role in the generation of energy.

Glucose tolerance   The ability of the body to maintain normal glucose levels when challenged with a carbohydrate load (see Impaired glucose tolerance below).

Glucoside   A glycoside that contains glucose as its carbohydrate (sugar) moiety (see Glycoside below).

Glutathione   A tripeptide consisting of glutamate, cysteine, and glycine. Glutathione is an endogenous intracellular antioxidant and is also required for some phase II biotransformation reactions

Glycemic index (GI)   An index of the blood glucose-raising potential of the carbohydrate in different foods. The GI is calculated as the area under the blood glucose curve after a test food is eaten, divided by the corresponding area after a control food (glucose or white bread) is eaten. The value is multiplied by 100 to represent a percentage of the control food (see Appendix 1).

Glycemic load (GL)   An index that simultaneously describes the blood glucose-raising potential of the carbohydrate in a food and the quantity of carbohydrate in a food. The GL of a food is calculated by multiplying the GI by the amount of carbohydrate in grams provided by a food and dividing the total by 100 (see Appendix 1).

Glycoside A compound containing a sugar molecule that can be cleaved by hydrolysis to a sugar and a nonsugar component (aglycone).

Glycosylated hemoglobin Glucose-bound hemoglobin. A test for glycosylated hemoglobin measures the percentage of hemoglobin that is glucose bound. Because glucose remains bound to hemoglobin for the life of a red blood cell (~120 days), glycosylated hemoglobin values reflect blood glucose control over the past 4 months.

HDL High-density lipoprotein. HDLs transport cholesterol from the tissues to the liver where it can be eliminated in bile. HDL cholesterol is considered good cholesterol because higher blood levels of HDL cholesterol are associated with lower risk of heart disease.

Heme Compounds of iron complexed in a characteristic ring structure known as a porphyrin ring.

Hemoglobin The oxygen-carrying pigment in red blood cells.

Hemoglobin A$_{1C}$ The main fraction of glycosylated (glucose-bound) hemoglobin. Because glucose remains bound to hemoglobin for the life of a red blood cell (~120 days), hemoglobin A$_{1C}$ values reflect blood glucose control over the past 4 months.

Hemolysis Rupture of red blood cells.

Hemorrhage Excessive or uncontrolled bleeding.

Hemorrhagic stroke A stroke that occurs when a blood vessel ruptures and bleeds into the brain.

Hepatitis Literally, inflammation of the liver. Hepatitis caused by a virus is known as viral hepatitis. Other causes of hepatitis include drugs, toxic chemicals, and alcohol abuse.

Hepatocellular carcinoma The most common type of primary liver cancer.

Heterodimer A dimer or complex of two different molecules, usually proteins.

Heterozygous Possessing two different forms (alleles) of a specific gene.

HIV Human immunodeficiency virus. HIV infection is the cause of acquired immunodeficiency syndrome (AIDS).

Homocysteine A sulfur-containing amino acid, which is an intermediate in the metabolism of methionine, another sulfur-containing amino acid. Elevated plasma homocysteine levels have been associated with increased risk of cardiovascular disease.

Homodimer A dimer or complex of two of the same molecule, usually a protein.

Homologous Having the same appearance, structure, or evolutionary origin.

Homozygous Possessing two identical forms (alleles) of a specific gene.

Hormone A chemical, released by a gland or a tissue, which affects or regulates the activity of specific cells or organs. Complex bodily functions, such as growth and sexual development, are regulated by hormones.

Hot flushes Sensations of heat in the skin, particularly the face, neck, and chest, also known as hot flashes. Hot flushes are most often related to declining estrogen levels during the perimenopause (period surrounding menopause).

Human papilloma virus (HPV) A group of viruses that may cause papillomas (growths or warts) on the skin or other parts of the body, including the genitals and the larynx. Infection with particular strains of HPV is associated with increased risk of cervical cancer.

Hydrolysis Cleavage of a chemical bond by the addition of water. In hydrolysis reactions, a large compound may be broken down into smaller compounds when a molecule of water is added.

Hydroxylation A chemical reaction involving the addition of a hydroxyl (-OH) group to a compound.

Hypertension High blood pressure. Hypertension is defined by the Joint National Committee on Prevention, Detection, Evaluation and Treatment of High Blood Pressure as a systolic blood pressure $\geq$ 140 mm Hg and/or a diastolic blood pressure $\geq$ 90 mm Hg.

Hyperthyroidism An excess of thyroid hormone, which may result from an overactive thyroid gland or nodule, or from taking too much thyroid hormone.

Hypokalemia Abnormally low serum potassium.

Hypothalamus An area at the base of the brain that regulates bodily functions, such as body temperature, hunger, and thirst.

Hypothesis An educated guess or proposition that is advanced as a basis for further investigation. A hypothesis must be subjected to an experimental test to determine its validity.

Hypothyroidism   A deficiency of thyroid hormone, which is normally made by the thyroid gland.

Idiopathic   Of unknown cause.

Ileostomy   A surgically created connection between the ileum (small intestine) and an opening in the abdominal wall (stoma) that allows for the evacuation of feces when a portion of the bowel has been removed.

Impaired glucose tolerance   A metabolic state between normal glucose regulation and overt diabetes. Impaired glucose tolerance is defined medically as a plasma glucose concentration between 140 and 199 mg/dL (7.8 to 11 mmol) 2 hours after the ingestion of 75 g of glucose during an oral glucose tolerance test.

Induction   Initiation of or increase in the expression of a gene in response to a physical or chemical stimulus (inducer).

Insulin   A peptide hormone secreted by the β-cells of the pancreas and required for normal glucose metabolism.

Insulin resistance   Impaired tissue responsiveness or sensitivity to insulin.

Insulin sensitivity   The capacity to increase cellular glucose uptake in response to insulin.

International normalized ratio (INR)   The preferred method for reporting prothrombin time, a measure of coagulation status that may be used to evaluate the therapeutic efficacy of anticoagulants, such as warfarin. The INR is a method for standardizing prothrombin time results to minimize variability between laboratories.

Intervention trial   An experimental study (usually a clinical trial) that tests the effect of a treatment or intervention on a health or disease outcome.

In vitro   Literally "in glass", referring to a test or research done in the test tube or in an artificial system.

In vivo   "Inside a living organism." An in vivo assay evaluates a biological process occurring inside the body.

Ion   An atom or group of atoms that carries a positive or negative electric charge as a result of having lost or gained one or more electrons.

Ion channel   A protein embedded in a cell membrane that allows for the regulated transfer of an ion or a group of ions across the membrane.

Irritable bowel syndrome (IBS)   A functional disorder of the intestines, characterized by episodes of abdominal pain or discomfort associated with a change in bowel movements, such as constipation or diarrhea.

Ischemia   A state of insufficient blood flow to a tissue.

Ischemic stroke   A stroke resulting from insufficient blood flow to an area of the brain, which may occur when a blood vessel supplying the brain becomes obstructed by a clot.

Isomers   Compounds that have the same number and types of atoms but differ in the way the atoms are arranged.

Kidney stone   A solid mass resulting from the crystallization of minerals and other compounds found in urine. Common types of kidney stones include those composed of calcium oxalate, calcium phosphate, and urate. Kidney stones may form in the kidney, ureters, or urinary bladder.

Larynx   The area of the throat (pharynx) that contains the vocal cords.

LDL   Low-density lipoprotein. LDLs transport cholesterol from the liver to the tissues of the body. Elevated serum LDL-cholesterol is associated with increased cardiovascular disease risk.

Leukocytes   White blood cells. Leukocytes are part of the immune system. Monocytes, lymphocytes, neutrophils, basophils, and eosinophils are different types of leukocytes.

Leukotrienes   Cell-signaling molecules involved in inflammation. Lipoxygenases catalyze the formation of leukotrienes from eicosanoids, such as arachidonic acid and eicosapentaenoic acid.

Lipid peroxidation   The process by which lipids are oxidized, so named because lipid hydroperoxides are formed in the process.

Lipids   A chemical term for fats. Lipids found in the human body include fatty acids, phospholipids, triglycerides, and cholesterol.

Lipoproteins   Particles composed of lipids and protein that allow for the transport of lipids through the bloodstream. A lipoprotein particle is composed of an outer layer of phospholipids, which renders it soluble in water, and a hydrophobic core that contains triglycerides and cholesterol esters. Different types of lipoproteins are distinguished by their surface proteins (apoproteins), their size, and the types and amounts of lipids they contain.

Lumbar spine The portion of the spine between the chest (thorax) and the pelvis. It is commonly referred to as the small of the back.

Lumen The channel within a tube, such as a blood vessel or the intestine.

Lymphocytes Leukocytes (white blood cells) that play important roles in the immune system. T lymphocytes (T cells) differentiate into cells that can kill infected cells or activate other cells in the immune system. B lymphocytes (B cells) differentiate into cells that produce antibodies.

Lysosome A cellular organelle that contains enzymes that are specialized for breaking down cellular debris. Lysosomal enzymes are separated from the rest of the cell by a lysosomal membrane and function optimally at an acid pH.

Macula A small area of the retina where vision is the sharpest. The macula is located in the center of the retina and provides central vision.

Malignant Cancerous.

Meta-analysis A statistical technique used to combine the results from different studies to obtain a quantitative estimate of the overall effect of a particular intervention or exposure on a defined outcome.

Metabolism The sum of the processes (reactions) by which a substance is assimilated and incorporated into the body or detoxified and excreted from the body.

Metabolite A compound derived from the metabolism of another compound is said to be a metabolite of that compound.

Metastasize To spread from one part of the body to another. Cancer is said to metastasize when it spreads from the primary site of origin to a distant anatomical site.

Methionine A sulfur-containing amino acid required for protein synthesis and other vital metabolic processes.

Methylation A biochemical reaction resulting in the addition of a methyl group ($-CH_3$) to another molecule.

Micelle An aggregate or cluster of amphipathic molecules in water. Amphipathic molecules have a polar or hydrophilic end and a nonpolar or hydrophobic end. In micelles, amphipathic molecules orient with their hydrophobic ends in the interior and their hydrophilic ends on the exterior surface, exposed to water.

Mitochondria Energy-producing structures within cells. Mitochondria possess two sets of membranes, a smooth continuous outer membrane and an inner membrane arranged in folds. Among other critical functions, mitochondria convert nutrients into energy via the electron transport chain.

mm Hg Millimeters of mercury; the unit of measure for blood pressure.

Moiety A portion of something, such as a functional group of a molecule.

Monomer A molecule that can be chemically bound as a unit of a polymer.

Monounsaturated fatty acid A fatty acid with only one double bond between carbon atoms.

Multifactorial Refers to diseases or conditions that are the result of interactions between multiple genetic and environmental factors.

Multiple sclerosis An autoimmune disorder, in which the myelin sheaths of nerves in the brain and spinal cord are damaged, resulting in progressive neurological symptoms.

Myocardial infarction (MI) Death (necrosis) of heart muscle tissue due to an interruption in its blood supply. Commonly known as a heart attack, an MI usually results from the obstruction of a coronary artery by a clot in people who have coronary atherosclerosis (heart disease).

Myocytes Muscle cells.

Necrosis Unprogrammed cell death in which cells break open and release their contents, promoting inflammation. Necrotic cell death may be the result of injury, infection, or infarction.

Nephropathy Kidney damage or disease.

Neurodegenerative disease A disease resulting from the degeneration or deterioration of nerve cells (neurons). Alzheimer's disease and Parkinson's disease are neurodegenerative diseases.

Neuropathy Nerve damage or disease.

Neurotransmitter A chemical that is released from a nerve cell and results in the transmission of an impulse to another nerve cell or organ (e. g., a muscle). Acetylcholine, dopamine, norepinephrine, and serotonin are neurotransmitters.

Neutrophil A type of leukocyte (white blood cell) that internalizes and destroys pathogens, such as bacteria.

NIH National Institutes of Health. Administered under the U.S. Department of Health and Human Services (HHS), the NIH is comprised of more than 20 separate institutes and centers devoted to medical research.

Nitric oxide A gaseous signaling molecule synthesized from the amino acid arginine by enzymes called nitric oxide synthases. In the vascular endothelium, nitric oxide promotes arterial vasodilation.

Nucleic acids DNA (deoxyribonucleic acid) and RNA (ribonucleic acid); long polymers of nucleotides.

Nucleotides Subunits of nucleic acids. Nucleotides are composed of a nitrogen-containing base (adenine, guanine, cytosine, uracil, or thymine), a 5-carbon sugar (ribose or deoxyribose), and one or more phosphate groups.

Nucleus A membrane-bound cellular organelle, which contains DNA organized into chromosomes.

Observational study A study in which no experimental intervention or treatment is applied. Participants are simply observed over time.

Organelles Specialized components of a cell, such as mitochondria or lysosomes, so named because they are analogous to organs.

Organic Refers to carbon-containing compounds, generally synthesized by living organisms.

Oropharynx A term used to describe the mouth and throat.

Osteoarthritis A degenerative joint condition that is characterized by the breakdown of articular cartilage (cartilage within the joint).

Osteoblasts Bone cells that are responsible for the formation of new bone mineral in the bone remodeling process.

Osteoclasts Bone cells that are responsible for the breakdown or resorption of bone in the bone remodeling process.

Osteoporosis A condition of increased bone fragility and susceptibility to bone fracture due to a loss of bone mineral density.

Oxidant A compound that oxidizes (removes electrons from) other compounds.

Oxidation A chemical reaction in which electrons are removed from an atom or molecule.

Oxidative stress A condition in which the effects of pro-oxidants (e.g., free radicals, reactive oxygen, and reactive nitrogen species) exceed the ability of antioxidant systems to neutralize them.

Pancreas A small organ located behind the stomach and connected to the duodenum (small intestine). The pancreas synthesizes enzymes that help digest food in the small intestine and hormones, including insulin, that regulate blood glucose levels.

Parkinson's disease A disease of the nervous system caused by degeneration of neurons in a part of the brain called the basal ganglia and by low production of the neurotransmitter dopamine. Symptoms include muscle rigidity, tremors, and slow voluntary movement.

Pathogen Disease-causing agents, such as viruses or bacteria.

Peptic ulcer disease A disease characterized by ulcers or breakdown of the inner lining of the stomach or duodenum. Common risk factors for peptic ulcer disease include the use of nonsteroidal anti-inflammatory drugs (NSAID) and infection with *Helicobacter pylori*.

Peptide A chain of amino acids. A protein is made up of one or more peptides.

Peptide hormones Hormones that are proteins, as opposed to steroid hormones, which are made from cholesterol. Insulin is an example of a peptide hormone.

Percutaneous transluminal coronary angioplasty (PTCA) A nonsurgical technique in which a balloon catheter is inserted into a peripheral artery and passed into an occluded coronary artery, where the balloon is inflated to dilate the artery.

Peripheral vascular disease Atherosclerosis of the vessels of the extremities, which may result in insufficient blood flow or pain in the affected limb, particularly during exercise.

pH   A measure of acidity or alkalinity.

Pharmacokinetics   The study of the absorption, distribution, metabolism, and elimination of drugs and other compounds.

Phase I clinical trial   Clinical trials in small groups of people aimed at determining bioavailability, optimal dose, safety, and early evidence of the efficacy of a new therapy.

Phase II clinical trial   Clinical trials designed to investigate the effectiveness of a new therapy in larger numbers of people and to further evaluate short-term side effects and safety of the new therapy.

Phenolic compounds   A class of chemical compounds consisting of a hydroxyl functional group (-OH) attached to an aromatic hydrocarbon group. An aromatic hydrocarbon has a ring structure like that of benzene.

Phospholipids   Lipid, in which phosphoric acid as well as fatty acids are attached to a glycerol backbone. Phospholipids are important structural components of cell membranes.

Phosphorylation   The creation of a phosphate derivative of an organic molecule. This is usually achieved by transferring a phosphate group ($-PO_4$) from ATP to another molecule.

Phytochemicals   Biologically active, non-nutrient compounds synthesized by plants.

Phytoestrogens   Compounds with estrogenic activity derived from plants.

Pigment   A compound that gives a plant or animal cell color by the selective absorption of different wavelengths of light.

Placebo   An inert treatment that is given to a control group while the experimental group is given the active treatment. Placebo-controlled studies are conducted to make sure that the results are due to the experimental treatment, rather than another factor associated with participating in the study.

Placenta   The organ that connects the fetus to the mother's uterus, allowing for the exchange of oxygen, carbon dioxide, nutrients, and waste between mother and fetus.

Plasma   The liquid portion of blood in which the cells are suspended. Plasma is separated from blood cells using a centrifuge. Unlike serum, plasma retains clotting factors because it is obtained from blood that is not allowed to clot.

Platelet   Irregularly shaped blood cell fragments that aggregate to help form blood clots.

Polymer   A large molecule formed by combining many similar smaller molecules (monomers) in a regular pattern.

Polymorphism   A variant form of a gene. Most polymorphisms are harmless and are part of normal human genetic variation, but some polymorphisms affect the function of the gene product (protein).

Polyunsaturated fatty acid   A fatty acid with more than one double bond between carbons.

Postprandial   After eating or after a meal.

Precursor   A molecule that is an ingredient, reactant, or intermediate in a synthetic pathway for a particular product.

Preeclampsia   A condition characterized by a sharp rise in blood pressure during the third trimester of pregnancy. High blood pressure may be accompanied by edema (swelling) and proteinuria (protein in the urine). In some cases, untreated preeclampsia can progress to eclampsia, a life-threatening situation for mother and child.

Prevalence   The proportion of a population with a specific disease or condition at a given point in time.

Procarcinogen   A carcinogen precursor that must be modified or metabolized to become an active carcinogen.

Prognosis   Predicted outcome based on the course of a disease.

Proliferation   Rapid cell division.

Pro-oxidant   An atom or molecule that promotes oxidation of another atom or molecule by accepting electrons. Examples of pro-oxidants include free radicals, reactive oxygen species (ROS), and reactive nitrogen species (RNS).

Prophylaxis   Prevention; often refers to a treatment used to prevent a disease.

Prospective cohort study   A study in which participants are initially enrolled, screened for risk factors or exposures (e. g., nutrient intake), and then followed up at subsequent times to determine their status with respect to a disease or health outcome.

Prostaglandins   Cell-signaling molecules involved in inflammation. Cyclooxygenases catalyze the formation of prostaglandins from eicosanoids, such as arachidonic acid and eicosapentaenoic acid.

Prostate   A gland in men, which is located at the base of the bladder and surrounds the urethra. The prostate produces fluid that forms part of semen. If the prostate becomes enlarged, it may exert pressure on the urethra and cause urinary symptoms. Prostate cancer is one of the most common types of cancer in men.

Prostate specific antigen (PSA)   A compound normally secreted by the prostate that can be measured in the blood. If prostate cancer is developing, the prostate secretes larger amounts of PSA. Blood tests for PSA are used to screen for prostate cancer and to follow-up on prostate cancer treatment.

Randomized controlled trial (RCT)   A clinical trial with at least one active treatment group and a control (placebo) group. In RCTs, participants are chosen for the experimental and control groups at random and are not told whether they are receiving the active or placebo treatment until the end of the study. This type of study design can provide evidence of causality.

RDA   Recommended dietary allowance. Established by the Food and Nutrition Board of the U. S. Institute of Medicine, the RDA is the average daily dietary intake level of a nutrient sufficient to meet the requirements of nearly all healthy individuals in a specific life stage and gender group.

Reactive oxygen species (ROS)   Highly reactive chemicals, containing oxygen, that react easily with other molecules, resulting in potentially damaging modifications.

Reactive nitrogen species (RNS)   Highly reactive chemicals, containing nitrogen, that react easily with other molecules, resulting in potentially damaging modifications.

Receptor   A specialized molecule inside or on the surface of a cell that binds a specific chemical (ligand). Ligand binding usually results in a change in activity with in the cell.

Recessive trait   A trait that is expressed only when two copies of the gene responsible for the trait are present.

Rectum   The last portion of the large intestine, connecting the sigmoid colon (above) to the anus (below). The rectum stores stool until it is evacuated from the body.

Redox reaction   Another term for an oxidation-reduction reaction. A redox reaction is any reaction in which electrons are removed from one molecule or atom and transferred to another. In such a reaction, one substance is oxidized (loses electrons), while the other is reduced (gains electrons).

Reduction   A chemical reaction in which a molecule or atom gains electrons.

Renal   Refers to the kidneys.

Residue   A single unit within a polymer, such as an amino acid within a polypeptide or protein.

Resorption   The process of breaking down or assimilating something. With respect to bone, resorption refers to the breakdown of bone by osteoclasts, resulting in the release of calcium and phosphate into the blood.

Response element   A sequence of nucleotides in a gene that can be bound by a protein. Proteins that bind to response elements in genes are sometimes called transcription factors or binding proteins. Binding of a transcription factor to a response element regulates the production of specific proteins by inhibiting or enhancing the transcription of genes that encode those proteins.

Restenosis   With respect to the coronary arteries, restenosis refers to the reocclusion of a coronary artery after it has been dilated using coronary angioplasty.

Retina   The nerve layer that lines the back of the eye. In the retina, images created by light are converted to nerve impulses, which are transmitted to the brain via the optic nerve.

Retrospective study   An epidemiological study that looks back in time. A retrospective study begins after the exposure and the disease have occurred. Most case-control studies are retrospective.

Rheumatoid arthritis   A chronic autoimmune disease, characterized by inflammation of the synovial lining of the joints. Rheumatoid arthritis may also affect other organs of the body, including the skin, eyes, lungs, and heart.

RNA   Ribonucleic acid; a single-stranded nucleic acid composed of many nucleotides. The nucleotides in RNA are composed of a nitrogen-containing base (adenine, guanine, cytosine, or uracil), a 5-carbon sugar (ribose), and a phosphate group. RNA functions in the translation of the genetic information encoded in DNA to proteins.

Saturated fatty acid A fatty acid with no double bonds between carbon atoms.

Scavenge (free radicals) To combine readily with free radicals, preventing them from reacting with other molecules.

Schizophrenia A debilitating brain disorder that affects about 1% of the world's population. Symptoms may include hallucinations, delusions, thought disorders, disorders of movement, cognitive deficits, flat affect, lack of pleasure, or impaired ability to speak, plan, or interact with others. Although its cause is not known, schizophrenia is thought to result from a combination of genetic and environmental factors.

Seizure Uncontrolled electrical activity in the brain, which may produce a physical convulsion, minor physical signs, thought disturbances, or a combination of symptoms.

Serotonin 5-Hydroxytryptamine. Serotonin is a neurotransmitter that also functions as a vasoconstrictor (substance that causes blood vessels to narrow).

Serum The liquid portion of blood in which the cells are suspended. Serum is separated from blood cells using a centrifuge. Unlike plasma, serum lacks clotting factors because it is obtained from blood that has been allowed to clot.

Signal transduction pathway A cascade of events that allows a signal outside a cell to result in a functional change inside the cell. Signal transduction pathways play important roles in regulating numerous cellular functions in response to changes in a cell's environment.

Small intestine The part of the digestive tract that extends from the stomach to the large intestine. The small intestine includes the duodenum (closest to the stomach), the jejunum, and the ileum (closest to the large intestine).

Status The state of nutrition of an individual with respect to a specific nutrient. Diminished or low status indicates inadequate supply or stores of a specific nutrient for optimal physiological functioning.

Stenosis Obstruction or narrowing of a passage. Coronary stenosis refers specifically to obstruction or narrowing of a coronary artery, which supplies blood to the heart muscle (myocardium).

Steroid A molecule related to cholesterol. Many important hormones, such as estrogen and testosterone, are steroids.

Stroke Damage that occurs to a part of the brain when its blood supply is suddenly interrupted (ischemic stroke) or when a blood vessel ruptures and bleeds into the brain (hemorrhagic stroke). A stroke is also called a cerebrovascular accident (CVA).

Substrate A reactant in an enzyme catalyzed reaction.

Supplement A nutrient or phytochemical supplied in addition to that which is obtained in the diet.

Synergistic When the effect of two treatments together is greater than the sum of the effects of the two individual treatments, the effect is said to be synergistic.

Systematic review A structured review of the literature designed to answer a clearly formulated question. Systematic reviews use systematic and explicitly predetermined methods to identify, select, and critically evaluate research relevant to the question, and to collect and analyze data from the studies that are included in the review. Statistical methods, such as meta-analysis, may be used to summarize the results of the included studies.

Systemic lupus erythematosus (SLE) A chronic autoimmune disease, characterized by inflammation of the connective tissue. SLE is more common in women than in men and may result in inflammation and damage to the skin, joints, blood vessels, lungs, heart, and kidneys.

Systolic blood pressure The highest arterial pressure measured during the heart beat cycle, and the first number in a blood pressure reading (e.g., 120/80).

Threshold The point at which a physiological effect begins to be produced.

Thyroid A butterfly-shaped gland in the neck that synthesizes and secretes thyroid hormones. Thyroid hormones regulate a number of physiological processes, including growth, development, metabolism, and reproductive function.

Topical   Applied to the skin or other body surface.

Total parenteral nutrition (TPN)   Intravenous feeding that provides patients with essential nutrients when they are too ill to eat normally.

Transcription   The process by which one strand of DNA is copied into a complementary sequence of RNA.

Transcription factor   A protein that functions to initiate, enhance, or inhibit the transcription of a gene. Transcription factors can regulate the formation of a specific protein encoded by a gene.

Translation   The process by which the sequence of nucleotides in a molecule of messenger RNA (mRNA) directs the incorporation of amino acids into a protein.

Triglycerides   Lipids consisting of three fatty acid molecules bound to a glycerol backbone. Triglycerides are the principal form of fat in the diet, although they are also synthesized endogenously. Triglycerides are stored in adipose tissue and represent the principal storage form of fat. Elevated serum triglycerides are a risk factor for cardiovascular disease.

Trimethylaminuria   A hereditary disorder characterized by increased urinary excretion of trimethylamine, a compound with a "fishy" or foul odor.

UL   Tolerable upper intake level. Established by the Food and Nutrition Board of the U.S. Institute of Medicine, the UL is the highest level of daily intake of a specific nutrient likely to pose no risk of adverse health effects in almost all individuals of a specified age.

Ulcerative colitis   A chronic inflammatory disease of the colon and rectum. Symptoms of ulcerative colitis include abdominal pain, cramping, and bloody diarrhea.

Unsaturated fatty acid   A fatty acid with at least one double bond between carbons.

Vascular endothelium   The single cell layer that lines the inner surface of blood vessels. Healthy vascular endothelium promotes vasodilation and inhibits platelet aggregation (clot formation).

Vasoconstriction   Narrowing of a blood vessel.

Vasodilation   Relaxation or opening of a blood vessel.

Ventricles   The two lower chambers of the heart that pump blood to the body (left) and the lungs (right).

Virus   A microorganism, which cannot grow or reproduce apart from a living cell. Viruses invade living cells and use the synthetic processes of infected cells to survive and replicate.

Xenograft   Transplant of tissue from a donor of one species to a recipient of another species.

Index

Page numbers followed by f or t indicate figures and tables respectively.